Urolithiasis
Medical and Surgical Management

Edited by

Margaret S Pearle, M.D., Ph.D
Department of Urology
University of Texas Southwestern Medical Center
Dallas, Texas, U.S.A.

and

Stephen Y Nakada, M.D.
Department of Urology
Clinical Science Center
University of Wisconsin
Madison, Wisconsin, U.S.A.

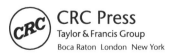

CRC Press
Taylor & Francis Group
Boca Raton London New York

CRC Press is an imprint of the
Taylor & Francis Group, an **informa** business

Urolithiasis
Medical and Surgical Management

Edited by

Margaret S Pearle, M.D., Ph.D
Department of Urology
University of Texas Southwestern Medical Center
Dallas, Texas, U.S.A.

and

Stephen Y Nakada, M.D.
Department of Urology
Clinical Science Center
University of Wisconsin
Madison, Wisconsin, U.S.A.

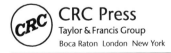

CRC Press
Taylor & Francis Group
Boca Raton London New York

CRC Press is an imprint of the
Taylor & Francis Group, an **informa** business

First published 2009 by Informa UK

Published 2019 by CRC Press
Taylor & Francis Group
6000 Broken Sound Parkway NW, Suite 300
Boca Raton, FL 33487-2742

© 2009 by Taylor & Francis Group, LLC
CRC Press is an imprint of Taylor & Francis Group, an Informa business

First issued in paperback 2019

No claim to original U.S. Government works

ISBN 13: 978-0-367-44602-4 (pbk)
ISBN 13: 978-1-84184-688-0 (hbk)

This book contains information obtained from authentic and highly regarded sources. While all reasonable efforts have been made to publish reliable data and information, neither the author[s] nor the publisher can accept any legal responsibility or liability for any errors or omissions that may be made. The publishers wish to make clear that any views or opinions expressed in this book by individual editors, authors or contributors are personal to them and do not necessarily reflect the views/opinions of the publishers. The information or guidance contained in this book is intended for use by medical, scientific or health-care professionals and is provided strictly as a supplement to the medical or other professional's own judgement, their knowledge of the patient's medical history, relevant manufacturer's instructions and the appropriate best practice guidelines. Because of the rapid advances in medical science, any information or advice on dosages, procedures or diagnoses should be independently verified. The reader is strongly urged to consult the relevant national drug formulary and the drug companies' and device or material manufacturers' printed instructions, and their websites, before administering or utilizing any of the drugs, devices or materials mentioned in this book. This book does not indicate whether a particular treatment is appropriate or suitable for a particular individual. Ultimately it is the sole responsibility of the medical professional to make his or her own professional judgements, so as to advise and treat patients appropriately. The authors and publishers have also attempted to trace the copyright holders of all material reproduced in this publication and apologize to copyright holders if permission to publish in this form has not been obtained. If any copyright material has not been acknowledged please write and let us know so we may rectify in any future reprint.

Visit the Taylor & Francis Web site at
http://www.taylorandfrancis.com

and the CRC Press Web site at
http://www.crcpress.com

A CIP record for this book is available from the British Library.
Library of Congress Cataloging-in-Publication Data

Typeset byC&M Digitals (P) Ltd, Chennai, India

Contents

III. Pediatric Stone Management

Contributors

Reem Al-Bareeq
Department of Urology
Department of Surgery
Schulich School of Medicine and Dentistry
The University of Western Ontario
London, Ontario, Canada

John R Asplin
Litholink Corporation
and Department of Medicine
University of Chicago Pritzker
    School of Medicine
Chicago, Illinois, U.S.A.

Dean G Assimos
Department of Urology
Wake Forest University School of Medicine
Winston-Salem, North Carolina, U.S.A.

Benjamin K Canales
Department of Urology
University of Florida
Gainesville, Florida, U.S.A.

Ralph Clayman
Department of Urology
University of California at Irvine
Irvine, California, U.S.A

Gary C Curhan
Harvard Medical School/Harvard School
    of Public Health
Channing Laboratory/Renal Division
Brigham and Women's Hospital
Boston, Massachusetts, U.S.A.

John D Denstedt
Department of Urology
Department of Surgery
Schulich School of Medicine and Dentistry
The University of Western Ontario
London, Ontario, Canada

Alana Desai
Department of Urology
Washington University School of Medicine
St Louis, Missouri, U.S.A.

Michael H Ferrandino
Division of Urologic Surgery
Comprehensive Kidney Stone Center
Duke University Medical Center
Durham, North Carolina, U.S.A.

Amy E Krambeck
Methodist Hospital Institute for Kidney
    Stone Disease
Indianapolis, Indiana, U.S.A.

James E Lingeman
Methodist Hospital Institute for Kidney
    Stone Disease
Indianapolis, Indiana, U.S.A.

Michael K Louie
Department of Urology
University of California at Irvine
Irvine, California, U.S.A.

Manoj Monga
University of Minnesota
Fairview, Minnesota, U.S.A.

Brian R Matlaga
James Buchanan Brady Urological Institute
The Johns Hopkins University School of
    Medicine
Baltimore, Maryland, U.S.A.

Stephen Y Nakada
Department of Urology
Clinical Science Center
University of Wisconsin
Madison, Wisconsin, U.S.A.

Gyan Pareek
The Warren Alpert Medical
    School of Brown University
Providence, Rhode Island, U.S.A.

Sangtae Park
Department of Surgery (Urology)
University of Chicago, Pritzker School of
    Medicine
Chicago, Illinois, U.S.A.

Corey M Passman
Department of Urology
Wake Forest University School of Medicine
Winston-Salem, North Carolina, U.S.A.

Bhavin N Patel
Department of Urology
Wake Forest University School of Medicine
Winston-Salem, North Carolina, U.S.A.

Margaret S Pearle
Department of Urology
University of Texas Southwestern Medical
    Center
Dallas, Texas, U.S.A.

Kristina Penniston
Department of Urology
Clinical Science Center
University of Wisconsin
Madison, Wisconsin, U.S.A.

Glenn M Preminger
Division of Urologic Surgery
Comprehensive Kidney Stone Center
Duke University Medical Center
Durham, North Carolina, U.S.A.

Khashayar Sakhaee
Department of Internal Medicine
Charles& Jane Pak Center for Mineral
    Metabolism & Clinical Research
University of Texas Southwestern Medical
    Center at Dallas
Dallas, Texas, U.S.A.

Bruce Slaughenhoupt
Division of Surgery
Clinical Science Center
University of Wisconsin
Madison, Wisconsin, U.S.A.

Olivier Traxer
Urology Department Tenon Hospital Pierre
    and Marie Curie University-Paris 6
Paris, France

Ramakrishna Venkatesh
Washington University School of Medicine
St. Louis to Division of Urology
University of Kentucky, Lexington
Kentucky, USA

Geoffrey R Wignall
Department of Urology
Department of Surgery
Schulich School of Medicine and Dentistry
The University of Western Ontario
London, Ontario, Canada

Elaine Worcester
Nephrology Section
Department of Medicine
University of Chicago
Chicago, Illinois, U.S.A.

1 | Epidemiology of stone disease

Gary C Curhan

INTRODUCTION

Nephrolithiasis is a complex disease, thus an understanding of the epidemiology, particularly the interactions among different factors, may help lead to approaches that reduce the risk of stone formation. Epidemiologic studies can also help quantify changes in patterns of burden of disease and identify risk factors. Uncovering new risk factors may provide insight into pathophysiologic processes related to stone formation. These types of studies also allow examination of genetic influences and gene–environment interactions.

PREVALENCE

Stone disease is common with the lifetime risk of stone formation in the United States exceeding 12% in men and 6% in women.(1, 2) However, the prevalence of nephrolithiasis, defined as a history of stone disease, varies by age, sex, and race. A history of nephrolithiasis increased in the last quarter of the 20th century for both men and women, and black and whites.(2) (See Figures 1.1 and 1.2) This increase may be due in part to increased detection of asymptomatic stones owing to the increasing use and sensitivity of imaging studies. Prevalence of stone disease has also increased in other parts of the world including Japan (3) and Germany.(4)

A history of stone disease in the United States varies by racial background (2, 5), being most common among older white males (~10%) and lowest in younger black females (~1%); rates for Asians and Hispanics are in between.

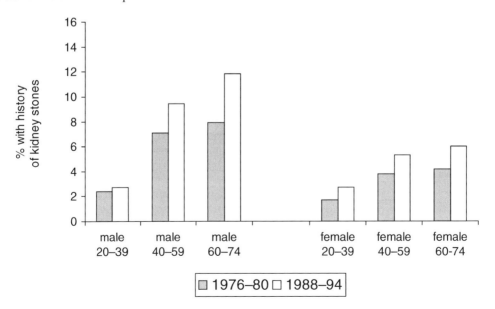

Figure 1.1 Prevalence of stone disease by sex and age.

Source: Reprinted from Stamatelou KK, Francis ME, Jones CA, Nyberg LM, Curhan GC. Time trends in reported prevalence of kidney stones in the United States: 1976–1994. Kidney International, 63, 1817–1823, Copyright 2003, with permission from Nature Publishing Group.

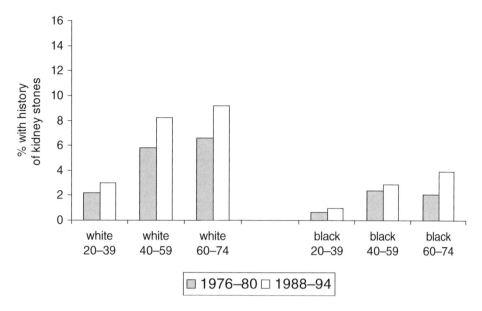

Figure 1.2   Prevalence of stone disease by race and age.

Source: Reprinted from Stamatelou KK, Francis ME, Jones CA, Nyberg LM, Curhan GC. Time trends in reported prevalence of kidney stones in the United States: 1976–1994. Kidney International, 63, 1,817–1,823, Copyright 2003, with permission from Nature Publishing Group.

Geographic variability was demonstrated in a study of more than 1 million individuals that found a north–south and west–east gradient; the highest prevalence of stone disease occurred in the Southeastern United States.(6)

A recent study raised the possibility of a change in the male-to-female ratio.(7) Based on hospital discharges for stone disease in the Nationwide Inpatient Survey between 1997 and 2002, the male-to-female ratio was 1.3:1. This study was based on hospital discharges; population-based studies are needed to confirm this interesting observation.

INCIDENCE

Several population-based studies have demonstrated that incidence rates, defined as onset of an individual's first kidney stone, vary by age, sex, and race. As with prevalence, the incidence rates are highest in white males. For men, the incidence begins to rise after age 20, peaks between 40 and 60 years at ~3/1000/year and then declines.(1, 8, 9) For women, incidence rates seem to be higher in the late 20s (2.5/1000/year) and then decrease to 1/1000/year by age 50, remaining relatively constant for the next several decades.(1, 9–11)

A recent study from Rochester, Minnesota, suggests that incidence rates may be decreasing. Compared to a study done 30 years earlier with the same methodology, which found increasing incidence rates in men and women between 1950 and 1974, the recent study observed that the incidence rates since 1990 may be falling in men and have reached a plateau in women. (12) Additional larger studies are needed to explore this important issue.

RECURRENCE RATES

Case series suggested that if left untreated the likelihood of forming another stone after the initial episode was 30–40% at 5 years.(1) Of course, the likelihood of recurrence depends on many factors including stone type and urinary composition. Encouragingly, randomized trials suggested that intervening can reduce recurrence rates by 50% or more.(13–16) These interventions emphasize that prevention of stone recurrence is possible.

RISK FACTORS

Information on the importance of a variety of risk factors for stone formation has increased substantially over the past several decades. Risk factors are generally divided into nondietary, dietary, and urinary.

Non-dietary

Family history

Studies of twins demonstrate that stone disease is heritable.(17) For the common type of stone disease, individuals with a family history of stone disease (18) have a two-fold higher risk of becoming a stone former. This higher risk is likely due to a combination of genetic predisposition as well as similar environmental exposures (e.g., diet). Although several genetic factors have been clearly associated with rare forms of nephrolithiasis, (e.g., cystinuria, Dent disease), information is still limited on genes that contribute to risk of the common forms of stone disease.

Race/ethnicity

A cross-sectional study of several racial and ethnic groups in Canada found that, compared to Europeans, higher risks were observed for individuals of Arabic, west Indian, west Asian, and Latin American descent.(19) Although in the general population African Americans have a lower frequency of stones, African Americans with end-stage renal disease had a higher than expected prevalence of stone.(20)

Systemic disorders

Traditionally considered a renal disorder, there is overwhelming evidence that nephrolithiasis is a systemic disorder. Primary hyperparathyroidism, renal tubular acidosis, and Crohn's disease are well-described conditions associated with higher risk of calcium-containing stones.

A number of other common conditions have recently been convincingly linked to nephrolithiasis. Increasing body size as assessed by weight, body mass index, or waistline is associated with an increasing risk of stone formation independent of other risk factors including diet (21), and the impact was larger in women than in men. For example, the risk of stone formation for individuals with a body mass index (BMI) $\geq 30 \text{ kg/m}^2$ compared to those with a BMI 21–23 was 30% higher among men but nearly two-fold higher among women. Weight gain also increases the risk of stone formation. Larger body size impacts urinary composition (e.g., higher urine oxalate, lower urine pH), changes that would increase risk for calcium oxalate or uric acid stones.(22)

In a U.S. national health survey, individuals with gout were 50% more likely to have a history of stones.(23) When examined prospectively, a history of gout was associated with a doubling of the risk of forming a stone, independent of diet, weight, and medications.(24) Possible mechanisms for this relation include insulin resistance and acidification defects.

Diabetes mellitus (DM Type II) increases risk of stone formation, independent of diet and body size.(25) Crosssectionally, individuals with a history of diabetes were more than 30% more likely also to have a history of nephrolithiasis. Prospectively, a history of DM increased the risk of stone formation by 30–50% in women but not in men.(26, 27)

ENVIRONMENTAL FACTORS

A hot working environment leads to higher insensible fluid losses and thus increases risk of stone formation.(28) Risk will be higher when individuals have restricted access to water or bathroom facilities, leading to lower fluid intake and lower urine volume.

Dietary Factors

Dietary intake influences the composition of the urine and thereby modifies the risk of nephrolithiasis. Nutrients that have been proposed to modify the risk of nephrolithiasis include calcium, animal protein (29), oxalate (30), sodium (31), sucrose (32), magnesium (33), and potassium.(34) Several challenges should be considered when evaluating studies of diet and stone risk. Individuals who develop stones may subsequently change their diet, thus studies that retrospectively assess diet may be hampered by recall bias. Because the composition of the urine does not completely predict risk and not all the components that modify risk are included in the calculation of supersaturation (e.g., urine phytate), care must be taken when the outcome is change in urine composition rather than actual stone formation. Thus, prospective studies are best suited for examining the associations between dietary factors and risk of actual stone formation.

Calcium

The first prospective studies of dietary factors and the risk of incident stone disease were performed in three large cohorts: Health Professionals Follow-up Study (HPFS) involving more than 45,000 male health professionals aged 40–75 years at baseline; Nurses' Health Study I (NHS I) involving more than 80,000 female nurses aged 34–59 at baseline; and NHS II involving more than 80,000 female nurses aged 27–44 at baseline.(8, 10, 11) Although dietary calcium had been strongly suspected of raising the risk of stone disease, individuals with a higher intake of dietary calcium actually had a *lower* risk of incident nephrolithiasis independent of other risk factors.(8, 10, 11) One possible mechanism to explain this association is that lower calcium intake increases dietary oxalate absorption and urinary oxalate excretion (35); individuals with lower calcium intake have higher 24-hour urine oxalate excretion. It is also possible that there is some other protective factor in milk (dairy products are the major source of dietary calcium in the United States). A subsequent study showed that low dietary calcium intake may increase the risk of stone formation, even among individuals with a family history of stones.(18)

These observational data were subsequently confirmed in a randomized trial by Borghi and colleagues. The investigators randomized men with elevated urine calcium and a history of calcium oxalate stones to one of two diets: a low calcium diet (400 mg/d) or a diet containing 1200 mg of calcium along with low sodium and low animal protein intake.(13) The rate of recurrence was reduced by 50% in the higher calcium intake group. There is now overwhelming evidence that calcium restriction is not beneficial and may in fact be harmful, both for stone formation and bone loss.

Supplemental calcium, in contrast to dietary calcium, does not appear to reduce risk and may in fact increase risk. In an observational study of older women, calcium supplement users were 20% more likely to form a stone than women who did not take supplements, after adjusting for dietary factors.(10) There was no association in younger women and men.(8, 11) The Women's Health Initiative randomized trial also demonstrated a 17% increased risk of stones with calcium supplementation (36), but these results should be interpreted cautiously as the participants were instructed to take their supplements with meals, and the supplements contained both calcium and vitamin D. The discrepancy between the risks from dietary calcium and calcium supplements may be due to the timing of calcium intake. In the cohort studies, calcium supplements were often taken in between meals, which would diminish binding of dietary oxalate.

Oxalate

Although urine oxalate is undoubtedly an important risk factor for calcium oxalate stone, the role of dietary oxalate in the pathogenesis of calcium oxalate nephrolithiasis is less clear.(37) The proportion of urinary oxalate derived from dietary oxalate is controversial; estimates range from 10 to 50%.(37) In part due to variable and often low bioavailability, much of the oxalate in food may not be readily absorbed. Urinary oxalate is also derived from the endogenous metabolism of glycine, glycolate, hydroxyproline, and vitamin C. Some individuals with calcium oxalate nephrolithiasis may have increased absorption of dietary oxalate, and in some cases a deficiency of oxalate degradation by the intestinal bacterium *Oxalobacter formigenes* could be the culprit. A recent study found that individuals with a history of calcium oxalate nephrolithiasis were less likely to be colonized with Oxalobacter.(38) The impact of dietary oxalate on risk of stone formation was only recently studied prospectively because of the lack of sufficient and reliable information on the oxalate content of many foods. However, recent reports using modern approaches to measure the oxalate content of food have allowed prospective studies of the impact of dietary oxalate.(39, 40) Surprisingly the impact of dietary oxalate was minimal in men and older women and not associated with stone formation in younger women.(41)

Other nutrients

Other nutrients have been implicated in stone formation, and some of the associations vary by age, sex, or (BMI). High animal protein intake leads to increased calcium and decreased urinary citrate (42), which could increase the risk of stone formation. However, when studied prospectively, animal protein was observed to increase risk in men but not women.(8, 10, 11) An increased risk of stone formation was observed for higher animal protein intake only among men with BMI < 25 kg/m².(43) Potassium supplementation reduces urine calcium excretion (34) and many potassium-rich foods increase urinary citrate due to their alkali content. Higher dietary potassium intake decreased risk in men and older women.(8, 10, 43) Higher intake of sodium (31) or sucrose (32) increases urinary calcium excretion independent of calcium intake. The prospective cohort studies found that sucrose was associated with an increased risk in women and fructose increased risk in men and women.(10, 11, 44) Phytate was observed to reduce risk of stone formation in younger women.(11)

Magnesium complexes with oxalate, thereby potentially reducing oxalate absorption in the gastrointestinal tract and decreasing calcium oxalate supersaturation in the urine. Randomized trials of magnesium supplements have not supported a protective effect on stone recurrence, but the dropout rates were high. In prospective observational studies, higher dietary magnesium was associated with a lower risk of stone formation in men (43) but not women.(10, 11)

Vitamin C (ascorbic acid) may be related to calcium oxalate stone formation because it can be metabolized to oxalate. Consumption of 1000 mg of supplemental vitamin C twice daily increased urinary oxalate excretion by 22%.(45) An observational study in men found that those who consumed 1000 mg or more per day of vitamin C had a 40% higher risk of stone formation compared to men who consumed less than 90 mg/day (the recommended dietary allowance). (43) Restricting *dietary* vitamin C is not appropriate (because foods high in vitamin C contain inhibitory factors such as potassium). However, calcium oxalate stone formers should be encouraged to avoid vitamin C supplements.

High doses of supplemental vitamin B6 (pyridoxine) may reduce oxalate production in selected patients with type 1 primary hyperoxaluria, but the use of vitamin B6 in other settings remains unclear. Based on observational data, high intake of vitamin B6 may reduce the risk of kidney stone formation in women (46) but not in men.(47)

Fluid Intake and Beverages

Urine volume is an important determinant of stone risk. When the urine output is less than 1 L/ day, risk of stone formation is markedly higher. Observational studies (8, 10, 11) and a randomized-controlled trial (48) have demonstrated that higher fluid intake reduces the likelihood of stone formation.

There are more data to advise patients with stone disease about which beverages they should and should not drink. Observational studies have found that coffee, tea, beer, and wine are associated with a *reduced* risk of stone formation.(49, 50) Although citrus juices theoretically could reduce the risk of stone formation by increasing urine citrate (51), the prospective studies found orange juice was not associated with stone formation and grapefruit juice was associated with a significantly higher risk.(49, 50) Although grapefruit juice affects several intestinal enzymes, the mechanism for the observed increased risk is unknown. Consumption of sugared soda was associated with a higher risk of stone formation.(49, 50) Milk intake also reduces the risk of calcium kidney stone formation.

Urinary Factors

The 24-hour urine chemistries provide important prognostic information and guide therapeutic recommendations for prevention. Traditionally, urine results have been categorized into "normal" and "abnormal", but recently there has been a greater appreciation of two important points. First, the urine values are continuous so the dichotomization into "normal" and "abnormal" is arbitrary and potentially misleading. Second, stone formation is a disorder of *concentration*, not just the absolute amount excreted. Although terms such as "hypercalciuria" are often used both clinically and scientifically, the limitations of these terms should be remembered.

Hypercalciuria has been traditionally defined as urine calcium excretion ≥ 300 mg/day in men and ≥ 250 mg/day in women (52) on a 1000-mg/day calcium diet (but a variety of definitions are in use). Based on the traditional definitions, ~20–40% of patients with calcium stone disease will have hypercalciuria. Allowing a higher cutoff value in males than females may be reasonable from a calcium balance perspective, but it does not seem appropriate for stone formation, given that 24-hour urine volumes are slightly higher in women than in men.(53)

Hyperoxaluria is typically defined as urinary oxalate excretion >45 mg/d. Elevated urinary oxalate excretion is three to four times more common among men (~40%) than in women (~10%).(53) Although mean urinary oxalate levels may not differ between cases and controls, oxalate does appear to be an important independent risk factor for stone formation (53) and the risk begins to increase well below the 45 mg/d level.

The relation between uric acid metabolism and calcium stone disease is unclear. Some studies have reported that *hyperuricosuria* (defined as greater than 800 mg/day in men or 750 mg/day in women) is more frequent in patients who form calcium stones than normal subjects. (54) However a recent study of more than 2200 stone formers and 1100 controls found that a higher urine uric acid was associated with a lower likelihood of being a stone former in men and there was no increase in risk for women.(53) Although allopurinol in a double-blind trial successfully decreased recurrence rates of calcium stones in patients with hyperuricosuria (14), it is possible that the beneficial effect was unrelated to the lowering of urine uric acid.

Hypocitraturia, typically defined as 24-hour excretion ≤ 320 mg/d, increases risk of stone formation (55) and is found in 5–11% of first time stone formers.(53) There is suggestive evidence that increasing urinary citrate into the high-normal range provides additional protection.

Low urine volume, for which a variety of definitions have been used, is a common and modifiable risk factor. When defined as 24-hour urine volume less than 1 L/day, 12–25% of first-time stone formers will have this abnormality.(53) Observational studies have demonstrated that the risk of stone formation decreases with increasing total urine volume (53), and a randomized trial confirmed the value of increasing urine volume.(48)

SUMMARY

Epidemiologic studies have expanded our understanding of the magnitude and risk factors for stone disease. A variety of dietary, nondietary and urinary risk factors contribute to the risk of stone formation and the importance of these varies by age, sex, and BMI. Scientifically, results from these studies have forced a reappraisal of our view of risk factors for stone disease. Importantly, the results from epidemiologic studies can be considered in the clinical setting when devising treatment plans for reducing the likelihood of stone formation.

REFERENCES

1. Johnson CM, Wilson DM, O'Fallon WM, Malek RS, Kurland LT. Renal stone epidemiology: a 25-year study in Rochester, Minnesota. Kidney Int 1979; 16: 624–31.
2. Stamatelou KK, Francis ME, Jones CA, Nyberg LM, Curhan GC. Time trends in reported prevalence of kidney stones in the United States: 1976-1994. Kidney Int 2003; 63: 1817–23.
3. Yoshida O, Okada Y. Epidemiology of urolithiasis in Japan: a chronological and geographical study. Urol Int 1990; 45: 104–11.
4. Hesse A, Brandle E, Wilbert D, Kohrmann KU, Alken P. Study on the prevalence and incidence of urolithiasis in Germany comparing the years 1979 vs. 2000. Eur Urol 2003; 44: 709–13.
5. Soucie JM, Thun MJ, Coates RJ, McClellan W, Austin H. Demographic and geographic variability of kidney stones in the United States. Kidney Int 1994; 46: 893–9.
6. Soucie J, Coates R, McClellan W, Austin H, Thun M. Relation between geographic variability in kidney stones prevalence and risk factors for stones. Am J Epidemiol 1996; 143: 487–95.
7. Scales CD Jr, Curtis LH, Norris RD et al. Changing gender prevalence of stone disease. J Urol 2007; 177: 979–82.
8. Curhan GC, Willett WC, Rimm EB, Stampfer MJ. A prospective study of dietary calcium and other nutrients and the risk of symptomatic kidney stones. N Engl J Med 1993; 328: 833–8.
9. Hiatt RA, Dales LG, Friedman GD, Hunkeler EM. Frequency of urolithiasis in a prepaid medical care program. Am J Epidemiol 1982; 115: 255–65.

10. Curhan G, Willett W, Speizer F, Spiegelman D, Stampfer M. Comparison of dietary calcium with supplemental calcium and other nutrients as factors affecting the risk for kidney stones in women. Ann Intern Med 1997; 126: 497–504.

11. Curhan GC, Willett WC, Knight EL, Stampfer MJ. Dietary factors and the risk of incident kidney stones in younger women: Nurses' Health Study II. Arch Intern Med 2004; 164: 885–91.

12. Lieske JC, Pena de la Vega LS, Slezak JM et al. Renal stone epidemiology in Rochester, Minnesota: an update. Kidney Int 2006; 69: 760–4.

13. Borghi L, Schianchi T, Meschi T et al. Comparison of two diets for the prevention of recurrent stones in idiopathic hypercalciuria. N Engl J Med 2002; 346: 77–84.

14. Ettinger B, Tang A, Citron JT, Livermore B, Williams T. Randomized trial of allopurinol in the prevention of calcium oxalate calculi. N Engl J Med 1986; 315: 1386–9.

15. Ettinger B, Pak CY, Citron JT et al. Potassium-magnesium citrate is an effective prophylaxis against recurrent calcium oxalate nephrolithiasis. J Urol 1997; 158: 2069–73.

16. Ettinger B, Citron JT, Livermore B, Dolman LI. Chlorthalidone reduces calcium oxalate calculous recurrence but magnesium hydroxide does not. J Urol 1988; 139: 679–84.

17. Goldfarb DS, Fischer ME, Keich Y, Goldberg J. A twin study of genetic and dietary influences on nephrolithiasis: a report from the Vietnam Era Twin (VET) Registry. Kidney Int 2005; 67: 1053–61.

18. Curhan G, Willett W, Rimm E, Stampfer M. Family history and risk of kidney stones. J Am Soc Nephrol 1997; 8: 1568–73.

19. Mente A, Honey RJ, McLaughlin JR, Bull SB, Logan AG. Ethnic differences in relative risk of idiopathic calcium nephrolithiasis in North America. J Urol 2007; 178: 1992–7; discussion 7.

20. Stankus N, Hammes M, Gillen D, Worcester E. African American ESRD patients have a high pre-dialysis prevalence of kidney stones compared to NHANES III. Urol Res 2007; 35: 83–7.

21. Taylor EN, Stampfer MJ, Curhan GC. Obesity, weight gain, and the risk of kidney stones. JAMA 2005; 293: 455–62.

22. Taylor EN, Curhan GC. Body size and 24-hour urine composition. Am J Kidney Dis 2006; 48: 905–15.

23. Kramer HM, Curhan G. The association between gout and nephrolithiasis: the National Health and Nutrition Examination Survey III, 1988-1994. Am J Kidney Dis 2002; 40: 37–42.

24. Kramer HJ, Choi HK, Atkinson K, Stampfer M, Curhan GC. The association between gout and nephrolithiasis in men: The Health Professionals' Follow-Up Study. Kidney Int 2003; 64: 1022–6.

25. Taylor EN, Stampfer MJ, Curhan GC. Diabetes mellitus and the risk of nephrolithiasis. Kidney Int 2005; 68: 1230–5.

26. Daudon M, Traxer O, Conort P, Lacour B, Jungers P. Type 2 diabetes increases the risk for uric acid stones. J Am Soc Nephrol 2006; 17: 2026–33.

27. Lieske JC, de la Vega LS, Gettman MT et al. Diabetes mellitus and the risk of urinary tract stones: a population-based case-control study. Am J Kidney Dis 2006; 48: 897–904.

28. Atan L, Andreoni C, Ortiz V et al. High kidney stone risk in men working in steel industry at hot temperatures. Urology 2005; 65: 858–61.

29. Robertson WG, Peacock M, Hodgkinson A. Dietary changes and the incidence of urinary calculi in the U.K. between 1958 and 1976. J Chron Dis 1979; 32: 469–76.

30. Larsson L, Tiselius HG. Hyperoxaluria. Miner Electrolyte Metab 1987; 13: 242–50.

31. Muldowney FP, Freaney R, Moloney MF. Importance of dietary sodium in the hypercalciuria syndrome. Kidney Int 1982; 22: 292–6.

32. Lemann J Jr, Piering WF, Lennon EJ. Possible role of carbohydrate-induced calciuria in calcium oxalate kidney-stone formation. N Engl J Med 1969; 280: 232–7.

33. Johansson G, Backman U, Danielson BG et al. Biochemical and clinical effects of the prophylactic treatment of renal calcium stones with magnesium hydroxide. J Urol 1980; 124: 770–4.

34. Lemann J Jr, Pleuss JA, Gray RW, Hoffmann RG. Potassium administration reduces and potassium deprivation increases urinary calcium excretion in healthy adults [corrected]. Kidney Int 1991; 39: 973–83.

35. Bataille P, Charransol G, Gregoire I et al. Effect of calcium restriction on renal excretion of oxalate and the probability of stones in the various pathophysiological groups with calcium stones. J Urol 1983; 130: 218–23.

36. Jackson RD, LaCroix AZ, Gass M et al. Calcium plus vitamin D supplementation and the risk of fractures. N Engl J Med 2006; 354: 669–83.

37. Holmes RP, Assimos DG. The impact of dietary oxalate on kidney stone formation. Urol Res 2004; 32: 311–6.

38. Kaufman DW, Kelly JP, Curhan GC et al. Oxalobacter formigenes may reduce the risk of calcium oxalate kidney stones. J Am Soc Nephrol 2008; 19: 1197–203.

39. Siener R, Honow R, Voss S, Seidler A, Hesse A. Oxalate content of cereals and cereal products. J Agric Food Chem 2006; 54: 3008–11.

40. Holmes R, Kennedy M. Estimation of the oxalate content of foods and daily oxalate intake. Kidney Int 2000; 57: 1662–7.

41. Taylor EN, Curhan GC. Oxalate intake and the risk for nephrolithiasis. J Am Soc Nephrol 2007; 18: 2198–204.
42. Breslau N, Brinkely L, Hill K, Pak C. Relationship of animal protein-rich diet to kidney stone formation and calcium metabolism. J Clin Endocrinol Metab 1988; 66: 140–6.
43. Taylor EN, Stampfer MJ, Curhan GC. Dietary factors and the risk of incident kidney stones in men: new insights after 14 years of follow-up. J Am Soc Nephrol 2004; 15: 3225–32.
44. Taylor EN, Curhan GC. Fructose consumption and the risk of kidney stones. Kidney Int 2008; 73: 207–12.
45. Traxer O, Huet B, Poindexter J, Pak CY, Pearle MS. Effect of ascorbic acid consumption on urinary stone risk factors. J Urol 2003; 170: 397–401.
46. Curhan GC, Willett WC, Speizer FE, Stampfer MJ. Intake of vitamins B6 and C and the risk of kidney stones in women. J Am Soc Nephrol 1999; 10: 840–5.
47. Curhan GC, Willett WC, Rimm EB, Stampfer MJ. A prospective study of the intake of vitamins C and B6, and the risk of kidney stones in men. J Urol 1996; 155: 1847–51.
48. Borghi L, Meschi T, Amato F et al. Urinary volume, water and recurrences in idiopathic calcium nephrolithiasis: a 5-year randomized prospective study. J Urol 1996; 155: 839–43.
49. Curhan GC, Willett WC, Rimm EB, Spiegelman D, Stampfer MJ. Prospective study of beverage use and the risk of kidney stones. Am J Epidemiol 1996; 143: 240–7.
50. Curhan GC, Willett WC, Speizer FE, Stampfer MJ. Beverage use and risk for kidney stones in women. Ann Intern Med 1998; 128: 534–40.
51. Wabner C, Pak C. Effect of orange juice consumption on urinary stone risk factors. J Urol 1993; 149: 1405–9.
52. Hodgkinson A, Pyrah LN. The urinary excretion of calcium and inorganic phosphate in 344 patients with calcium stone of renal origin. Br J Surg 1958; 46: 10–8.
53. Curhan GC, Taylor EN. 24-h uric acid excretion and the risk of kidney stones. Kidney Int 2008; 73: 489–96.
54. Coe FL. Hyperuricosuric calcium oxalate nephrolithiasis. Kidney Int 1978; 13: 418–26.
55. Pak CY. Citrate and renal calculi: an update. Miner Electrolyte Metab 1994; 20: 371–7.

2 | Pathogenesis of renal calculi
Brian R Matlaga

HISTORICAL THEORIES OF STONE PATHOGENESIS

Archaeological explorations have unearthed findings confirming that ancient man suffered from urinary lithiasis: in one expedition, a renal calculus dating to approximately 4200 BC was found among the bones of a young egyptian.(1) Ancient records similarly confirm that stone disease was present among the Greek and Roman civilizations. As a disease dating back at least to antiquity, physicians and scientists of the time offered differing theories on the origin urinary calculi. Hippocrates presented one of the earliest hypotheses on the etiology of urinary lithiasis, when he observed that many patients with calculi had sandy sediment in their urine, and suggested that stone formation was a consequence of the consumption of water rich in lime or silt.(2) Galen, the Roman physician, postulated that gout and rheumatism were related to calculi, and suggested that the pathophysiology of these processes was intertwined. Ancient Indian physicians presented an alternative theory on stone pathogenesis, describing four unique types of calculi, variously formed by phlegm, vapour, bile, and semen.(3) The type of stone could be divined by the physician following examination of its morphology. In later centuries, medieval physicians hypothesized that urinary calculi arose as a consequence of excessive dietary salt, exposure to excessive heat, or the presence of obstructing matter in the urinary tract.

As science progressed, an increased appreciation of the anatomy of the urinary tract and renal physiology gave rise to more informed theories on stone pathogenesis. Importantly, stones arising in the urinary bladder were considered to be different from stones arising in the kidney. Delet, a sixteenth century French physician, reported that "stones found in the kidneys are formed by fine sands and assume the shape of the pelvis. Bladder calculi look like river pebbles ... and are formed not with sand, but by an almost solid matter." (3) In the seventeenth century, Von Heyden reported on the ultrastructure of urinary calculi; subsequently Schele further advanced our understanding of stone composition when he isolated uric acid from a stone.(4) Our understanding of stone composition was refined in the nineteenth century, when oxalate, cystine, calcium carbonate, phosphate, struvite were identified and characterized as components of calculi.

The advent of modern analytic techniques and technology has fostered a greater understanding of stone ultrastructure and composition. As a result, investigators in the twentieth century have endeavored to define the site of stone formation in the kidney and the mechanisms by which stones grow. Among the many different theories on stone pathogenesis that were presented at this time, Alexander Randall reported in the 1930s that renal papillary calcifications were a precursor lesion to stone formation.(5) The development of the renal papillary plaque, he hypothesized, was a tripartite process: first, the plaques appeared in the basement membrane of the collecting tubules; in the second stage plaque became visible on the papillary surface; the third stage is characterized by calcium oxalate overgrowth on the papillary plaque.

Although more recently published studies appear to corroborate much of Randall's work, the field of stone pathogenesis is one replete with many incompletely answered questions. It is likely that there is no single, universal process of stone pathogenesis that applies to all stone compositions and all stone formers. However, the basic processes by which a mineral comes out of solution and is retained in the kidney to become a clinically evident calculus, may be parallel, to some extent, among different stone-forming phenotypes.

PHYSICAL CHEMISTRY OF STONE FORMATION

Saturation

In order for a urinary calculus to form, the urine must contain an excess of the crystalline material that can generate a stone. That is to say, the urinary environment must be supersaturated

Table 2.1 Zones of Urinary Saturation.

Unstable Zone	Nuclei form, grow, and aggregate
• Calcium Oxalate SS > 8	
• Brushite SS > 2.5	
• Uric Acid SS > 2	
Metastable Upper Limit	First solid phase formation
• Formation Product	
Metastable Zone	No spontaneous nucleation
• Calcium Oxalate 1 < SS < 8	Crystals already present can grow
• Brushite 1 < SS < 2.5	Inhibitors can prevent crystallization
• Uric Acid 1 < SS < 2	
Equilibrium Point	Crystals neither grow nor dissolve
• SS = 1	
Undersaturation Zone	Nuclei may dissolve
• SS < 1	

with these stone-forming crystals. To better elucidate this concept, it is instructive to consider urinary saturation (Table 2.1).(6) For all solutions, urine included, there is a maximum amount of dissolved salt that can be kept in a stable solution. The concentration at which urine becomes saturated with the dissolved salt and crystallization begins is known as the thermodynamic solubility product (*Ksp*). *Ksp* is a mathematical expression, equal to the product of the concentration of the pure chemical components of the solute at the point of saturation. For example, the *Ksp* for sodium chloride is $[Na+][Cl-]$. When the concentration of the salt in a solution is less than the solubility product, the solution is said to be undersaturated. No spontaneous crystallization will occur in an undersaturated solution; therefore, in undersaturated urine, stones will not form. As the concentration of the salt increases above its solubility product, there will be a second point encountered where the solution becomes unstable with respect to the salt and crystallization will spontaneously begin; this point is termed the formation product. The region between the solubility product and the formation product is known as the metastable region. When a solution is metastable with respect to a salt, de novo crystallization is unlikely to occur, although growth may occur on existing crystals.(7)

Nucleation

Nucleation is the establishment of the smallest unit lattice of a crystal species, the first step in crystal formation. There are two types of nucleation: homogeneous nucleation and heterogeneous nucleation. When a solution is pure, the nucleation process is homogeneous. In human urine, though, the chemical environment is diverse, and homogeneous nucleation is unlikely to occur; rather, a heterogeneous nucleation process, by which crystal nuclei can form on structures such as cellular material, urinary crystals, and urinary casts occurs.(8) In fact, most urinary stones are a mixture of more than one crystal type suggesting that a process of heterogeneous nucleation is responsible for the formation of most stones. In general, thermodynamic forces require a higher level of urinary supersaturation for a homogeneous nucleation process than for a heterogeneous nucleation process, favoring the heterogeneous process in the human urinary environment.(9)

AGGREGATION

Crystal nuclei bind to one another to form larger particles, a process known as aggregation. (10) In the urinary environment, chemically or electrically induced forces can promote crystal aggregation; once crystals have aggregated to one another, they are held in place by strong intermolecular forces, and cannot be easily separated. Crystal aggregation is likely an important mechanism in stone formation, as a single crystal will never be large enough to be retained in the urinary collecting system.(11) Rather, ultrastructural analyses of stones typically demonstrate highly aggregated structural arrangements.(12)

Epitaxy

Most stones are composed of more than one crystal type, but the process by which a multicomponent stone forms is not well understood. Certainly heterogeneous nucleation accounts for the initiation of the process. However, it is likely that epitaxy, or the process by which one crystal lattice overgrows another crystal lattice, also has a contributory role.(13) For epitaxy to occur, the crystal lattices of the constituent components must be compatible and supportive.(14) Intermolecular forces, particularly ionic bonds, account for the strength of attachment of one lattice to another.

Retention

For a stone to form, crystal retention is necessary; if nucleated and aggregated crystals passed out of the renal collecting system with normal urinary flow, a clinically evident kidney stone would never form. Therefore, stone formation hinges on the retention of crystal material in the kidney until it achieves a size great enough that it is a clinical renal calculus. There have been two mechanisms proposed to account for crystal retention: the free particle hypothesis and the fixed particle hypothesis.(15, 16) In the free particle scenario, the process of nucleation occurs entirely in the tubular lumen. As crystals move through the renal tubules, nucleation followed by rapid aggregation generates a crystalline structure large enough to be retained at the level of the papillary collecting duct. Although the free particle theory is plausible from a purely thermodynamic perspective, Finlayson ultimately disproved this hypothesis as it relates to stone disease when he reported that the flow of ultrafiltrate through the renal tubule was so rapid as to prohibit the formation of such an obstructing crystalline mass.(17)

The alternative fixed particle hypothesis relies on the adherence of crystals to a surface point within the renal collecting system, such as renal epithelial cells.(18) Although normal urothelium is resistant to crystal adhesion, chemically injured urothelium will promote crystal adherence.(19) It may also be that cell surface molecules, so-called crystal-binding molecules such as phosphatidylserine, sialic acid, osteopontin, and hyaluronan, promote this process as well.(20–24)

INHIBITORS OF CRYSTAL GROWTH

Although urinary supersaturation is important in the formation of calcium oxalate calculi, other urinary factors may be equally important, for the urine of non-stone-formers is quite often supersaturated with respect to calcium oxalate yet no stone forms in these patients. There are a number of urinary molecules that modulate the process of crystal nucleation and aggregation, and it may be that different urinary concentrations of these molecules will affect the likelihood of stone formation. For example, repletion of the urine with citrate will reduce the likelihood of calcium oxalate stone formation; citrate acts to reduce both the spontaneous and heterogeneous nucleation of calcium oxalate. Other inhibitory molecules include magnesium, pyrophosphate, nephrocalcin, Tamm-Horsfall protein, uropontin, crystal matrix protein, prothrombin fragment one, lithostathine, inter-alpha-trypsin inhibitor molecule/uronic acid-rich protein (bikunin), albumin, RNA and DNA fragments, glycosaminoglycans, and calgranulin.(6) The exact mechanism of action and effect of many of these inhibitors remain to be elucidated.

ROLE OF PROTEINS/MATRIX

All kidney stones contain organic matrix, generally comprising 2–3% of the dry weight of the stone (excluding the rare predominantly matrix stone that occurs in the setting of chronic urinary tract infection). (25, 26) From an anatomic standpoint, matrix has been localized to intercrystal regions, suggesting that matrix acts as a crystal-to-crystal attachment mediator. (27) Compositional assays have found matrix to be composed of lipids, glycosaminoglycans, carbohydrates, and proteins.(28) Approximately two-thirds of matrix is composed of proteinaceous material, but as matrix is poorly soluble, many of these proteins have yet to be identified. (29) Although the role of noncrystalline, organic matrix in the pathogenesis of renal calculi has not been definitively characterized, it is likely that matrix does play a significant role in the process of stone formation. It may be that stone matrix is derived from the incorporation of urinary macromolecules during the process of crystal aggregation.(30) Future efforts devoted to the proteomic characterization of renal calculi and their associated matrix will likely advance our knowledge of this subject.

THEORIES OF STONE PATHOGENESIS

Crystal-Induced Renal Injury

Crystal retention is required for kidney stone formation; one proposed mechanism that will allow crystal retention to occur centers on the concept of tubular cell injury. In certain animal and tissue culture models, it is possible to induce cellular injury that will then serve as a site for crystal attachment.(31) In general, this has been accomplished by creating a hyperoxaluric state through the administration of oxalate directly or a metabolic precursor of oxalate.(19) When hyperoxaluria occurs, there is a resulting increase in the production of reactive oxygen species, which cause lipid peroxidation and cellular injury.(32) Confirmatory studies in these models have reported an increase in the excretion of enzymes associated with renal epithelial cell injury, such as N-acetyl-β-glucosaminidase, gamma-glutamyl transpeptidase, and alkaline phosphatase.(33) Additionally certain macromolecules that may promote crystal to cell attachment are also present. Although there are natural defenses to reactive oxygen species, generally in these models of hyperoxaluria the oxalate levels are so great that they will overwhelm the protective systems.(34) When cellular crystal adherence does occur, an inflammatory cascade is initiated. Intersitital tumor necrosis factor alpha increases, with a resultant rise in the levels of several matrix metalloproteinases.(32) Matrix metalloproteinases may induce the erosion of subepithelial crystal deposits present at the renal papillary surface, which can create a nidus for stone formation.(35)

Although these animal and tissue models have reliably induced calcium oxalate crystalluria, they do have a number of shortcomings. In the ethylene glycol-induced animal model, in which calcium oxalate calculi are well documented to occur, there are a number of changes that also occur which are not encountered in the human calcium oxalate stone former. For example, other organ systems often demonstrate effects of elevated circulating oxalate levels, and the treated animals generally exhibit a metabolic acidosis.(36, 37) Furthermore, the levels of oxalate found in these animal models are supraphysiologic, in some cases by several orders of magnitude. Importantly, at a physiologic dose of dietary oxalate, Holmes and associates have reported no evidence of renal injury or oxidative stress.(38) Another flaw in the tissue culture models described herein is that they have only demonstrated crystal adherence to injured renal epithelial cells; no study has yet reported crystal attachment to healthy inner medullary collecting duct cells.(39)

Free Particle Formation

It has been proposed that nucleation and aggregation may occur within the tubular lumen, resulting in crystal retention at the papillary collecting duct. This free particle hypothesis has generated a body of discordant literature. Finlayson and Reid have reported that there was insufficient time for the formation of a lumen-obstructing crystal mass, due to the rapid flow of ultrafiltrate through the tubular network.(17) However, other investigators have suggested that given certain nephron dimensions, saturation levels, and crystal growth rates, it may be theoretically possible to form retainable crystals.(15)

Robertson has used mathematical modeling analyses to find that it is unlikely that individual crystals can grow large enough to be trapped in the renal collecting system.(40) Therefore, if the free particle hypothesis is correct, there must be an alternative supporting explanation. Robertson has suggested that three hydrodynamic factors may influence stone formation: (1) fluid drag close to the tubule walls (2), the drag effect of tubular walls on particles traveling close to the tubule walls, and (3) the effect of gravity on particles traveling in upward-draining sections of tubule. Applying these assumptions to the mathematical models, Roberston has found that the free particle model of calcium stone formation remains theoretically possible.

Intravascular Phenomenon

Stoller has suggested that renal calculi may develop as a consequence of an intravascular phenomenon within the vasa recta, at the innermost portion of the renal papilla.(41, 42) Injury to the papillary microvasculature at this location, with subsequent repair of the injury, may yield an atherosclerotic-like reaction with calcification. This pathologic calcification may ultimately erode into the renal papillary collecting ducts and serve as a nidus for calculus formation. Furthermore, the authors note that free and esterified cholesterol have been identified within kidney stones, a finding which may support this theory of stone formation. Although the intravascular hypothesis of stone formation relies on epidemiological, clinical, physiological, and anatomical observations, true confirmatory pathologic evidence from living human stone formers is lacking. In fact, in tissue from living human stone formers that has been analyzed by Evan and associates, there are no such abnormalities present in the papillary microvasculature.(18)

Nanobacteria

Nanobacteria are cytotoxic, gram-negative, atypical bacteria detected in bovine and human blood that have been implicated in a variety of disease states, such as atherosclerotic heart disease, periodontal disease, and renal cystic disease.(43–48) Several investigations have speculated that nanobacteria may play a role in the formation of renal calculi, as they may nucleate carbonate apatite on their surfaces.(49–52) In an *in vitro* study, Ciftcioglu and colleagues demonstrated the presence of nanobacteria in human kidney stones, and *in vitro* and animal studies have reported stone formation induced by nanobacteria as well.(43) Despite these supportive basic science reports, the role of nanobacteria in stone pathogenesis is controversial. Cisar and colleagues demonstrated that biomineralization previously attributed to nanobacteria may in fact be initiated by macromolecules, rather than a living organism.(53)

Stasis

There are likely certain clinical situations where the stasis of urine may contribute to stone formation, such as ureteropelvic junction obstruction, calyceal diverticulum, horseshoe kidney, hydronephrosis, and medullary sponge kidney.(54, 55) The impaired drainage of urine from the upper urinary tract in these situations may result in the retention of crystalline material. It is unclear if urinary stasis alone is sufficient to induce stone formation, as some have reported that metabolic abnormalities may also contribute to stone development in these settings.(56–58) Matlaga and associates have demonstrated that urinary risk profiles of patients who had diverticular calculi were similar to those of calcium oxalate stone formers, suggesting a metabolic etiology of diverticular stones.(59) However, these authors also found that the supersaturation of urine aspirated directly from the diverticular cavity was significantly lower than that of the urine found in the renal pelvis, suggesting an effect of urinary stasis in the pathogenesis of calyceal diverticular calculi. It may be that a combination of both metabolic abnormalities and urinary stasis influence stone formation in patients who have anatomic abnormalities of the kidney that impair urine drainage.

Randall's Plaque

Over six decades ago, Alexander Randall conducted a detailed examination of the papillae of more than 1,000 nonselected cadaveric renal units.(5) He observed calcium salt deposits in the tip of the renal papillum in 19.6% of individuals studied. These deposits, which he termed plaque, were interstitial in location, composed of calcium phosphate, and not observed in the tubular lumen. Randall hypothesized that these areas of plaque would be an ideal site for an overgrowth of calcium oxalate to develop into a calculus. Since Randall's observations, reported in 1940, little progress has been made in defining the role of plaque in the pathogenesis of kidney stone disease, for the most part because of a lack of appropriate in vivo data, but perhaps also aided by the fact that Randall tried to expand his hypothesis to fit all stone formers, and the great risk of a universal theory is that it only requires one exception to disprove the rule.

Kuo and associates, however, have reported on the safety of performing renal papillary and cortical biopsies at the time of percutaneous nephrolithotomy (PNL).(60) Subsequent data derived from the tissue of living, well-characterized human stone-formers have demonstrated

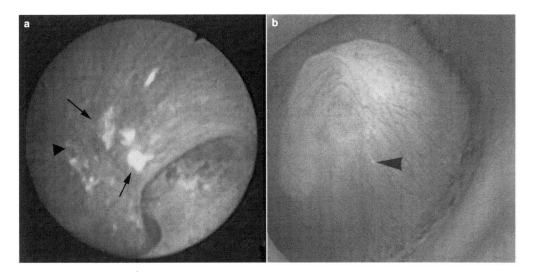

Figure 2.1   A. An example of a papilla from a calcium oxalate stone former that was video recorded at the time of the mapping. Several sites of Randall's plaque (arrows) appear as irregular white areas beneath the urothelium in this calcium oxalate patient. In addition, a plaque site that lacks an urothelial layer (arrowhead) may be a site where a stone had been attached to the papilla. B. An example of a papilla from a nonstone former that was video recorded at the time of the mapping. No distinct sites of Randall's plaque are noted on the papilla of the nonstone former; instead, a nodular appearing structure (arrowhead) is seen along the side of the papilla. Reprinted from Matlaga et al., The Role of Randall's Plaques in the Pathogenesis of Calcium Stones, Journal of Urology, 177:31, 2006, with permission from Elsevier.

a prominent role for Randall's plaque in the pathogenesis of stone disease.(61) Metabolic and surgical pathologic findings in four distinct groups of stone formers have clearly shown that "the histology of the renal papilla from a stone former is particular to the clinical setting."(62)

THE PATHOGENESIS OF IDIOPATHIC CALCIUM OXALATE STONE FORMERS

In defining the pathogenesis of stone disease, the first question to be answered is that of crystal deposition: where, and due to what forces, are crystals initially deposited that will lead to a kidney stone. To answer this question requires a study of the living, human, idiopathic calcium oxalate stone former. Idiopathic calcium oxalate stone formers, a condition defined as those patients in whom calcium oxalate stones form without any systemic cause other than idiopathic familial hypercalciuria, are the most common type of stone former.(63) Therefore, they represent an ideal initial group in which to define the pathogenesis of renal calculous disease. When examined with high-resolution digital endoscopic imaging, the renal papillae in all such patients were noted to have sites of Randall's plaques, which were manifest as irregular, whitish lesions generally located on the papillary tip, just as Randall initially described (Figure 2.1a).(5) A cohort of nonstone-forming patients served as a control population and when the papillary surfaces of these patients were examined, only rare sites of Randall's plaques were identified (Figure 2.1b). The renal papillae in the stone former and nonstone former groups were carefully mapped to quantify the papillary surface area covered by plaque. The fractional plaque coverage in stone formers was significantly higher than that in control (nonstone former) patients.(64)

Histological examination of the papillary tissue demonstrated that plaque was composed of calcium salts, as defined by the Yasue metal substitution technique (Figure 2.2a). (62) Furthermore, the plaque areas originated in the basement membranes of the thin loops of Henle, and these deposits were localized to the inner medullary interstitial space and followed the thin loops of Henle to the basal urothelium (Figure 2.2.b and c). Higher power imaging demonstrated that crystalline deposits as small as 50 nm could be identified in the basement membrane of otherwise normal-appearing thin loops of Henle, where they were

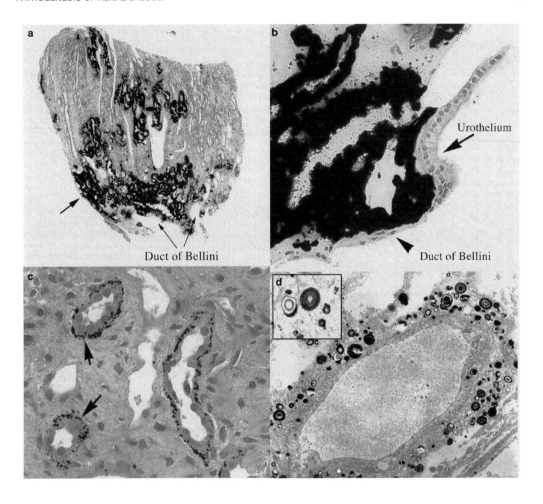

Figure 2.2 A. A low-power light microscopic image of a papillary biopsy specimen from a calcium oxalate patient is shown; the sites of calcium deposits (arrows) were stained black by the Yasue metal substitution method for calcium histochemistry. B. A light micrograph shows large regions of crystal deposits in the interstitial tissue surrounding the ducts of Bellini (arrowhead), proceeding up to the urothelium of a papillary tip (arrow), and progressing up the inner medulla. C. A higher power light micrograph shows sites of crystalline material (arrows) in the basement membranes. D. A transmission electron micrograph demonstrates sites of crystal material in the basement membranes. The insert image confirms the location of the crystals is associated with the collagen of the thin loops of Henle. Magnification, x100 (A); x600 (B); x1,000 (C); x25,000 (D). Reprinted from Matlaga et al., The Role of Randall's Plaques in the Pathogenesis of Calcium Stones, Journal of Urology, 177:31, 2006, with permission from Elsevier.

closely associated with type I collagen bundles in the interstitial space of the papillary tip (Figure 2.2d). Two techniques were used to determine and verify the mineral composition of the interstitial deposits. Micro Fourier transformed infrared microspectroscopy demonstrated that in all cases the primary spectral band of the crystalline deposits was hydroxyapatite. These results were confirmed with electron diffraction analysis and the investigators concluded that the hydroxyapatite was biological apatite, and calcium oxalate was not detected in any specimen. These results to a great extent confirm much that Randall initially stated many years previously, namely that plaque is interstitial and composed of hydroxyapatite.(5) The aforementioned investigations also demonstrate that in the process of stone formation there is no evidence of cellular injury or inflammation. Rather, the smallest of lesions can be traced back to the basement membranes of the thin loops of Henle. Such findings can be explained, in that the basement membrane and large fields of type I collagen present an ideal matrix to attract calcium and phosphate.

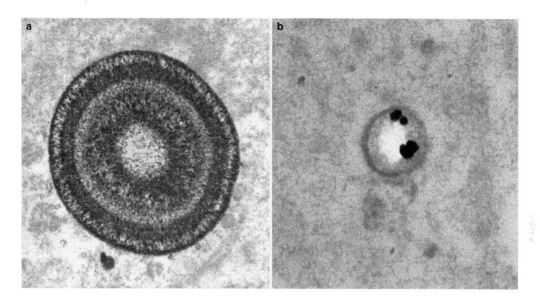

Figure 2.3 This set of transmission electron micrographs shows the initial sites of crystal deposition in a calcium oxalate stone former. A. The deposits are single spheres with a multilaminated internal morphology consisting of a central light region of crystalline material surrounded by a dark layer of matrix material. These layers alternate as many as six to seven times, and are clearly seen in the high magnification transmission electron micrograph. B. Immunoelectron microscopic localization of osteopontin; immunogold label, indicating osteopontin localization within single crystals found in the basement membrane of loops of Henle. Magnification, x70,000 (A); x50,000 (B). Reprinted from Matlaga et al., The Role of Randall's Plaques in the Pathogenesis of Calcium Stones, Journal of Urology, 177:31, 2006, with permission from Elsevier.

The calcium phosphate, or hydroxyapatite, deposits range from single crystals in the basement membranes of the thin loops of Henle to dense interstitial collections forming a syncytium of mineral deposit islands in a sea of organic material. Transmission electron microscopy showed the single deposits were generally spherical in shape, as small as 50 nm and laminated with mineral and organic molecules layered over each other (Figure 2.3a). All crystals were coated with organic material, and no uncoated crystals were observed. Osteopontin was present in the organic layer, positioned on the outer surface of the crystal and the overlying organic molecular layer, as confirmed by immunohistochemical techniques, suggesting that osteopontin is involved in plaque biology (Figure 2.3b).(65)

Metabolic and clinical evidence also supports that Randall's plaques are integral to the process of stone formation. Kuo and associates measured papillary plaque surface area in a cohort of idiopathic calcium oxalate stone formers undergoing percutaneous nephrolithotomy and then compared these data to metabolic data derived from two 24-hour urine measurements in each patient.(64) They found independent correlations between plaque surface area and urine volume (inverse), urine pH (inverse) and urine calcium (direct) (Figure 2.4). These results lend support to the idea that interstitial plaque deposits arise from driving forces that are reflected in urine calcium excretion and urine volume. Furthermore, the finding that plaque coverage is inversely related to urine pH may reflect the reality that lower urine pH is associated with a higher delivery of bicarbonate to the deep medulla, a finding that would account for an increased interstitial pH and foster the development of calcium phosphate plaque.

Kim and associates provided further evidence supporting a clinical effect of Randall's plaque when they assessed whether a simple count of stones formed in a patient correlated with the fraction of renal papillae covered by plaque.(66) In a group of idiopathic calcium oxalate stone formers who underwent endoscopic mapping of the renal papilla during percutaneous stone removal, these authors found that mean plaque surface area correlated significantly with the number of stone events (Figure 2.5). When corrected for the duration of stone disease, plaque coverage maintained a significant and independent correlation with the number of stones.

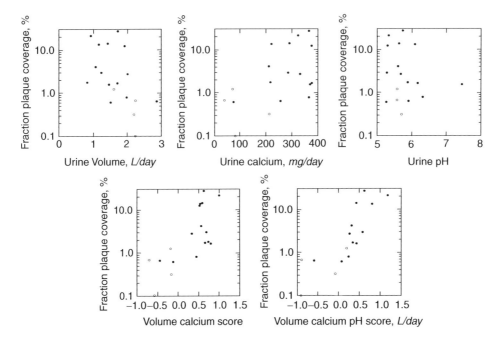

Figure 2.4 Fractional plaque coverage per papillum varies inversely with urine volume (upper left panel) among stone formers (closed circle) and nonstone-forming control subjects (open circle). Plaque coverage varies with urine calcium excretion (upper middle panel) and is inverse to urine pH (upper right panel). A composite multivariate regression score using urine volume and calcium excretion (lower left panel) and one that includes urine pH as well (lower right panel) strongly correlate with plaque coverage. Reprinted from Matlaga et al., The Role of Randall's Plaques in the Pathogenesis of Calcium Stones, Journal of Urology, 177:31, 2006, with permission from Elsevier.

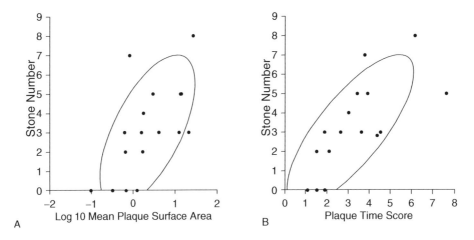

Figure 2.5 A. Number of stones vs log transformed mean plaque surface area. Nonparametric ellipse of containment includes 2 standard deviations. B. Number of stones vs multivariate regression equation from general linear model, including stone disease duration and plaque surface. Plaque time score x 1.788 + 1.386 x log 10 mean plaque surface area + 0.082 x time. Reprinted from Matlaga et al., The Role of Randall's Plaques in the Pathogenesis of Calcium Stones, Journal of Urology, 177:31, 2006, with permission from Elsevier.

To support Randall's hypothesis that calcium oxalate calculi begin as small attached stones to the renal papillae at sites of plaque, Matlaga and associates investigated the prevalence of attached stones in calcium oxalate stone formers.(67) In approximately half of this cohort of patients, papilla-attached stones were observed. In all patients, Randall's plaque was

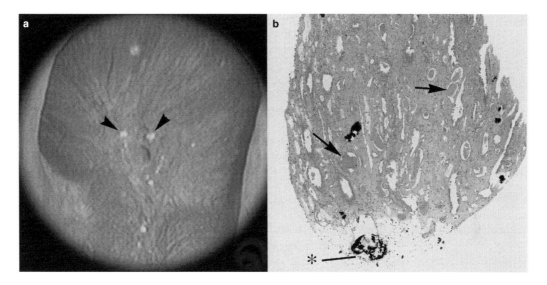

Figure 2.6 A. An example of a papilla from an intestinal-bypass stone former that was video recorded at the time of the mapping. Distinct sites of Randall's plaque material are not found in the papilla of the intestinal-bypass patient; instead, several nodular-appearing structures (arrowheads) were noted near the opening of the ducts of Bellini. B. A low magnification light microscopic image of a papillary biopsy specimen from an intestinal-bypass patient is shown. Crystal deposition was only found in the lumens of a few collecting ducts as far down as the ducts of Bellini (*). A large site of crystal material was seen in a duct of Bellini. No other sites of crystal deposits were noted. Note dilated collecting ducts (arrows) with cast material and regions of fibrosis around crystal-deposit-filled collecting ducts. Magnification, x 100 (B). Reprinted from Matlaga et al., The Role of Randall's Plaques in the Pathogenesis of Calcium Stones, Journal of Urology, 177:31, 2006, with permission from Elsevier.

present. These findings suggest that the attached stone is likely a common early stage in the formation of calcium oxalate stones.

Intestinal Bypass Stone Formers

Patients who undergo jejunal-ileal bypass surgery for bariatric reasons have been reported to form calcium oxalate kidney stones, likely as a consequence of metabolic derangements induced by the procedure. Evan and associates studied a cohort of patients who had previously undergone jejunal-ileal bypass procedures and subsequently formed kidney stones.(62) These patients underwent the same rigorous set of studies as idiopathic calcium oxalate stone formers; endoscopically the renal papillae in these patients showed no evidence of Randall's plaques. Rather, these patients were noted to harbor small nodular deposits projecting off of the urothelium, close to the openings of the ducts of Bellini (Figure 2.6a). Histologic examination of the papillary biopsies revealed Yasue positive deposits only in the lumens of a few inner medullary collecting ducts as far down as the terminal collecting ducts (Figure 2.6b). No crystalline deposits were found in the interstitium or around the thin loops of Henle. Light microscopic examination and transmission electron microscopic imaging found crystals attached to the apical surfaces of the collecting duct cells, and in some cases completely filling the tubular lumen, associated with extensive cell injury and death. Similar to idiopathic calcium oxalate stone-forming patients, crystal deposits on micro Fourier transformed infrared and electron diffraction analysis were confirmed to be hydroxyapatite, and no calcium oxalate was detected in any papillary or cortical biopsies.

Taken all together, the histopathological findings in patients with intestinal bypass demonstrated findings different from the idiopathic calcium oxalate stone fomers. There was no evidence of Randall's plaque; rather there were intraluminal crystal deposits, suggesting a pathogenesis of stone formation that is distinct from that in idiopathic calcium oxalate stone formers. Remarkably crystals in tissue biopsies from patients with intestinal bypass were hydroxyapatite, an unexpected finding as the patients in this study cohort were significantly hyperoxaluric.

Brushite Stone Formers

Approximately 15% of stone formers produce predominantly calcium phosphate stones and about a quarter of these patients form stones containing brushite (calcium monohydrogen phosphate). The incidence of calcium phosphate stone disease may be increasing, as Parks and associates have noted an increase in the prevalence of calcium phosphate stones and Mandel and associates have noted an increase in the prevalence of brushite stone disease.(68, 69) The endoscopic examination of the renal papillae in brushite stone formers has consistently demonstrated three types of deposits. The first pattern was sites of Randall's plaques, as seen in idiopathic calcium oxalate cases (Figure 2.7a). The second pattern was large, yellow deposits projecting from the opening of the ducts of Bellini into the urinary collecting space (Figure 2.7a). The third pattern was suburothelial yellow deposits on the sides of the papillary tip and clearly within the lumina of inner medullar collecting ducts (Figure 2.7b). Histopathological techniques confirmed the sites of interstitial crystal deposits as well as the inner medullary collecting ducts and ducts of Bellini, which contained crystalline deposits (Figure 2.7c). Papillae in brushite stone formers were noted to be covered with depressions or pits, which were most commonly associated with dilated terminal collecting ducts, but occasionally were found on the sides of a papilla.

Histological examination of the crystal-filled medullary collecting ducts of brushite stone formers has demonstrated extensive cell injury surrounded by interstitial fibrosis; some tubules altogether lacked viable cells. Interstitial changes were also detected in cortical biopsies along with advanced glomerulosclerosis, tubular atrophy and interstitial fibrosis (Figure 2.8). However, there was no evidence of inflammation in any tissue samples, confirming that this process was not the consequence of dystrophic calcification.

Cystine Stone Formers

Cystinuria is an autosomally recessive heritable disease characterized by a defect in the dibasic amino acid transporter. Evan and associates have reported on the gross and microscopic pathology of the renal papilla, medulla, and cortex of cystine stone formers.(70) Endoscopically, the renal papilla of a cystinuric stone former is characterized by dilated terminal collecting ducts, in many cases with grossly evident cystine crystal plugging. Histologically, the renal papilla reveal evidence of inner medullary collecting duct dilation and surrounding interstitial fibrosis. Epithelial injury is evident, and ranges from minor flattening to more severe, complete necrosis. The amount of interstitial Randall's plaque was not significantly different from that found in nonstone formers.

It may be that cystine crystallizes in the terminal collecting ducts, with likely resulting cellular injury, interstitial reaction, and nephron obstruction. The finding of cystine crystals in the terminal collecting ducts is not unexpected, as water extraction is complete at this point in the nephron, and cystine concentrations are likely comparable to that in urine. It is plausible that chronic collecting duct obstruction from cystine crystal plugs can induce cortical changes.

Distal Renal Tubular Acidosis

Distal renal tubular acidosis (dRTA) is a metabolic disorder characterized by a nonanion gap metabolic acidosis, accompanied by an alkaline urinary pH that does not fall appropriately during an exogenous acid challenge. Hypokalemia is always present, due to renal potassium losses. Evan and associates reported on a series of patients with dRTA who formed, as expected, calcium phosphate calculi.(71) Many patients with dRTA have extensive renal calcifications; in this report, most of these calcifications were surgically removable stones, rather than calcified renal tissue. Endoscopically, this cohort of patients with dRTA exhibited varying degrees of disease; some patients had minimal changes of the renal papilla, whereas the papilla of other patients were pitted, with mineral plugs protruding from dilated collecting ducts. Only rare regions of interstitial Randall's plaque were encountered. The dilated collecting ducts were filled with calcium phosphate, and there was extensive fibrosis surrounding these obstructed ducts. Cortical biopsies demonstrated some degree of nephron loss and cortical interstitial fibrosis.

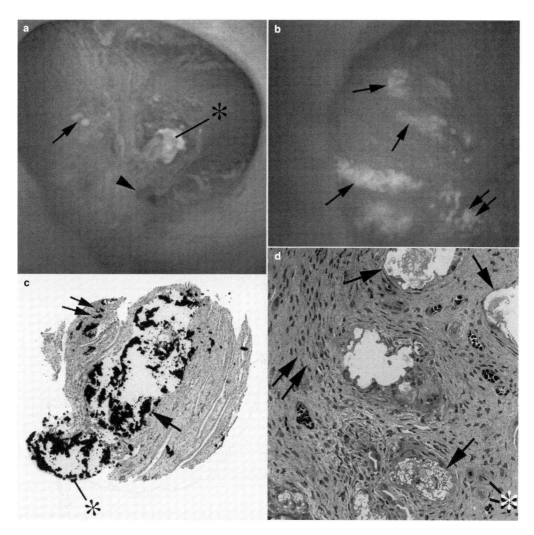

Figure 2.7   A. An example of a papilla from a brushite stone former that was video recorded at the time of the mapping. This papilla shows the irregular white areas of crystalline deposits (arrow) (type I crystal pattern) beneath the urothelium previously described for calcium oxalate patients. In addition, the papilla from the brushite patient possesses sites of a yellowish crystalline deposit at the opening of the ducts of Bellini (*). A large pit (arrowhead) is seen along the side of the papilla. B. During endoscopic examination, other papilla exhibited a pattern of yellowish mineral deposition within the lumens of medullary collecting ducts, just like that described for the type 2 pattern, except that these collecting ducts are located just beneath the urothelium. Certain papilla harbored large areas of crystal deposition, forming a spoke and wheel-like pattern around the circumference of the papilla (arrows). These papilla also showed the type 1 pattern of whitish crystal deposition that correlates with interstitial sites of Randall's plaque (double arrow). C. Low power magnification light microscopic images, in which the sites of calcium deposits were stained black by the Yasue metal substitution method, demonstrate an enormous amount of Yasue-positive material within the ducts of Bellini (arrows). The crystalline material is seen protruding from the opening of the duct of Bellini and also in an associated inner medullary collecting duct (*). In addition, Yasue positive material is in the interstitium of the renal papilla surrounding thin loops of Henle (double arrows), as previously described for calcium oxalate stone formers. D. Extensive cellular damage is noted in several inner medullary collecting ducts (arrows) where the mineral has been chemically removed. Extensive regions of interstitial fibrosis surround the injured collecting tubules (double arrows). Entrapped injured thin loops of Henle and vasa recta (*) are also noted in these fields of interstitial fibrosis. Magnification, x90 (C), x1,100 (D). Reprinted from Matlaga et al., The Role of Randall's Plaques in the Pathogenesis of Calcium Stones, Journal of Urology, 177:31, 2006, with permission from Elsevier.

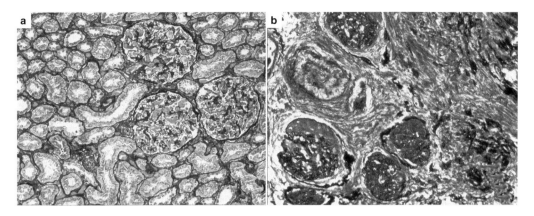

Figure 2.8   A. Cortical tissue from a normal individual. B. The cortex of a brushite stone former, demonstrating glomerular opalescence, tubular atrophy, and interstitial fibrosis. Magnification, x1,000 (A), x1,000 (B). Reprinted from Matlaga et al., The Role of Randall's Plaques in the Pathogenesis of Calcium Stones, Journal of Urology, 177:31, 2006, with permission from Elsevier.

REFERENCES

1. Shattock S. A prehistoric or predynastic Egyptian calculus. Trans Path Soc 1905; 61: 275–90.
2. Butt A. Historical Survey. In: Butt A, ed. Etiologic factors in renal lithiasis. Springfield: Charles C. Thomas; 1956: 3–47.
3. Murphy L. The History of Urology. Springfield: Charles C. Thomas; 1972.
4. Resnick MI, Boyce WH. Aetiological theories of renal lithiasis - A Historical Review. In: Wickham J, ed. Urinary Calculus Disease. Edinburgh: Churchill Livingstone; 1979.
5. Randall A. Papillary pathology as a precursor of primary renal calculus. J Urol 1940; 44: 580.
6. Coe FL, Evan A, Worcester E. Kidney stone disease. J Clin Invest 2005; 115(10): 2598–608.
7. Asplin JR, Bushinsky DA, Singharetnam W et al. Relationship between supersaturation and crystal inhibition in hypercalciuric rats. Kidney Int 1997; 51(3): 640–5.
8. Khan SR. Calcium phosphate/calcium oxalate crystal association in urinary stones: implications for heterogeneous nucleation of calcium oxalate. J Urol 1997; 157(1): 376–83.
9. Garside J. Nucleation. In: Nancollas G, ed. Biological mineralization and demineralization. Heidelberg: Springer-Verlag; 1982: 23–5.
10. Chung H, Abrahams HM, Meng MV, Stoller ML. Theories of stone formation. In: Stoller ML, Meng, MV, ed. Urinary Stone Disease: A Practical Guide to Medical and Surgical Management. Totowa: Humana Press, Inc.; 2007.
11. Kok DJ, Papapoulos SE, Bijvoet OL. Crystal agglomeration is a major element in calcium oxalate urinary stone formation. Kidney Int 1990; 37(1): 51–6.
12. Iwata H, Nishio S, Wakatsuki A, Ochi K, Takeuchi M. Architecture of calcium oxalate monohydrate urinary calculi. J Urol 1985; 133(2): 334–8.
13. Mandel N, Mandel GS. Epitaxis in renal stones. In: Wickham J, Colin-Buck, A, ed. Renal Tract Stone: Metabolic Basis and Clinical Practice. Edinburgh: Churchill Livingstone; 1990: 87–101.
14. Lonsdale K. Epitaxy as a growth factor in urinary calculi and gallstones. Nature 1968; 217(5123): 56–8.
15. Kok DJ, Khan SR. Calcium oxalate nephrolithiasis, a free or fixed particle disease. Kidney Int 1994; 46(3): 847–54.
16. Vermeulen CW, Lyon ES. Mechanisms of genesis and growth of calculi. The Am J Med 1968; 45(5): 684–92.
17. Finlayson B, Reid F. The expectation of free and fixed particles in urinary stone disease. Invest Urol 1978; 15(6): 442–8.
18. Evan A, Lingeman J, Coe FL, Worcester E. Randall's plaque: pathogenesis and role in calcium oxalate nephrolithiasis. Kidney Int 2006; 69(8): 1313–8.
19. Khan SR. Calcium oxalate crystal interaction with renal tubular epithelium, mechanism of crystal adhesion and its impact on stone development. Urol Res 1995; 23(2): 71–9.
20. Bigelow MW, Wiessner JH, Kleinman JG, Mandel NS. Surface exposure of phosphatidylserine increases calcium oxalate crystal attachment to IMCD cells. Am J Physiol 1997; 272: F55–62.
21. Lieske JC, Toback FG, Deganello S. Sialic acid-containing glycoproteins on renal cells determine nucleation of calcium oxalate dihydrate crystals. Kidney Int 2001; 60(5): 1784–91.

22. Verkoelen CF, van der Boom BG, Kok DJ, Romijn JC. Sialic acid and crystal binding. Kidney Int 2000; 57(3): 1072–82.

23. Verkoelen CF, Van Der Boom BG, Romijn JC. Identification of hyaluronan as a crystal-binding molecule at the surface of migrating and proliferating MDCK cells. Kidney Int 2000; 58(3): 1045–54.

24. Yamate T, Kohri K, Umekawa T et al. Interaction between osteopontin on madin darby canine kidney cell membrane and calcium oxalate crystal. Urol Int 1999; 62(2): 81–6.

25. Williams JC Jr, Zarse CA, Jackson ME, Witzmann FA, McAteer JA. Variability of protein content in calcium oxalate monohydrate stones. J Endourol 2006; 20(8): 560–4.

26. Allen TD, Spence HM. Matrix stones. J Urol 1966; 95(3): 284–90.

27. Khan SR, Hackett RL. Role of organic matrix in urinary stone formation: an ultrastructural study of crystal matrix interface of calcium oxalate monohydrate stones. J Urol 1993; 150(1): 239–45.

28. Malek RS, Boyce WH. Intranephronic calculosis: its significance and relationship to matrix in nephrolithiasis. J Urol 1973; 109(4): 551–5.

29. Kumar V, Lieske JC. Protein regulation of intrarenal crystallization. Curr Opin Nephrol Hypertens 2006; 15(4): 374–80.

30. Jones WT, Waterhouse RL, Resnick MI. The evaluation of urinary protein patterns in a stone-forming animal model using two-dimensional polyacrylamide gel electrophoresis. J Urol 1991; 145(4):868–74.

31. Khan SR. Animal models of kidney stone formation: an analysis. World J Urol 1997; 15(4): 236–43.

32. Khan SR. Crystal-induced inflammation of the kidneys: results from human studies, animal models, and tissue-culture studies. Clin Exp Nephrol 2004; 8(2): 75–88.

33. Khan SR, Shevock PN, Hackett RL. Urinary enzymes and calcium oxalate urolithiasis. J Urol 1989; 142(3): 846–9.

34. Khan SR. Renal tubular damage/dysfunction: key to the formation of kidney stones. Urol Res 2006; 34(2): 86–91.

35. de Water R, Leenen PJ, Noordermeer C et al. Cytokine production induced by binding and processing of calcium oxalate crystals in cultured macrophages. Am J Kidney Dis 2001; 38(2): 331–8.

36. Robinson M, Pond CL, Laurie RD et al. Subacute and subchronic toxicity of ethylene glycol administered in drinking water to Sprague-Dawley rats. Drug Chem Toxicol 1990; 13(1): 43–70.

37. Poldelski V, Johnson A, Wright S, Rosa VD, Zager RA. Ethylene glycol-mediated tubular injury: identification of critical metabolites and injury pathways. Am J Kidney Dis 2001; 38(2): 339–48.

38. Holmes RP, Ambrosius WT, Assimos DG. Dietary oxalate loads and renal oxalate handling. J Urol 2005; 174(3): 943–7; discussion 7.

39. Bhandari A, Koul S, Sekhon A et al. Effects of oxalate on HK-2 cells, a line of proximal tubular epithelial cells from normal human kidney. J Urol 2002; 168(1): 253–9.

40. Robertson WG. Kidney models of calcium oxalate stone formation. Nephron 2004; 98(2): 21–30.

41. Low RK, Stoller ML. Endoscopic mapping of renal papillae for Randall's plaques in patients with urinary stone disease. J Urol 1997; 158(6): 2062–4.

42. Stoller ML, Meng MV, Abrahams HM, Kane JP. The primary stone event: a new hypothesis involving a vascular etiology. J Urol 2004; 171(5): 1920–4.

43. Ciftcioglu N, Bjorklund M, Kuorikoski K, Bergstrom K, Kajander EO. Nanobacteria: an infectious cause for kidney stone formation. Kidney Int 1999; 56(5): 1893–8.

44. Kajander EO, Ciftcioglu N, Miller-Hjelle MA, Hjelle JT. Nanobacteria: controversial pathogens in nephrolithiasis and polycystic kidney disease. Curr Opin Nephrol Hypertens 2001; 10(3): 445–52.

45. Dorrell S. Nanobacteria linked to kidney disease. Mol Med Today 1999; 5(9): 373.

46. Jelic TM, Malas AM, Groves SS et al. Nanobacteria-caused mitral valve calciphylaxis in a man with diabetic renal failure. South Med J 2004; 97(2): 194–8.

47. Wood HM, Shoskes DA. The role of nanobacteria in urologic disease. World J Urol 2006; 24(1): 51–4.

48. Ciftcioglu N, McKay DS, Kajander EO. Association between nanobacteria and periodontal disease. Circulation 2003; 108(8): e58–9; author reply e–9.

49. Kajander EO, Ciftcioglu N. Nanobacteria: an alternative mechanism for pathogenic intra- and extracellular calcification and stone formation. Proc Natl Acad Sci U S A 1998; 95(14): 8274–9.

50. Kajander EO, Ciftcioglu N, Aho K, Garcia-Cuerpo E. Characteristics of nanobacteria and their possible role in stone formation. Urol Res 2003; 31(2): 47–54.

51. Vogel G. Bacteria to blame for kidney stones? Science (New York), NY 1998; 281(5374): 153.

52. Shiekh FA, Khullar M, Singh SK. Lithogenesis: induction of renal calcifications by nanobacteria. Urol Res 2006; 34(1): 53–7.

53. Cisar JO, Xu DQ, Thompson J et al. An alternative interpretation of nanobacteria-induced biomineralization. Proc Natl Acad Sci U S A 2000; 97(21): 11511–5.

54. Liatsikos EN, Bernardo NO, Dinlenc CZ, Kapoor R, Smith AD. Caliceal diverticular calculi: is there a role for metabolic evaluation? J Urol 2000; 164(1): 18–20.

55. Gambaro G, Fabris A, Puliatta D, Lupo A. Lithiasis in cystic kidney disease and malformations of the urinary tract. Urol Res 2006; 34(2): 102–7.

56. Raj GV, Auge BK, Assimos D, Preminger GM. Metabolic abnormalities associated with renal calculi in patients with horseshoe kidneys. J Endourol 2004; 18(2): 157–61.
57. Hsu TH, Streem SB. Metabolic abnormalities in patients with caliceal diverticular calculi. J Urol 1998; 160(5): 1640–2.
58. Matin SF, Streem SB. Metabolic risk factors in patients with ureteropelvic junction obstruction and renal calculi. J Urol 2000; 163(6): 1676–8.
59. Matlaga BR, Miller NL, Terry C et al. The pathogenesis of calyceal diverticular calculi. Urol Res 2007; 35(1): 35–40.
60. Kuo RL, Lingeman JE, Evan AP et al. Endoscopic renal papillary biopsies: a tissue retrieval technique for histological studies in patients with nephrolithiasis. J Urol 2003; 170: 2186–9.
61. Evan AP, Coe FL, Lingeman JE, Worcester E. Insights on the pathology of kidney stone formation. Urol Res 2005; 33(5): 383–9.
62. Evan AP, Lingeman JE, Coe FL et al. Randall's plaque of patients with nephrolithiasis begins in basement membranes of thin loops of Henle. J Clin Invest 2003; 111(5): 607–16.
63. Coe FL, Parks JH, Asplin JR. The pathogenesis and treatment of kidney stones. New Engl J Med 1992; 327(16): 1141–52.
64. Kuo RL, Lingeman JE, Evan AP et al. Urine calcium and volume predict coverage of renal papilla by Randall's plaque. Kidney Int 2003; 64(6): 2150–4.
65. Evan AP, Coe FL, Rittling SR et al. Apatite plaque particles in inner medulla of kidneys of calcium oxalate stone formers: osteopontin localization. Kidney Int 2005; 68(1): 145–54.
66. Kim SC, Coe FL, Tinmouth WW et al. Stone formation is proportional to papillary surface coverage by Randall's plaque. J Urol 2005; 173(1): 117–9; discussion 9.
67. Matlaga BR, Williams JC Jr, Kim SC et al. Endoscopic evidence of calculus attachment to Randall's plaque. J Urol 2006; 175(5): 1720–4; discussion 4.
68. Parks JH, Worcester EM, Coe FL, Evan AP, Lingeman JE. Clinical implications of abundant calcium phosphate in routinely analyzed kidney stones. Kidney Int 2004; 66(2): 777–85.
69. Mandel N, Mandel I, Fryjoff K, Rejniak T, Mandel G. Conversion of calcium oxalate to calcium phosphate with recurrent stone episodes. J Urol 2003; 169(6): 2026–9.
70. Evan AP, Coe FL, Lingeman JE et al. Renal crystal deposits and histopathology in patients with cystine stones. Kidney Int 2006; 69(12): 2227–35.
71. Evan AP, Lingeman J, Coe F et al. Renal histopathology of stone-forming patients with distal renal tubular acidosis. Kidney Int 2007; 71(8): 795–801.

3 | Basic metabolic evaluation for nephrolithiasis

Michael N Ferrandino and Glenn M Preminger

EVALUATION OF PATIENTS WITH NEPHROLITHIASIS

The goal of the physician when evaluating patients with nephrolithiasis should be to provide a simple, financially acceptable work-up which yields information that can be directly applied to directed medical and dietary therapies.(1) Most would agree that stone prevention should be primary goal of treating patients with recurrent nephrolithiasis. Yet, debate continues as to which to patients should undergo metabolic evaluation and to what extent the evaluation should be performed.

While certain general guidelines have been agreed upon, it is clear that not all stone formers will benefit either medically and/or financially from undergoing a metabolic evaluation and subsequent treatment. However, beyond medical recommendations based on recurrence rates and cost-effectiveness, the patients themselves should be included in the decision to perform a metabolic evaluation. Due to the discomfort associated with symptomatic stone disease, patients at even low risk for recurrence may elect to undergo metabolic evaluation. In fact, it has been shown that almost 90% of stone formers, either first-time or recurrent, report a willingness to undergo a metabolic evaluation with resultant dietary or medical modifications. (2) Despite significant patient willingness to undergo metabolic evaluation, there are subsets of patients that will have increased benefit from a formal diagnostic work-up.

Patient Selection

The question of who should undergo a metabolic evaluation often begins with first-time stone formers. Studies have reported varying stone recurrence rates, from 26% to 50%, following the first presentation of symptomatic nephrolithiasis.(3, 4) Clearly, not all first-time stone formers require an in-depth metabolic evaluation. In fact, dietary modification alone has been shown to decrease the overall rate of recurrence in 58% of patients with a variety of metabolic risk factors.(5) More specifically, one study demonstrated a 71% and 47% reduction in stone formation for patients with hypercalciuria and hyperuricosuria, respectively, while on high fluid intake and avoidance of dietary excess of either dairy products or meats.

The lack of new stone formation, however, does not imply that patients on dietary modifications do not have metabolic risk factors for recurrence. The presence of an existing stone burden may be indicative of significant underlying systemic medical diseases, such as osteoporosis or osteopenia, hyperparathyroidism, renal tubular acidosis (RTA), or sarcoidosis. Metabolic evaluation, combined with selective medical therapy will also help to prevent systemic effects of associated medical disorders. Generally, first-time stone formers who are at high risk for recurrence should undergo metabolic evaluation. These high-risk categories include patients with family history of stones, intestinal disease/chronic diarrhea, urinary tract infections, gout, osteoporosis, and skeletal fractures (Table 3.1).

First-time stone formers at low risk may still benefit from a "simplified" work-up. Such an evaluation may help to elucidate any of the aforementioned underlying medical illnesses in addition to providing clinicians information with which to direct conservative measures. The listed "simplified" protocol (Table 3.2) is a straight-forward, single office visit evaluation which should be readily acceptable to patients and clinicians, alike. This protocol avoids the use of 24-hour urine analyses which are the corner stone of the basic and extensive metabolic work-up.

Some authors suggest that patients with stones composed of uric acid, cystine, and struvite should undergo metabolic evaluation. However, this same subset of stone compositions has been used to identify patients which may not benefit from further evaluation.(6) Additionally, recommendations have been put forth which include metabolic evaluation of patients with difficult-to-treat stones, as well as patients with a solitary kidney or nephrocalcinosis.(7)

Table 3.1 Risk factors for high risk of recurrence.

Strong Family History of Stones
Intestinal Disease (particularly chronic diarrhea)
Pathologic Skeletal Fractures
Osteoporosis
History of Urinary Tract Infection with Calculi
Personal History of Gout
Infirm Health (unable to tolerate repeat stone episodes)
Solitary Kidney
Anatomic Abnormalities
Renal Insufficiency
Stones Composed of: cystine, uric acid, struvite

Table 3.2 "Simplified" evaluation of single stone formers.

HISTORY

Underlying predisposing conditions (as per Table 3.1)
Medications (Ca, Vit C, Vit D, acetazolamide, steroids)
Dietary excesses, inadequate fluid intake or excessive fluid loss

MULTICHANNEL BLOOD SCREEN

Basic Metabolic Panel (Sodium, Potassium, Chloride, CO_2, BUN, Creatinine)
Calcium
Intact Parathyroid Hormone (if serum Ca^{++} elevated)
Uric Acid

URINE

Urinalysis
  pH > 7.5: infection lithiasis
  pH < 5.5: uric acid lithiasis
  Sediment for crystalluria
Urine culture
  Urea-splitting organisms: suggestive of infection lithiasis
Qualitative Cystine

X-RAY

Radiopaque stones:	Calcium oxalate, calcium phosphate, magnesium ammonium phosphate (struvite), cystine.
Radiolucent stones:	Uric acid, xanthine, triamterene
IVP:	Radiolucent stones, anatomic abnormalities

STONE ANALYSIS

Racial differences of stone formation and recurrence rates have previously been used to support the use of routine metabolic evaluation in African Americans. Yet, recent studies suggest that African Americans, Asians, and Hispanics have similar rates of metabolic abnormalities, as Caucasians.(8, 9) Mente et al, confirm ethnic diversity in stone occurrence. Compared to Europeans, Arabic, West Indian, West Asian, and Latin American patients had a higher relative risk of calcium nephrolithiasis whereas East Asian and African patients had decreased relative risk.(10) Unlike previously reported studies, these authors found differing urinary profiles for a variety of the ethnicities reported when compared to Europeans. However patients of African ancestry demonstrated no significant differences in urinary metabolites. Based on the decreased rates of stone formation in African Americans but similar metabolic abnormalities it is reasonable to perform metabolic evaluations for African-American patients following their first stone presentation.

Children with nephrolithiasis are a clear indication for metabolic evaluation. Young patients with nephrolithiasis are at similar risk of metabolic disturbances as adults.(11) The increased risk of detrimental effects of repeated episodes of obstruction, urinary tract infections, and the need for surgical intervention strengthen the recommendation for metabolic evaluation and management of children with nephrolithiasis. Furthermore, questions regarding repeated radiographic imaging and radiation exposure for children are currently being raised. By limitation of stone recurrences via thorough metabolic evaluation and selective medical therapy in children, physicians may potentially minimize lifetime radiation exposure.

Extensive Diagnostic Evaluation

Historically, in patients with a high risk for stone recurrence and in those with difficult-to-treat stones, an exhaustive diagnostic evaluation had been performed in an attempt to identify the underlying cause of stone formation. This comprehensive metabolic evaluation was initially described by Pak et al. in 1980 and has been repeatedly modified.(1)

The extensive diagnostic evaluation included a history and physical, radiographic evaluation, two 24-hr urinalyses on random diet, an additional 24-hour collection on a restricted diet (low calcium and sodium) and a subsequent calcium fast and load test. Serum chemistry was analyzed for parathyroid hormone, calcium, uric acid, and creatinine as well as a complete blood count. During the evaluation, patients were instructed to discontinue use of any medication or supplement which interfered with blood and urinary levels of calcium, uric acid, and/or oxalate. Generally this evaluation could be performed over two outpatient visits. The 24-hour urine collection, during the calcium/sodium restricted diet was performed to standardize the results of the random collections and to prepare patients for the fast and load test and to help identify those patients with absorptive hypercalciuria Type II. The calcium fast and load test requires patients to be on a restricted calcium diet and fast for 12 hours before beginning the test. Patients would then be hydrated and urine collected before ingestion of a calcium load. After ingestion of 1gram of calcium in a synthetic meal, urine was collected and evaluated for milligrams calcium excreted relative to urinary creatinine. The purpose of the calcium fast and load test was to differentiate between absorptive hypercalciuria and renal leak hypercalciuria.

However, as selective medical therapy for patients with absorptive hypercalciuria is currently not available, and the treatment of these diagnoses is now similar with both groups of patients being treated with thiazide diuretics, most clinicians are no longer performing the calcium fast and load evaluation.

Rarely is this extensive metabolic evaluation performed today, because of the time, expense, and diminished clinical benefit involved. More commonly, a basic evaluation is performed which does include many of these studies but lacks the restricted diet 24-hour urinalysis, and the calcium fast and load test.

Basic Metabolic Evaluation

The basic metabolic evaluation begins as any physician–patient interaction should – with a thorough history and physical exam. As previously mentioned, key points in the history should include: medical illnesses and surgical procedures (Table 3.3) which may contribute to stone formation, family history of nephrolithiasis, evaluation of medications and dietary supplements, as well as dietary habits. Evaluation of general hydration and activity levels are important to consider. Assessment of the patients' social history including employment may yield important insight into the cause of stone formation – physical labor, prolonged sun exposure, dehydration, etc...

Serum chemistries (basic metabolic panel) should be performed in an attempt to identify hypercalcemia, hypokalemia, or metabolic acidosis. Hypercalcemia may be indicative of hyperparathyroidism and would warrant further evaluation with a parathyroid hormone assay. The presence of hypokalemia and metabolic acidosis is highly associated with distal renal tubular acidosis. Additionally, if clinical history suggests possible derangement of purine metabolism serum uric acid may be confirmatory.

Urine studies should include urinalysis with pH, urine culture and sensitivities (if clinically indicated), and review of urinary sediment. Variation in urine pH may point to particular diagnoses. A pH greater than 7.5 is correlated with urinary infection whereas a pH less than 5.5 supports the diagnosis of gouty diathesis. High-normal urine pH (6.7–7.2) may indicate renal tubular acidosis. Care should be taken, however, not to rely too heavily on a single urine pH value from the urinalysis, as alterations of the patients' diet may be reflected instead of

Table 3.3 Medical and Surgical risk Factors for Nephrolithiasis.

MEDICAL

Hyperparathyroidism
Sarcoidosis
Inborn Errors of Metabolism
Lesch-Nyan Syndrome
Gout
Inflammatory Bowel Disease
Obesity (Metabolic Syndrome)
Medullary Sponge Kidney
Granulomatous Diseases
Immobilization (prolonged)
Multiply Myeloma
Metastatic Bone Disease
Paget's Disease

SURGICAL

Roux-en-Y Gastric Bypass
Total colectomy (or other intestinal surgeries leading to chronic diarrheal states)

underlying metabolic disorders.(12) Urine cultures are valuable if the patient demonstrates signs and symptoms of infection. Cultures positive for *Klebsiella pneumonia*, *Proteus mirabilis*, *Pseudomonas aeruginosa* or other urea-splitting organisms may indicate the presence of struvite stone. Additionally, clinical and surgical management will vary depending upon the presence or absence of infection. Inspection of sediment is likely to yield clues about stone composition. Calcium oxalate calculi demonstrate "envelopes" crystals, whereas struvite crystals are generally rectangular ("coffin lid"), while hexagonal crystals confirm cystinuria.

Radiographic imaging is a standard part of the metabolic evaluation which should not be overlooked. Although the utility of imaging is greater as a clinical management tool, there are insights which can be gleaned from plain films, intravenous pyelograms, and computed tomography (CT). In addition to assessing residual stone burden, radio-opacity/radiolucency of stones on plain films, as compared to CT, can indicate presence of uric acid, xanthine, and triamterene calculi. An intravenous pyelogram permits appraisal of anatomic anomalies and filling defects.

CT scanning is currently the gold standard for the diagnosis of urolithiaisis.(13, 14) Multiple researchers have reported using CT to ascertain stone composition based on measurement of Hounsfield units.(15–20) Unfortunately, this technique is not yet perfected and offers little clinical benefit. Currently, the technique of dual energy CT is under investigation and delineation between uric acid, calcareous, struvite, and cystine stone compositions has been demonstrated in vitro.(21, 22) The reproducibility and clinical utility of the dual energy CT technique is yet to be determined.

The remainder of the basic metabolic evaluation relies on the performance of two 24-hour urine collections with the patient on a random diet. Generally, it is not necessary to undertake all of the collections and analyses performed during the extensive metabolic evaluation (three – 24-hour urine collections and a calcium fast/load assay). Although performing an extensive work-up for nephrolithiasis may provide superior diagnostic accuracy, such a comprehensive metabolic evaluation is often time consuming and difficult for patients to reliably perform. The extensive evaluation requires two or three office visits and differentiates between various hypercalciuric causes. Patients and clinicians, alike, are more apt to adhere to a time and cost-efficient method which continues to provide basic information on stone formation and how to prevent recurrent nephrolithiasis.

In lieu of extensive evaluations which utilize two 24-hour urine specimens on a random diet, a 24-hour urinalysis on a restricted diet and fasting and calcium load testing, basic protocols have been developed which obviate the restricted diet urine collection and the calcium fast and loading tests. One such simplified approach includes the performance of a urinalysis, urine culture, comprehensive metabolic serum assessment and serum parathyroid hormone, and two 24-hour urine collections – one on a restricted diet and one on a random diet.(23) This approach avoids the inconvenience of a fast and loading test, but does require adherence

Table 3.4 Commercial Providers of 24-hour Urinary Stone Risk Profiles.

Dianon (Stratford, CT)
LabCorp (Burlington, NC)
LithoLink (Chicago, IL)
ARUP Laboratories (Salt Lake City, UT)
Quest Diagnostics (Madison, NJ)
Mission Pharmacal (San Antonio, TX)

to dietary calcium restriction. In an attempt to further simplify the metabolic evaluation, Pak described the adequacy of a single 24-hr urine collection without a second 24-hr collection or calcium fast/load testing.(24) After reviewing the stone risk profile data on 225 patients with nephrolithiasis, no significant difference in the urinary calcium, oxalate, uric acid, citrate, pH, total volume, sodium, potassium, sulfate, or phosphorous was noted between two random samples. However, most investigators suggest that two 24-hour urine collections are better than one. One group found that, although there was excellent correlation of stone-forming risk factors between individual collections, the variance found within one standard deviation could easily lead to misdiagnosis and inappropriate treatment.(25) It is currently our routine to have our patients perform two 24-hour urine samples while on random diet.

The ability to preserve 24-hour urine specimens and analyze small aliquots of the overall sample has permitted these collections to be performed as outpatients in virtually any settings, therefore avoiding proximity to research institutions and stone centers. Currently, multiple companies provide the ability for patients to collect their 24-hour urine samples at home. Some of the more commonly used commercial companies are listed in Table 3.4. These companies extrapolate data on 24-hour urine collections from a small well-preserved sample. Generally, a list of all urinary constituents is provided, along with a graphic representation of factors promoting and reducing the risk of stone formation. Unfortunately, these analyses will not differentiate between the causes of hypercalciuria – Type I, Type II and renal leak – on random diet. Discrimination of specific causes of hypercalciuria may not alter further medical management thereby making the distinction moot. Additionally, the limits of acceptable normal values may not be accurately represented by the 3rd party diagnostic laboratories. Physicians, therefore, must review all reported results and critically evaluate patient's risk factors, rather than rely on the diagnosis provided by these laboratory reports.

A further simplification of metabolic stone evaluation avoids 24-hour urine collection altogether, excluding patients who are at high risk for stone formation. This protocol uses a basic metabolic evaluation to assess the risk of systemic disorders.(26) Hesse and Straub further support avoidance of 24-hour urine collection except in patients at high risk for stone recurrence. This evaluation strategy is based on EAU-Guidelines, the 1st International Consultation on Stone Disease, and literature review.(27) Hesse and Straub identify high-risk stone formers as those with: ≥3 stones in 3 years, infection stones, uric acid stones, children, cystinuria, primary hyperoxaluria, RTA type I, cystic fibrosis, brushite stones, hyperparathyroidism, gastrointestinal diseases, solitary kidneys, nephrocalcinosis, vast stone burden bilaterally, and family history.

Though differing in exact protocols, none of the current varying basic evaluation regimens utilize calcium fast and load tests. While these additional tests help to differentiate absorptive from renal hypercalciuria, we do not have differing therapeutic options for managing these two conditions. Currently, our practice is to offer all patients, with any risk factors for recurrence, two 24-hour urine collections while on random diet, basic metabolic profile and serum PTH testing if serum calcium is elevated.

Stone Analysis in Metabolic Evaluation

Before determining specific stone composition, the supersaturation of urinary crystals has been shown to accurately track and predict stone composition.(28) The information on particular crystal supersaturation is useful because it can aid the physician when following patients on therapy. If supersaturation is prognostic of stone formation, then by assessing supersaturation rates, physicians can tailor metabolic treatment to prevent stone recurrence. An additional study suggests that determination of urinary supersaturation of various stone-forming salts is

Table 3.5 Stone composition as a clue to metabolic diagnosis.

Stone analysis	Possible metabolic abnormalities
Uric acid	Gouty diathesis
Cystine	Cystinuria
Struvite	
Carbonate apatite	Infection lithiasis
Magnesium ammonium phosphate	
Hydroxyapatite	Distal renal tubular acidosis
	Primary hyperparathyroidism

predictive of stone composition and implies that supersaturation during treatment is indicative of stone composition while on medical therapy.(29)

The ability to analyze urinary stone composition is questioned as an integral part of the initial metabolic evaluation. Most investigators suggest that the majority of the metabolic evaluation be based in urine and serum chemistries with decreased importance given to the analysis of stone composition.

Despite the fact that stones are not always collected, valuable information can be gained from analysis of stone composition. By utilizing the stone analysis to focus the physician on specific metabolic and pathogenic features, clinicians can more readily reach the appropriate diagnosis and begin medical management.(6) For patients with less common stones – cystine, pure struvite, and pure uric acid – minimal to no further evaluation may be required and treatment regimens can begin immediately. Patients with calcium phosphate stones are at significant risk of renal tubular acidosis or primary hyperparathyroidism, whereas patients with calcium oxalate stone formation may have a mixture of metabolic diagnoses. Table 3.5 illustrates potential diagnoses based on results of stone analysis.

The importance of stone analysis is promoted by Pak et al.(30) By analyzing the stone composition in almost 1400 patients, this study suggests a significant increase in the rate of RTA as the percentage of calcium phosphate was increased in calcareous stones. Of pure calcium oxalate stone formers, only 5% had RTA as compared to 18%, 39%, and 44% for patients with calcium oxalate–calcium apatite, calcium apatite, and brushite, respectively. Notably, >50% of patients with RTA did form calcium oxalate stone during their follow-up. All patients with cystine stone composition were diagnosed with cystinuria on metabolic evaluation. Gouty diathesis was found to have a strong association with uric acid stone composition, both pure and as a mixture. Of struvite stone formers, 59% of patients were found to have infection; however hypocitraturia and absorptive hypercalciuria were also commonly associated diagnoses.

Though struvite stones are strongly associated with infection, these stones are not always correlated with additional metabolic abnormalities, as has been previously suggested. One study found that when stone composition demonstrated pure struvite stones, rarely were additional metabolic abnormalities identified.(31) Yet, when composition was mixed (ie., struvite plus calcium-based calculi), all patients had underlying metabolic abnormalities elucidated.

Beyond its contribution to the metabolic evaluation, the role of stone analysis, if known beforehand, may play a contributory role to surgical management. As calcium oxalate monohydrate and cystine calculi are notoriously resistant to fragmentation during shock wave lithotripsy (SWL), knowledge of specific stone composition could be used to better select shock wave lithotripsy or endoscopic-based stone removal. Numerous authors have attempted to utilize imaging to document stone composition and/or subsequent treatment success with SWL.(16, 18, 19, 32–36) The results of these publications have not yielded highly applicable guidelines because of the inaccuracy of imaging in foretelling stone composition. Currently, attaining and analyzing stone fragments for composition may provide clinicians with an increased ability to predict success and failure of various surgical interventions, should patients require treatment for recurrent calculi.

METABOLIC EVALUATION CLASSIFICATION

The goal of a basic metabolic stone evaluation is to determine the underlying cause(s) of stone formation. Upon completion of the work-up, patients may be diagnosed with one or more of

Table 3.6 Classification of nephrolithiasis.

	Percent	
	Sole Occurrence	Combined Occurrence
Absorptive Hypercalciuria	20	40
Type I		
Type II		
Renal Hypercalciuria	5	8
Primary Hyperparathyroidism	3	8
Unclassified Ca Nephrolithiasis	15	25
Hyperoxaluric Ca Nephrolithiasis	2	15
Enteric Hyperoxaluria		
Primary Hyperoxaluria		
Dietary Hyperoxaluria		
Hypocitraturic Ca Nephrolithiasis	10	50
Distal Renal Tubular Acidosis		
Chronic Diarrheal Syndrome		
Thiazide-Induced		
Idiopathic		
Hypomagnesiuric Ca Nephrolithiasis	5	10
Gouty Diathesis	15	30
Cystinuria	<1	
Infection Stones	1	5
Low Urine Volume	10	50
No Disturbance and Miscellaneous	<3	
	100	

Adapted from: Levy, F. L., B. Adams-Huet, et al. (1995). "Ambulatory evaluation of nephrolithiasis: an update of a 1980 protocol." Am J Med 98(1): 50–9.

13 separate diagnostic categories. The diagnostic categories are listed in Table 3.6. Assessment of the various metabolic abnormalities may lead to unique or overlapping causes for stone formation. A thorough description of the pathophysiology and management of these metabolic abnormalities will be presented in subsequent chapters.

Calcium-based nephrolithiasis

Stones with calcium components develop as a result of various metabolic derangements and oftentimes patients are found to have a combination of risk factors. The most prevalent diagnoses in calcium stone formers are absorptive hypercalciuria (Types I and II), unclassified calcium nephrolithiasis, gouty diathesis, and low urinary volumes. However, low urinary volumes may contribute to uric acid stone formation, cystinuria, and infectious stones; while gouty diathesis may also predispose patients to uric acid stone formation.

The remaining diagnoses commonly found in calcium stone formers include hypocitraturia, hypomagnesuria, renal leak hypercalciuria, primary hyperparathyroidism, and hyperoxaluria. Again, these diagnoses are not necessarily exclusive and can often be found in combination with each other.

Uric Acid–based nephrolithiasis

Patients with pure uric acid nephrolithiasis inevitably have a low urinary pH (< 5.5) and are therefore determined to have gouty diathesis. As previously mentioned, patients with the diagnosis of gouty diathesis may form calcium stones in conjunction with uric acid stone formation. Occasionally, uric acid stones may result from myeloproliferative disorders or errors of inborn metabolism (see Chapter 8).

Cystine-based nephrolithiasis

Cystine nephrolithiasis is the result of an autosomal recessive trait which disrupts the transepithelial transport of cystine, ornithine, lysine, and arginine. The concentrations of cystine rise to levels above the saturation point and as a consequence cystine crystals precipitate.(37, 38) Of note, even though cystine stone formers all have elevated urinary cystine levels, they may also have a number of additional metabolic risk factors. One study demonstrated the presence of hypocitraturia, hyperuricosuria, and hypercalciuria in 44.4%, 22.2%, and 18.5%, respectively, of patients with cystine stones.(39)

Infectious nephrolithiasis

High urinary pH (usually pH of >7.2) is associated with the presence of urinary tract infection and the formation of infectious calculi. The presence of urea-splitting organisms leads to an increase in the ammonia concentration which further promotes struvite stone formation.(40, 41) Struvite stones compose the majority of staghorn calculi. The presence of metabolic defects in patients with struvite stones and the concurrent need for metabolic evaluation are arguable. As noted previously, no further metabolic evaluation is necessary in patients with pure struvite nephrolithiasis. However, if struvite stone formers demonstrate a mixed composition, with calcium-based components, a metabolic evaluation is likely to yield additional metabolic abnormalities contributing to their stone formation.(31)

COST-EFFECTIVENESS OF METABOLIC EVALUATION FOR NEPHROLITHIASIS

As of 2000, the estimated annual cost attributed to nephrolithiasis was $2.1 billion dollars accounting for the second most expensive cause of urologic disorders.(42) This cost estimation includes initial diagnosis, emergent and surgical intervention, and metabolic evaluation. Clearly, any optimization in this expense would be beneficial to the overall financial state of health care. To this end, multiple authors have analyzed the cost-effectiveness of metabolic evaluation. Although metabolic evaluations and medical therapy have been shown to reduce the risk of recurrent episodes of symptomatic nephrolithiasis, these findings do not imply a direct cost-benefit for the health-care system.(43)

Early publications on the cost-effectiveness of metabolic evaluation maintained that the financial benefit of selective medical therapy outweighed the burden of medical evaluation. (44–47) Although these initial publications demonstrated a cost-benefit of comprehensive metabolic evaluation, the studies were based on recurrence rates and the risk reduction of medical therapy. The inclusion of dietary management in medical therapy, the small percentage of patients requiring surgical intervention for recurrent stone disease, and the absence of empiric therapy were not included in any of these early analyses.

Because of the absence of these key factors, recent authors have downplayed the financial benefit of comprehensive metabolic evaluation of recurrent nephrolithiasis. One study performed an analysis comparing the cost of medical prophylaxis to clinical management of recurrent stone episodes in an attempt to determine the recurrence rate at which the two treatment modalities become cost equivalent.(48) This study represented an international cost survey of 10 countries, where the costs for medical management of nephrolithiasis were: initial limited metabolic evaluation, drug therapy, follow-up visits every six months, which included a 24-hr urinalysis, and yearly radiographic imaging of the urinary tract. Alternatively, the management of the recurrent stone episode included: emergency room visit, computerized tomography for stone identification, and outpatient treatment of stones with shock wave lithotripsy or ureteroscopy for those stones that did not pass spontaneously. A number of assumptions on rates of symptomatic recurrence, percentage of patients requiring subsequent urologic intervention, as well as the remission rate of medical prophylaxis were gleaned from review of urologic literature. The author determined that only at a recurrence rate of 0.3–4 stones per year does medical evaluation and treatment become equivalent to surgical management of recurrent episodes. The range of recurrence rates necessary for equivalence is due to the varying health-care costs between the countries. This report concluded that medical management of a first stone episode is not cost-effective and that the decision to perform a metabolic evaluation should be individualized for specific health-care plans.

Further evidence against routine metabolic evaluation and directed medical therapy for first-time stone formers has been suggested in another financial analysis.(49) This group similarly performed an international cost comparison analysis utilizing the urologic literature on stone recurrence to support their assumptions. A decision tree model was generated to assess the cost-effectiveness of empiric medical therapy, conservative (dietary) therapy, or directed medical therapy based on a comprehensive metabolic evaluation. Results were reported for both first-time and recurrent stone formers. For first-time stone formers, the recurrence rate on conservative therapy (diet and fluids) was determined to be 0.07 stones/patient/year. The authors identified a 20-fold increase in the cost for drug therapy compared to conservative management. However, drug therapy yielded a 80% reduction in stone recurrence rates. Conservative therapy was also found to be the least costly option for recurrent stone formers but was associated with the highest rate of recurrence (0.3 stones/patient/year) compared to empiric and directed medical therapy (0.06 and 0.084 stones/patient/year, respectively). In agreement with Chandhoke, the authors concluded that first-time stone formers should initially be treated conservatively. These studies suggest that recurrent stone formers, however, should undergo a simplified metabolic evaluation due to the high rate of recurrence associated with conservative therapy. It should be noted that many investigators suggest that the decision to perform a comprehensive metabolic evaluation ultimately falls to discussions between the physician and patient.

While these studies attempt to assess costs to the health-care system associated with metabolic evaluation vs expectant management of recurrent stone episodes, these investigations do not evaluate a number of factors. These studies do not account for the costs associated with lost wages and productivity, costs of ancillary medication requirements, and other associated personal expenses. Additionally, patients' pain and suffering, though not a financial burden, should be taken into account when deciding to undertake a metabolic evaluation and associated reduction in recurrence of stone episodes. It is likely that the pain experienced by patients explains the 92% and 99% willingness to collect 24-hr urine samples for first-time and recurrent stone formers, described by some investigators.[2] Indeed, others have demonstrated, with a patient decision analysis, that patients perceive long-term management with medical therapy a desirable option.[50] Additionally, in this analysis, only shock wave lithotripsy ranked higher in patients' decisions and patients appreciated medical therapy the longer they complied with recommendations. For these reasons, the decision to undertake a metabolic evaluation is one reached by patient and physician consensus, with the understanding of all the diagnostic/therapeutic benefits and limitations.

CONCLUSIONS

The goal of the basic metabolic evaluation is to provide a simple, readily acceptable, cost-effective method to determine the specific cause of stone disease in a particular patient. Although debate continues regarding the utility of evaluating a low-risk stone former, there are clear benefits for those patients who are at high risk or those who have demonstrated a propensity for recurrent stone formation. Our current practice is to perform a basic serum chemistry (including uric acid), urine analysis, urine culture, two random diet 24-hr urinalyses, radiographic work-up, stone analysis (when available), and standard history and physical exam. This diagnostic assessment is generally satisfactory to both patient and clinician with a high degree of diagnostic accuracy.

REFERENCES

1. Pak CY, Britton F, Peterson R et al. Ambulatory evaluation of nephrolithiasis. Classification, clinical presentation and diagnostic criteria. Am J Med 1980; 69: 19.
2. Grampsas SA, Moore M, Chandhoke PS. 10-year experience with extracorporeal shockwave lithotripsy in the state of Colorado. J Endourol 2000; 14: 711.
3. Ljunghall S, Danielson BG. A prospective study of renal stone recurrences. Br J Urol 1984; 56: 122.
4. Ahlstrand C, Tiselius HG. Recurrences during a 10-year follow-up after first renal stone episode. Urol Res 1990; 18: 397.
5. Hosking DH, Erickson SB, Van den Berg CJ et al. The stone clinic effect in patients with idiopathic calcium urolithiasis. J Urol 1983; 130: 1115.
6. Kourambas J, Aslan P, Teh CL et al. Role of stone analysis in metabolic evaluation and medical treatment of nephrolithiasis. J Endourol 2001; 15: 181.

7. Chandhoke PS. Evaluation of the recurrent stone former. Urol Clin North Am 2007; 34: 315.
8. Sarmina I, Spirnak JP, Resnick MI. Urinary lithiasis in the black population: an epidemiological study and review of the literature. J Urol 1987; 138: 14.
9. Maloney ME, Springhart WP, Ekeruo WO et al. Ethnic background has minimal impact on the etiology of nephrolithiasis. J Urol 2005; 173: 2001.
10. Mente A, Honey RJ, McLaughlin, JR et al. Ethnic differences in relative risk of idiopathic calcium nephrolithiasis in North America. J Urol 2007; 178: 1992.
11. Bartosh SM. Medical management of pediatric stone disease. Urol Clin North Am 2004; 31: 575.
12. Reddy ST, Wang CY, Sakhaee K et al. Effect of low-carbohydrate high-protein diets on acid-base balance, stone-forming propensity, and calcium metabolism. Am J Kidney Dis 2002; 40: 265.
13. Yilmaz S, Sindel T, Arslan G et al. Renal colic: comparison of spiral CT, US and IVU in the detection of ureteral calculi. Eur Radiol 1998; 8: 212.
14. Teichman JM. Clinical practice. Acute renal colic from ureteral calculus. N Engl J Med 2004; 350: 684.
15. Bellin MF, Renard-Penna R, Conort P et al. Helical CT evaluation of the chemical composition of urinary tract calculi with a discriminant analysis of CT-attenuation values and density. Eur Radiol 2004; 14: 2134.
16. Deveci S, Coskun M, Tekin MI et al. Spiral computed tomography: role in determination of chemical compositions of pure and mixed urinary stones--an in vitro study. Urology 2004; 64: 237.
17. Mitcheson HD, Zamenhof RG, Bankoff MS et al. Determination of the chemical composition of urinary calculi by computerized tomography. J Urol 1983; 130: 814.
18. Mostafavi MR, Ernst RD, Saltzman B. Accurate determination of chemical composition of urinary calculi by spiral computerized tomography. J Urol 1998; 159: 673.
19. Motley G, Dalrymple N, Keesling C et al. Hounsfield unit density in the determination of urinary stone composition. Urology 2001; 58: 170.
20. Zarse CA, McAteer JA, Tann M et al. Helical computed tomography accurately reports urinary stone composition using attenuation values: in vitro verification using high-resolution micro-computed tomography calibrated to fourier transform infrared microspectroscopy. Urology 2004; 63: 828.
21. Graser A, Johnson TR, Bader M et al. Dual energy CT characterization of urinary calculi: initial in vitro and clinical experience. Invest Radiol 2008; 43: 112.
22. Boll DT, Patil PN, Paulson EK et al. A Pilot-Study assessing Renal Stones with Dual Energy MDCT and advanced Postprocessing Techniques: Improved Characterization of Stone Composition. Radiology, Ahead of Print, 2008.
23. Rivers K, Shetty S, Menon M. When and how to evaluate a patient with nephrolithiasis. Urol Clin North Am 2000; 27: 203.
24. Pak CY, Peterson R, Poindexter JR. Adequacy of a single stone risk analysis in the medical evaluation of urolithiasis. J Urol 2001; 165: 378.
25. Parks JH, Goldfisher E, Asplin JR et al. A single 24-hour urine collection is inadequate for the medical evaluation of nephrolithiasis. J Urol 2002; 167: 1607.
26. Lifshitz DA, Shalhav AL, Lingeman JE et al. Metabolic evaluation of stone disease patients: a practical approach. J Endourol 1999; 13: 669.
27. Hesse A, Straub M. Rational evaluation of urinary stone disease. Urol Res 2006; 34: 126.
28. Parks JH, Coward M, Coe FL. Correspondence between stone composition and urine supersaturation in nephrolithiasis. Kidney Int 1997; 51: 894.
29. Asplin J, Parks J, Lingeman J et al. Supersaturation and stone composition in a network of dispersed treatment sites. J Urol 1998; 159: 1821.
30. Pak CY, Poindexter JR, Adams-Huet B et al. Predictive value of kidney stone composition in the detection of metabolic abnormalities. Am J Med 2003; 115: 26.
31. Lingeman JE, Siegel YI, Steele B. Metabolic evaluation of infected renal lithiasis: clinical relevance. J Endourol 1995; 9: 51.
32. Newhouse JH, Prien EL, Amis ES Jr et al. Computed tomographic analysis of urinary calculi. AJR Am J Roentgenol 1984; 142: 545.
33. Saw KC, McAteer JA, Monga AG et al. Helical CT of urinary calculi: effect of stone composition, stone size, and scan collmation. AJR Am J Roentgenol 2000; 175: 329.
34. Sheir KZ, Mansour O, Madbouly K et al. Determination of the chemical composition of urinary calculi by noncontrast spiral computerized tomography. Urol Res 2005; 33: 99.
35. Zhong P, Preminger GM. Mechanisms of differing stone fragility in extracorporeal shockwave lithotripsy. J Endourol 1994; 8: 263.
36. Saw KC, McAteer JA, Fineberg NS et al. Calcium stone fragility is predicted by helical CT attenuation values. J Endourol 2000; 14: 471.
37. Thier SO, Segal S, Fox M et al. Cystinuria: Defective Intestinal Transport of Dibasic Amino Acids and Cystine. J Clin Invest 1965; 44: 442.
38. Pak CY, Fuller CJ. Assessment of cystine solubility in urine and of heterogeneous nucleation. J Urol 1983; 129: 1066.

39. Sakhaee K, Poindexter JR, Pak CY. The spectrum of metabolic abnormalities in patients with cystine nephrolithiasis. J Urol 1989; 141: 819.

40. Nemoy NJ, Staney TA. Surgical, bacteriological, and biochemical management of "infection stones". JAMA 1971; 215: 1470.

41. Healy KA, Ogan K. Pathophysiology and management of infectious staghorn calculi. Urol Clin North Am 2007; 34: 363.

42. Pearle MS, Calhoun EA, Curhan GC. Urologic diseases in America project: urolithiasis. J Urol 2005; 173: 848.

43. Pearle MS, Roehrborn CG, Pak CY. Meta-analysis of randomized trials for medical prevention of calcium oxalate nephrolithiasis. J Endourol 1999; 13: 679.

44. Tiselius HG. Comprehensive metabolic evaluation of stone formers is cost effective. Presented at the Urolithiasis; 2000.

45. Parks JH, Coe FL. The financial effects of kidney stone prevention. Kidney Int 1996; 50: 1706.

46. Robertson WG. Is prevention of stone recurrence financially worthwhile? Urol Res 2006; 34: 157.

47. Strohmaier WL. [Economic aspects of evidence-based metaphylaxis]. Urologe A 2006; 45: 1406.

48. Chandhoke PS. When is medical prophylaxis cost-effective for recurrent calcium stones? J Urol 2002; 168: 937.

49. Lotan Y, Cadeddu JA, Pearle MS. International comparison of cost effectiveness of medical management strategies for nephrolithiasis. Urol Res 2005; 33: 223.

50. Kuo RL, Aslan P, Abrahamse PH et al. Incorporation of patient preferences in the treatment of upper urinary tract calculi: a decision analytical view. J Urol 1999; 162: 1913.

4 | Role of diet in stone prevention

Kristina Penniston

INTRODUCTION

Diet influences kidney stone disease by inhibiting or promoting lithogenesis. Specific nutrients as well as non-nutrient food components play roles at different stages of the process.(1, 2) Certain combinations of foods, comprising discrete dietary patterns, appear to influence the course of the disease.(3, 4) Current nutrition recommendations and mechanisms by which specific nutrients, foods, and dietary patterns affect urolithiasis risk, particularly those of calcium and uric acid composition, are described in this chapter. The clinical application of nutrition therapy to patients is also addressed.

DEFINITION OF MEDICAL NUTRITION THERAPY

Nutrition intervention to reduce risk factors for urolithiasis in recurrent stone formers is recognized as a key aspect of prevention. Medical nutrition therapy (MNT) is the application of "nutritional diagnostic, therapy, and counseling services for the purpose of disease management which are furnished by a Registered Dietitian or nutrition professional."(5) Whereas pharmacotherapy is the treatment of a disease with appropriate drugs, MNT is the practice of treating and managing diseases with specific foods, nutrients, dietary supplements, and combinations thereof. MNT is driven by the existence of clinical and/or biochemical derangements or risk factors for a specific condition or disease. MNT is physician directed, meaning that a patient's physician makes a referral to a Registered Dietitian for therapy. MNT can be directed at primary, secondary, or tertiary prevention of disease. As of 2002, the U.S. Medicare program commenced coverage and reimbursement of MNT as treatment for individuals with diabetes and pre-renal disease.(5) Currently, the U.S. Congress is considering the inclusion of MNT coverage for other diseases.

STATUS OF NUTRITION RESEARCH IN UROLITHIASIS

There is general consensus that well-controlled studies on the effects of diet on urolithiasis risk and incidence, particularly those that are randomized and prospective, are lacking. In contrast to other chronic diseases with nutritional effectors, such as diabetes, asthma, and hypertension, for example, there are currently no published meta-analyses on diet and renal stones. Information to date on dietary factors and the effects of dietary changes on renal stone risk and incidence are largely from epidemiological investigations (Table 4.1), retrospective reviews, and small studies of variable control in both stone formers and nonstone formers. Most studies are focused on individual nutrients and food components and not whole dietary patterns. A few studies have addressed patient compliance with and adherence to nutrition recommendations to reduce stone risk.(6–9) Few, if any, studies have adequately assessed patient understanding of the recommendations provided in the clinical management of stone disease. No studies have linked medical management or nutritional management of stone disease with patients' quality of life. Few studies have rigorously evaluated the "stone clinic effect," i.e., sum of medical management strategies, which may change over time depending on the patient's risk factors, to reduce stone risk and incidence.

SPECIFIC DIETARY INHIBITORS OF LITHOGENESIS

Fluids and beverages. A consistently high fluid intake is most effective in reducing urinary supersaturation.(10) Daily urine output greater than 2 L is targeted, but more may be required

Table 4.1   Major epidemiological studies on diet and urolithiasis incidence and/or risk factors from 1985 to 2008.

Lead Author, Year, and Journal[1]	Diet, Food Component or Supplement Studied	Primary Outcome Measure	Major Findings and Associations of Interest[2]	Comment(s) *(e.g., gender, study design, cohort)*[5–10]
Shuster J, 1985, J Chronic Dis(22)	Beverages, general	Stone prevalence	Regular soda, + Beer, - Coffee, -	Men (*n*=2,295), 2 geographical regions in United States.
Curhan GC, 1996, Am J Epidemiol(11)	Beverages, general	Stone incidence, symptomatic	Coffee, - Decaf coffee, - Tea, - Wine, - Beer, - Apple juice, + Grapefruit juice, +	HPFS, prospective, 6 y follow-up
Curhan GC, 1998, Ann Intern Med(12)	Beverages, general	Stone incidence, symptomatic	Total fluids, - Coffee, - Decaf coffee, - Tea, - Wine, - Grapefruit juice, +	NHS, prospective, 8 y follow-up
Choi HK, 2004, Arthritis Rheum(25)	Beverages, alcoholic	Serum uric acid	Beer, + Liquor, + Wine, NA	NHANES III
Curhan GC, 1998, J Am Soc Nephrol(64)	Body size	Stone incidence, symptomatic	Body weight, + [3] BMI, + [3]	NHS and HPFS, prospective, 14 and 8 y follow-up, respectively
Taylor EN, 2005, JAMA(65)	Body size	Stone incidence, symptomatic	Body mass, + [3] BMI, + [3] Weight gain, + [3] Waist circumference, + [3]	HPFS, NHS, and NHS II, prospective
Taylor EN, 2006, Am J Kidney Dis(66)	Body size	Association of BMI with 24-h urinary risk factors	Urinary oxalate, + [3] Urinary uric acid, + Urinary Na, + Urinary P, + Urine pH, -	HPFS, NHS, and NHS II, stone formers vs. non stone formers
Choi HK, 2007, Arthritis Rheum(165)	Coffee, tea, caffeine	Serum uric acid	Coffee, - Decaffeinated coffee, - Tea, NA Total caffeine, NA	NHANES III
Choi HK, 2007, Arthritis Rheum(166)	Coffee, caffeine	Gout incidence	Coffee, - Decaffeinated coffee, - Total caffeine, NA	HPFS, prospective, 12 y follow-up
Curhan GC, 1993, N Engl J Med(34)	Diet factors, various	Stone incidence, symptomatic	Supplemental calcium, NA Dietary calcium, - Potassium, - Total fluids, - Animal protein, +	HPFS, prospective, 4 y follow-up
Curhan GC, 1997, Ann Intern Med(35)	Diet factors, various	Stone incidence, symptomatic	Supplemental calcium, + Dietary calcium, - Potassium, - Sodium, + Sucrose, + Total fluids, -	NHS, prospective, 12 y follow-up
Hirvonen T, 1999, Am J Epidemiol(63)	Diet factors, various	Stone incidence	Magnesium, - Calcium, NA Fiber, + Beer, -	ATBC study, prospective, 5 y follow-up

(Continued)

Table 4.1 (Continued)

Lead Author, Year, and Journal[1]	Diet, Food Component or Supplement Studied	Primary Outcome Measure	Major Findings and Associations of Interest[2]	Comment(s) (e.g., gender, study design, cohort)[5–10]
Taylor EN, 2004, J Am Soc Nephrol[1]	Diet factors, various	Stone incidence, symptomatic	Fluids, - Potassium, - Calcium, - [4] Magnesium, - Vit. C, +	HPFS, prospective, 14 y follow-up
Curhan GC, 2004, Arch Intern Med(59)	Diet factors, various	Stone incidence, symptomatic	Supplemental calcium, NA Dietary calcium, - Phytate, - Animal protein, - Total fluids, - Sucrose, +	NHS II, prospective, 12 y follow-up
Goldfarb DS, 2005, Kidney Int(167)	Diet factors, various	History of kidney stones	Coffee, - Milk, - Rice, - Alcohol, -	VET Registry (cotwin control study)
Taylor EN, 2005, Am J Kidney Dis(126)	Fatty acids	Stone incidence, symptomatic	Arachidonic acid, NA Linoleic acid, NA n-3 fatty acids, NA	HPFS, NHS, NHS II, prospective, 36 y combined follow-up
Gao X, 2007, Hypertension(20)	Fructose/ sugar-sweetened beverages	Serum uric acid	Added sugar, + (men only) Sugar-sweetened beverages, + (men only)	NHANES 2001-2002
Taylor EN, 2008, Kidney Int(21)	Fructose/ other carbohydrates (CHOs)	Stone incidence, symptomatic	Total fructose, + Free fructose, + Non-fructose CHOs, NA	HPFS, NHS, NHS II, prospective, 48 y combined follow-up
Choi HK, 2008, BMJ(19)	Fructose/ sugar-sweetened beverages	Gout incidence	Sugar-sweetened soda, + Fructose, + Diet soda, NA	HPFS, prospective, 12 y follow-up
Choi JW, 2008, Arthritis Rheum(18)	Fructose/ sugar-sweetened beverages	Serum uric acid	Sugar-sweetened soda, + Diet soda, NA	NHANES III
Taylor EN, 2007, J Am Soc Nephrol(110)	Oxalate intake	Stone incidence, symptomatic	Dietary oxalate, + / NA [3,4] Spinach, + / NA [3,4]	HPFS, NHS, NHS II, prospective, 44 y combined follow-up
Choi HK, 2004, N Engl J Med(81)	Purines, protein	Gout incidence	Meat, + Seafood, + Dairy, - Total protein, NA Purine-rich vegetables, NA	HPFS, prospective, 12 y follow-up
Choi HK, 2005, Arthritis Rheum(80)	Purines, protein	Serum uric acid	Meat, + Seafood, + Dairy, - Total protein, NA	NHANES III
Curhan GC, 1996, J Urol(53)	Vitamins B6, C	Stone incidence, symptomatic	Vit. B6, NA Vit. C, NA	HPFS, prospective, 6 y follow-up
Curhan GC, 1999, J Am Soc Nephrol(54)	Vitamins B6, C	Stone incidence, symptomatic	Vit. B6, - Vit. C, NA	NHS, prospective, 14 y follow-up

1 Superscripted numbers correspond to numbered literature references.
2 NA, no association; +, positive association; -, inverse association
3 Some gender differences in associations were reported
4 Some age differences in associations were reported
5 NHANES III, Third National Health and Nutrition Examination Survey, 1988–1994, males and females 2 months of age and older
6 HPFS, Health Professionals Follow-Up Study, initiated in 1986, male health professionals only
7 NHS, Nurses' Health Study, original cohort initiated in 1976 for female registered nurses between 30 and 55 years of age
8 NHS II, Nurses' Health Study II, initiated in 1989 for female registered nurses between 25 and 42 years of age
9 ATBC, Alpha-Tocopherol, Beta-Carotene Cancer Prevention Study, 1984-1988, 27,001 Finnish male smokers between 50 and 69 years
10 VET Registry, Vietnam Era Twin Registry, ~7,500 male-male twin pairs born between 1939 to 1955 with both twins having served in the military from 1965 to 1975

in most individuals to maintain urine saturation within acceptable limits. In general, this requires drinking at least 2.5 L of fluids/day, distributed throughout the day, including at bedtime to promote nighttime urine dilution. More fluids must be consumed if there is excessive sweating, diarrhea, or vomiting. Patients whose urinary risk factors cannot be completely controlled with targeted nutrition and/or pharmacologic therapy should be advised that a higher urine output, exceeding the 2 L/day cutoff, is necessary to maintain suitably low urine supersaturation in the face of excessive crystal promoters and/or suboptimal crystal inhibitors. Similarly, patients on medications known to increase risk for urinary stones should aim for a higher urine output as a "trade off" for the elevated risk conferred by the medication. While the intake of almost all beverages are associated with reduced risk for kidney stones (11, 12), fruit juices and other beverages known to enhance urinary oxalate (13–17), beverages high in sodium (e.g., tomato juice), and beverages sweetened with fructose, which has been associated with hyperuricosuria and hyperuricemia (18–21), should be avoided. Caffeinated beverages, while not usually necessary to avoid completely, and in fact associated with a protective effect against stones prevalence (22) and incidence (11, 12), should comprise a minority of the fluids consumed during the day as caffeine may enhance urinary calcium excretion, via enhanced bone resorption, in some individuals.(23, 24) Alcoholic beverages, beer and wine specifically, are also associated with reduced urinary stone risk factors (11, 12, 22, 25), but it would make sense to recommend a moderate intake of alcohol, if at all, as it may enhance serum uric acid (26) and, at 7 kilocalories per gram, confers a relatively high caloric load.

Citrate-containing fruits and beverages. Certain fruit juices are rich in citric acid and other bicarbonate precursors and have been explored for their ability to enhance fluid intake as well as urinary citrate excretion. The juices of lemons and limes are most concentrated with citric acid (27) and also contain some potassium. Lemon juice ingestion has been reported in some studies (27–29) but not others (30) to increase urinary citrate excretion. Lemonade, commercially prepared, is usually only 15% lemon juice and usually heavily sweetened with sucrose and/or fructose, which may offset clinical benefits. In one study, while no adverse effects were reported, intake of commercially prepared lemonade did not increase urinary citrate excretion. (31) Other fruit juices also contain appreciable citric acid and more potassium than lemon or lime juice, which may further enhance urinary citrate excretion due to their alkali load; these include orange, grapefruit, apple, and blackcurrant juice. However, orange, grapefruit, and apple juice also raise urinary oxalate (14–17), potentially offsetting the crystal inhibitory effect of the citric acid. Moreover, fruit juices generally provide ample carbohydrates, fructose, and kilocalories, excessive intake of which should be avoided to maintain appropriate weight and to reduce the risk of hypercalciuria and other metabolic derangements.

Dietary calcium. In 1938, Grossmann conjectured that a diet containing vegetable material coupled with a deficiency of calcium-containing dairy foods contributed to the calcium oxalate "stone wave" that occurred in Eastern Europe after World War I.(32) In 1969, Zarembski and Hodgkinson reported enhanced urinary oxalate excretion in stone-forming individuals when they consumed controlled diets low in calcium.(33) Nonetheless, low calcium intakes were traditionally recommended for individuals forming calcium oxalate or calcium phosphate stones and particularly those with hypercalciuria. Two large epidemiologic investigations in the United States in the 1990s showed an inverse relationship between dietary calcium intake and the relative risk for calcium oxalate stones.(34, 35) Studies using isotopic tracer methodology confirmed that calcium reduces oxalate absorption in the gastrointestinal tract.(36) Thus, an appropriate calcium intake, such as per the Adequate Intake (AI) as defined within the Dietary Reference Intakes, appears necessary for most individuals to provide optimum gastrointestinal binding of oxalate. (In general, although there are gender and age distinctions, this is around 1000–1200 mg calcium daily for adults, ingested in distributed dosages to ensure intermittent presence of calcium in the GI tract.(37)) Table 4.2 lists major food sources of calcium. Recently, results from other studies have added improvements in blood pressure, bone strength, and weight management to the benefits of an adequate calcium intake.(38, 39) When calcium is bound to oxalate in the GI tract, neither the calcium nor the oxalate is absorbed. Due to the presence of fat malabsorption from bowel disease or alterations in gut physiology, resulting in the complexation of calcium with fat to form fatty acid soaps instead of calcium with oxalate, some patients may need to ingest calcium in amounts that exceed the AI in order to effect appropriate oxalate binding in the gut.(40–42) In these individuals, the amount of calcium ingested daily, and its timing, should be individually derived based on serial 24-h urine profiles and progression of stone disease. It

Table 4.2 Major selected food sources of calcium.[1,2]

Food	Amount/ preparation	Mg calcium
Collard greens	1 cup, cooked	350
Rhubarb	1 cup, cooked	350
Calcium-fortified breakfast cereals, ready-to-consume	1 serving (per nutrition label of individual cereals)	300–1000
Milk	8 fluid ounces	300
Spinach	1 cup, cooked	300
Yogurt	8 ounces	200–400
Calcium-fortified fruit juices	8 fluid ounces	200–300
Calcium-fortified soy/ rice milk	8 fluid ounces	200–300
Cheese	1 ounce	200–300
Kale	1 cup, cooked	200
Cottage cheese	1 cup	200

1 Data compiled from the U.S. Department of Agriculture, Agricultural Research Service, 2007. USDA National Nutrient Database for Standard Reference, Release 20. Nutrient Data Laboratory Home Page, http://www.ars.usda.gov/ba/bhnrc/ndl, accessed 06/09/2008.
2 Calcium bioavailability is not accounted for in this table. Thus, food sources rich in calcium but also rich in oxalate (e.g., collard greens, rhubarb, spinach) would not yield highly bioavailable calcium.

should be noted that excessive calcium intake may promote the formation of calcium renal stones in susceptible individuals, particularly those in whom intestinal calcium absorption is enhanced, as in absorptive hypercalciuria, or whose reabsorption of renal tubule calcium is decreased.(43) Age-related differences in risk with calcium intake have been reported.(1)

Supplemental calcium. Results are mixed with respect to supplemental calcium with some studies showing an inverse and others a positive relationship with risk factors for urinary stones and stone formation.(34, 35, 44) Although more research is clearly needed to define the formulation(s) of calcium supplements that are most or least beneficial (e.g., calcium citrate, calcium carbonate), it seems clear that calcium supplements may be useful in reducing urinary oxalate excretion in calcium oxalate stone formers and that the timing of supplemental calcium ingestion is key. When timed with meals or snacks, particularly those providing oxalate, supplemental calcium has been shown to decrease oxalate absorption, with a concomitant reduction in urinary oxalate excretion, and either no increase in urinary calcium excretion or no increase in urine calcium oxalate supersaturation.(44, 45) Calcium supplements, timed with meals, may be especially important for patients whose calcium needs are high or in those whose dietary calcium intake is low. Calcium citrate appears to be superior to calcium carbonate, not because it binds oxalate any better, but because it may also enhance urinary citrate excretion.(46) As additional urinary citrate appears useful in maintaining the solubility of calcium in urine, it is logical that calcium citrate supplements would be the first choice recommendation. Calcium citrate, as well as other calcium supplement formulations, are available over-the-counter. Calcium citrate tablets tend to be larger than the tablets of other calcium supplements, making them contraindicated in patients with swallowing difficulties, and chewable or dissolvable formulations are lacking. Thus, a patient's ability to tolerate calcium citrate supplements should be individually determined. The amount of calcium to be supplemented should be titrated against the patient's usual dietary calcium intake.

Potassium. Dietary potassium is associated with decreased incidence of stones.(1, 35, 36) Urinary potassium concentration is linked with reduced stone formation after extracorporeal shock wave lithotripsy (ESWL).(47) Many American adults fail to meet the AI for potassium (48), which is 4700 mg/day.(37) There is some evidence that the dietary sodium:potassium ratio may be higher in stone formers than in nonstone formers.(49) Low potassium status results in enhanced urinary calcium excretion, due to decreased renal tubular reabsorption, and hypokalemia, which has a potent hypocitraturic effect. Potassium in foods is supplied by most fruits and vegetables, milk, yogurt, fish, meat, and poultry. Of these, the potassium in fruits and vegetables is usually complexed with bicarbonate precursors in the form of organic acids, and these alkali potentiate the urinary excretion of citrate. In contrast, certain animal sources of potassium confer a dietary acid load, owing to the presence of methionine and other sulfur-containing amino acids, which may reduce urinary citrate excretion. Table 4.3 lists major selected food sources of potassium.

Table 4.3   Major selected food sources of potassium.[1]

Food	Amount/ preparation	Mg potassium
Dried fruits (dates, raisins, prunes)	1 cup	800–1200
Potatoes, white and sweet	1 medium	800–1000
Beans (white, soy, lima, baked, pinto, kidney navy, lentils, black)	1 cup, cooked	600–1200
Squash, winter	1 cup, cooked	895
Plantains	1 cup, cooked	700
Bulgur, barley	1 cup, raw/dry	550
Banana	1 medium	540
Fruit & vegetable juices (grapefruit, prune, carrot, tomato, orange)	6 fluid ounces	500–1000
Canned tomato products	1 cup	500–1000
Yogurt	8 ounces	500–600
Brussels sprouts	1 cup, cooked	500
Orange juice	8 fluid ounces	500
Fish (halibut, rockfish, haddock, salmon, tuna, cod, flounder, sole)	½ fillet, cooked (about 160 grams)	400–900
Corn	1 cup, coked	400
Milk (chocolate, white)	8 fluid ounces	360–420
Fruits (pear, peach, mango, papaya, melon)	1 cup, 1 med. fruit, or 1 wedge	300–400

1 Data compiled from the U.S. Department of Agriculture, Agricultural Research Service, 2007. USDA National Nutrient Database for Standard Reference, Release 20. Nutrient Data Laboratory Home Page, http://www.ars.usda.gov/ba/bhnrc/ndl, accessed 06/09/2008.

Table 4.4   Major selected food sources of magnesium.[1]

Food	Amount/ preparation	Mg magnesium
Whole flour (buckwheat, wheat, cornmeal)	1 cup, dry	150–300
Whole grains (bulgur, oat bran, barley)	1 cup, dry/ raw	160–230
Fish, halibut	½ fillet (about 160 grams)	170
Spinach	1 cup, cooked	160
Seeds (pumpkin, squash)	1 ounce, roasted	150
Soybeans	1 cup, cooked	150
Beans (white, black, navy, lima)	1 cup, cooked	100–130
Brazil nuts	1 ounce, dried	100
Artichokes	1 cup, cooked	100
Greens (beet, okra)	1 cup, cooked	100
Nuts (almonds, cashews, pine)	1 ounce	70–80
Fortified breakfast cereals, ready-to-consume	1 serving (per nutrition label of individual cereals)	50–110

1 Data compiled from the U.S. Department of Agriculture, Agricultural Research Service, 2007. USDA National Nutrient Database for Standard Reference, Release 20. Nutrient Data Laboratory Home Page, http://www.ars.usda.gov/ba/bhnrc/ndl, accessed 06/09/2008.

Magnesium. Dietary magnesium has been associated with lower stone-forming risk in men but not in women.(1, 35, 36) Many Americans fail to achieve the Recommended Dietary Allowance (RDA) for magnesium (50), which is 320 and 420 mg/day for adult women and men, respectively.(37) In theory, a higher magnesium intake should confer a reduced risk for calcium oxalate stones. Magnesium binds oxalate in the gastrointestinal tract, forming an insoluble complex, and reduces its absorption. In urine, magnesium forms a soluble complex with oxalate, which could reduce the availability of urinary oxalate supersaturation, assuming that other factors involved with supersaturation remain constant. Foods rich in magnesium include whole grains, halibut, beans, some nuts and seeds, and spinach (Table 4.4). It is not known whether urinary magnesium interferes with the actions of other urinary inhibitors, e.g., citrate, or whether enhanced urinary magnesium might increase the risk for struvite stones, if urine conditions are otherwise favorable for struvite crystallization.

Table 4.5 Major selected food sources of phytate.[1]

Food	Example(s)
Cereal germ	Corn germ, wheat germ
Cereal bran	Wheat bran, oat bran
Whole grain cereals	Corn, wheat, rice, oats, barley, sorghum
Beans and lentils	Whole beans, bean flours, bean pastes
Nuts and seeds	Peanuts, Brazil nuts, sesame seeds

1 Data compiled from literature references (168) and (169).

Vitamin B6. Pyridoxine is a cofactor for the enzyme [L-alanine:glyoxalate aminotransferase (AGT)] involved in the hepatic peroxisomal conversion of glyoxalate, a substrate of oxalate, to glycine. Supplementation with vitamin B6 is thus useful in a subsection of patients with primary hyperoxaluria type 1 (51), who lack this enzyme and perhaps in those whose intake of vitamin B6 is deficient.(52) However, it is not clear whether vitamin B6 supplementation in vitamin B6–replete individuals is effective in reducing oxalate biosynthesis. Epidemiologic studies have shown no association in men of vitamin B6 with kidney stone risk (53) but an inverse association in young women.(54) In theory, pyridoxine reduces oxalate biosynthesis by participating as a cofactor in the enzymatic conversion of glyoxalate to glycine. Supraphysiological dosages of 100–200 mg/day or more have been used clinically; results have not been well characterized. It may be that supplemental pyridoxine works in the subset of patients whose enzymatic cleavage of glyoxalate is suboptimal, due to genetic variations. Although vitamin B6 is water soluble and usually safe at intakes up to 200 mg/day in adults, hypervitaminosis has been documented in individuals taking supplements. Vitamin B6 toxicity can damage sensory nerves, causing numbness in the hands and feet as well as difficulty in walking. Other symptoms may include poor coordination, staggering, numbness, decreased tactile sensation, chronic fatigue.(55) The RDA for vitamin B6 for adults is between 1.3 and 1.7 mg/day, with the exact requirement differing slightly with respect to age and gender.(37)

Phytate. Also known as inositol hexaphosphate, phytate, the salt of phytic acid, is a non-nutrient richly expressed in certain plant foods, notably, beans, nuts, and whole grains. Certain baking and cooking processes degrade phytate. Estimates of daily phytate intake vary widely from 150–1400 mg for mixed diets to 2000–2600 mg or higher for vegetarian diets as well as diets of rural populations in developing countries whose caloric intake is largely plant based.(56) Animal and *in vitro* studies demonstrate a potent inhibitory potential for calcium stones as phytate forms a soluble complex with calcium in urine and perhaps acts as an inhibitor via intrapapillary mechanisms as well.(57) The urinary concentrations of phytate in stone formers have been reported to be low compared to non-stone formers, and dietary intake of phytate does correlate well with urinary excretion.(58) Observational studies show both an inverse and null relationship between dietary phytate and risk of lithogenesis.(1, 59) As a diet rich in fruits and vegetables is associated with a protective effect against urolithiasis, the increased phytate content of a plant-based diet may be a key factor. Phytate binds strongly to divalent cations, decreasing their absorption. Table 4.5 lists some food sources of phytate commonly consumed in the United States.

Fiber. Fiber binds calcium in the gastrointestinal tract and may therefore reduce or regulate calcium absorption. Fiber is also an essential component of a healthy diet and one that reduces circulating lipids and risk for cardiovascular disease. Most American adults fail to achieve the AI for fiber, which is between 21 and 38 g per day, depending on gender and age. (37) A high fruit and vegetable intake is associated with reduced urolithiasis risk.(60) While fruits and vegetables contain multiple bioactive chemicals, the high fiber component of these foods may account for some of the favorable effects observed. Fiber is well known to reduce intestinal transit time, which may reduce the amount of time available for oxalate absorption. Fiber may also bind to calcium in the GI tract and reduce its absorption. Some studies have shown an inverse association of dietary fiber with stone risk (57, 61) whereas others have shown a positive association.(62, 63) It is unclear whether certain fibers are more protective against kidney stone formation than others.

SPECIFIC DIETARY PROMOTERS OF LITHOGENESIS

Excessive kilocalories. Overweight and obesity occur from an imbalance between kilocalories ingested and those expended. Excessive caloric intake leading to overweight and obesity is independently associated with higher risk for kidney stone formation.(64–66) Stone episodes and stone risk factors are reportedly higher in overweight and obese vs. normal weight patients.(67)Putative mechanisms responsible for these relationships include increased urinary excretion of stone promoters in overweight and obese patients (68–70), reduced urine pH (71), reduced excretion of urinary citrate (72), and reduced kidney function.(3)

Dietary animal protein. A positive association between kidney stone formation and animal protein intake has been shown.(34, 73–75) There are four factors that explain the association between animal protein and urolithiasis: (1) **dietary acid load**, (2) **uric acid precursors**, (3) **oxalate precursors**, and (4) **cysteine precursors**. These factors will be addressed individually.

(1.) **Dietary acid load.** Animal protein is rich in methionine, an amino acid which is not synthesized in humans and therefore considered essential. It is abundant in all foods of animal origin, whereas it is often a limiting amino acid in plant foods. Methionine contains sulfur, which generates sulfuric acid during metabolism, representing an acid load that increases urinary calcium excretion and enhances renal reabsorption of citrate. Among hypercalciuric stone formers, the calciuric effects of a high animal protein intake may be exaggerated.(76) The acid load increases calcium resorption from bone, resulting in higher urinary calcium (77), and also reduces urine pH (71), abetting the crystallization of uric acid, which may provide a nidus for calcium oxalate stone disease. Foods with the highest potential renal acid load (PRAL) are cheese, eggs, meat, fish, and poultry.(78) Grains confer a much lower PRAL but contribute to the dietary acid load nonetheless. The only foods with a net negative PRAL (alkaline load) are fruits and vegetables. A few fruits and vegetables are slightly acidic, but avoidance of these few (e.g., corn, lentils, cranberries, etc.) is likely unnecessary for the vast majority of patients who may lower their dietary PRAL by simply reducing the highest acid-load foods. Interestingly, milk and yogurt appear to be much less acidic than their other animal food counterparts and actually convey only a slight PRAL.(78)

(2.) **Uric acid precursors.** Meat, fish, seafood, and poultry are rich in uric acid precursors. Siener et al. showed the strongest decrease in urinary risk factors for uric acid stones in stone formers who followed either a lacto-ovo-vegetarian diet or a balanced omnivorous diet that was rich in fruits and vegetables and moderate for animal flesh protein.(79) Dairy foods, although of animal origin, may offer some protection against uric acid biosynthesis, evidenced by a recent study in men with gout (80); the mechanisms for this observation remain unclarified. While few nonanimal foods also provide ample uric acid precursors (e.g., lentils and legumes), the majority of purine intake is from animal sources.(74) Moreover, a study in men with gout revealed that purine-rich vegetables did not exacerbate the disease.(81)

(3.) **Oxalate precursors.** Recent evidence suggests that meat may provide oxalate precursors in the form of hydroxyproline, an amino acid present in collagen.(82) Hydroxyproline metabolism in the hepatocytes and renal proximal tubule cells results in glyoxalate, a substrate for oxalate biosynthesis. Dietary sources of hydroxyproline include collagen-containing meat products and foods containing gelatin.(83) Dietary hydroxyproline ingestion has been shown to increase the urinary oxalate excretion of rats, pigs, and, recently, humans.(83) This would explain earlier findings of increased urinary oxalate from a high meat intake (82, 84) and also the hyperoxaluria clinically observed in patients whose vegetable material intake, and, hence, oxalate intake, is not high. The endogenous synthesis of oxalate from foods that are low in oxalate warrants further attention.

(4.) **Cysteine precursors.** The degradation of methionine generates cysteine, which can be cleaved to form cystine, which is then excreted in urine in an insoluble form at a normal and acid urine pH. Thus, low-methionine diets have been recommended to cystine stone formers.(85) The efficacy of and compliance with low-methionine diets for cystine stone formers is questionable. A strict methionine restriction should not be rigorously pursued in pediatric cystine stone formers as methionine is required for growth. Foods with the highest methionine concentrations include: fish, meat, poultry, eggs, milk, cheese, nuts, legumes, wheat flour, and soy flour.

The RDA for protein for adults is 0.8 g protein per kg body weight (37), which usually amply meets the normal healthy adult's need to maintain homeostasis. The average protein intake by adult men and women in the United States exceeds the RDA, although the extent of overconsumption is body weight dependent. There are subsections of the population with low protein intakes. Recommendations on limiting animal protein intake may need to be individually titrated against expression of urinary risk factors in the form of uric acid, calcium, pH, and phosphorus. In other words, the need to reduce animal, fowl, and fish protein intake may vary from patient to patient, depending on his/her urinary risk profile and stone history. While for some it may be helpful to simply reduce protein intake to the RDA, or at least reduce the percentage of which comes from animal flesh, it may be necessary in others to attempt an even lower animal protein intake. It is important to note that as dairy and yogurt are not associated with hyperuricosuria and do not confer a high dietary acid load (78), and as they are also important calcium sources, which may be used to bind dietary oxalate and thereby reduce the risk of calcium oxalate stone formation and growth, they should be separated from the general recommendation to limit animal flesh, poultry, fish, and seafood.

Dietary carbohydrates. Excessive carbohydrate intake is associated with an increased urinary calcium excretion.(86, 87) This effect is thought to be mediated at least in part by insulin.(89) The intake of sucrose, a disaccharide composed of glucose and fructose, was associated in one study with new kidney stone formation in women (35) but not in men. Fructose, about half of which comes from sucrose (table sugar) in the typical American diet (34), is associated with increased stone risk factors in both men and women.(21) Specifically, it is associated with hyperuricemia and hyperuricosuria, possibly due to enhanced uric acid biosynthesis from fructose metabolism and degradation. In this sense, fructose may be considered a possible uric acid precursor as well as a potent contributor to excessive kilocalories and overweight. In addition to sucrose, common fructose sources include foods sweetened with fructose, fruit juices, and fruits. It makes sense to recommend a reduction in the intake by stone formers of both sucrose and fructose, focusing on sweets, baked goods, sweetened beverages and fruit juices, snack foods, and processed foods.

Dietary fats. The average American obtains more than 30% of his/her kilocalorie intake from fat, about one-third of that as saturated fat.(88) At an average 9 kilocalories per gram, excessive dietary fat provides ample kilocalories and is often associated with weight gain, which is independently associated with increased risk for urolithiasis.(65) Excessive fat intake is associated with the dietary habits of stone formers vs. nonstone formers.(62, 90, 91) Oxalate absorption may be enhanced by the presence of certain fatty acids in the intestinal tract.(84) While no studies have shown that oxalate absorption is increased by fat intake, it is logical to recommend reduced kilocalories from fat, especially saturated fat, in oxalate stone-forming patients. This recommendation may enhance ability to maintain an appropriate weight as well as enhance the cardiovascular and overall health profile of stone formers. The role of specific fatty acids on stone risk is unclear. Arachidonic acid, a polyunsaturated omega-6 fatty acid, has been linked with increased stone risk, possibly by increasing the intestinal absorption of oxalate and increasing the renal clearance of oxalate.(92–94)

Salt (sodium chloride). The human adult requires approximately 200 mg sodium/day. (95) The AI for sodium for adults is 1200–1500 mg/day (37) (the amount of sodium in 1/2 to 2/3 of a teaspoon of table salt). The average American consumes 2300–6900 mg sodium daily (86), which exceeds the Tolerable Upper Intake Level for sodium (2300 mg/day) set by the Food and Nutrition Board of the Institute of Medicine. Most dietary sodium comes from sodium chloride; only a small percentage (10–15%) comes from that which is added to foods during cooking or at the table.(96) The vast majority is obtained from processed and canned foods, such as luncheon meats, canned vegetables and soups, cheese, potato chips and other salty snacks, breads and other baked goods, breakfast cereals, and condiments (Table 4.6). (97) Because of the high intake of sodium relative to the body's need, the 24-h urine collection is 90–99% reflective of intake, except in individuals whose sweat losses are inordinately high. A high sodium chloride intake increases urinary calcium excretion by expansion of the renal extracellular volume and perhaps by increased calcium resorption from bone (98), reduces urinary citrate excretion, and promotes crystallization of urate-induced calcium oxalate stones. (99) Studies confirm an increase in daily urinary calcium of 40 mg and a decrease in urinary citrate of 50 mg with every 2300 mg increase in sodium intake.(99) Sodium enhances the urinary excretion of cystine and for this reason should be limited in cystine stone formers.(100) As

Table 4.6 Major selected food sources of sodium.[1]

Food	Amount/ preparation	Mg sodium
Miso	1 cup	2563
Salt, table	1 teaspoon	2325
Submarine sandwich with cold cuts	1 sandwich, 6" roll	1651
Sauerkraut, canned	1 cup, solids and liquids	1560
Potato salad, home-prepared	1 cup	1323
Bacon cheeseburger on bun	1 sandwich, with condiments	1314
Tomato sauce, canned	1 cup	1284
Baking soda	1 teaspoon	1259
Cured ham	3 ozs., roasted	1128
Baked beans, canned, with meat	1 cup	1106–1114
Macaroni and cheese, canned entrée	1 cup	1061
Cottage cheese, 1% and 2%	1 cup	918
Soy sauce	1 tablespoon	902
Tunafish salad	1 cup	824
Hamburger on bun	1 sandwich, with condiments	824
Salami, beef and pork	2 slices (57 ozs.), cooked	822
Pretzels, hard, salted	10 pretzels (60 ozs.)	814
Soups, canned	1 cup	600–1000
Frozen entrée, variable, major brands	1 meal	500–2500
Bread, pita, white	6-½" pita	322
Canned vegetables, with salt	1 cup	300–800
Hotdog/ frankfurter, made from various meats	1 frank (about 45 ozs.)	300–400
Buttermilk	8 fluid ounces	257
Bagel, English muffin	4" bagel or 1 muffin	215–400
Pizza, with cheese and various toppings, and with variable crust thickness	1 slice	200–1000
Breads (various), rolls, biscuits, muffin	1 slice or serving	200–400
Luncheon meats, various, packaged	1 oz.	200–400
Snacks, e.g., potato chips, salted nuts, Chex mix	1 oz.	200–300
Catsup	1 tablespoon.	167
Chocolate milk, reduced fat	8 fluid ozs.	165
Pickle relish	1 tablespoon	164
Cheese, various types	1 oz.	150–400
Salad dressings, various	1 tablespoon	100–250
Cereals, ready-to-consume	1 serving (generally ¾ to 1 cup)	0–350

1 Data compiled from the U.S. Department of Agriculture, Agricultural Research Service, 2007. USDA National Nutrient Database for Standard Reference, Release 20. Nutrient Data Laboratory Home Page, http://www.ars.usda.gov/ba/bhnrc/ndl, accessed 06/09/2008.

a subsection of stone formers are hypertensive, a reduction is sodium intake may reduce risk factors for both stone disease as well as cardiovascular disease. Also, as hypercalciuric stone formers are at increased risk for premature bone loss (101), a reduced sodium chloride intake may address this risk factor as well.

Phosphorus. Hyperphosphaturia as a risk factor among stone formers has not been adequately addressed. While excessive urinary phosphorus excretion obviously increases urine supersaturation for calcium phosphate (102, 103), other factors, such as alkaline urine and hypercalciuria, must also be present for the formation and growth of calcium phosphate stones. Phosphorus is ample in the typical American diet as it is provided in almost all foods of animal origin, including meat and dairy, and also legumes. Deficiency in the United States is uncommon (86), and most American adults easily achieve the RDA for phosphorus, which is 700 mg/day.(37) In theory, a phosphorus deficiency would cause a concomitant increase in GI calcium absorption, potentially leading to hypercalciuria. Thus, a phosphorus deficiency would be a promoter of calcium stone disease. On the other hand, excessive dietary phosphorus could lead to hyperphosphaturia and increased risk of calcium phosphate and possibly struvite stones, if other urinary conditions are favorable. If the source of urinary phosphate is from bone resorption in addition to intestinal absorption of dietary phosphorus, then measures

Table 4.7 Food sources of oxalate containing ≥30 mg oxalate per serving.[1,2]

Food Group	Food Item	Serving Size
Fruits	Raspberries	1 cup
Vegetables	Baked potato with skin	1 medium
	Bamboo shoots	1 cup
	Beets	½ cup
	French fries	4 ozs. (1/2 cup)
	Navy beans	½ cup
	Okra	½ cup
	Rhubarb	½ cup
	Rutabaga	½ cup, mashed
	Spinach, cooked	½ cup
	Spinach, raw	1 cup
	Turnip	½ cup, mashed
	Yams	½ cup, cubed
Grains	Brown rice flour	1 cup
	Buckwheat groats	1 cup, cooked
	Bulgur	1 cup, cooked
	Corn grits	1 cup
	Cornmeal	1 cup
	Millet	1 cup, cooked
	Rice bran	1 cup
	Soy flour	1 cup
	Wheat berries	1 cup, cooked
Nuts	Almonds	1 oz. (about 22)
	Cashews	1 oz. (about 18)
	Mixed nuts with peanuts	1 oz.
	Walnuts	1 cup
	Candies with nuts (e.g., Snickers)	1 bar
Soups, sauces	Chocolate syrup	2 Tbsp.
	Lentil	1 cup
	Miso	1 cup
Beverages	Hot cocoa	1 cup
Cereals, ready-to-consume	Bran Flakes	1 cup
	Bran Flakes with Raisins	1 cup
	Fruit & Fiber Dates, Raisins & Walnuts	1 cup
	Honey Nut Shredded Wheat Bite Size	1 cup
	Raisin Bran	1 cup
	Raisin Squares Mini Wheats	¾ cup
	Shredded Wheat	2 biscuits
	Shredded Wheat & Bran	1–1/4 cup
	Spoonsize Shredded Wheat	1 cup

1 Data compiled from the Harvard School of Public Health and the Brigham and Women's Hospital Nutrition Department's File Download Site, https://regepi.bwh.harvard.edu/health/nutrition.html, accessed 06/09/2008.

2 Oxalate bioavailability and urinary excretion is not accounted for in the foods listed in this table. Thus, food sources rich in oxalate but not necessarily associated with an increase in urinary oxalate excretion are noted.

to control bone resorption are usually necessary. These may include a reduction in the acid load of the diet and reduced sodium chloride intake.

Oxalate from foods. Consumption of oxalate-rich foods increases oxalate excretion in susceptible individuals, especially those with suboptimal calcium intake.(104) However, no studies to date have shown that a dietary oxalate restriction results in either reduced urinary risk factors for stones or reduced stone incidence. Although many plant foods contain oxalate (Table 4.7), acquired through the soil during growth and maturation, only a few foods are known to cause high urinary excretion. These include spinach, Swiss chard, okra, rhubarb, beet greens and roots, certain nuts and seeds, cocoa powder, black and green tea, concentrated wheat bran, and soy.(105–109) Spinach, in one study, accounted for >40% of total dietary oxalate intake.(110) It should be noted, however, that the oxalate content of foods varies with soil conditions, plant maturity, and other factors.(105) Cooking may or may not have much of an effect on the oxalate ingested from a food.(111) Moreover, data on the oxalate content of foods suffer from variability because of differences in analytical methods. Oxalate absorption from foods is highly variable and is influenced by the form of oxalate in the food (soluble or insoluble) and gut factors, which primarily include the amount of calcium and magnesium available to bind dietary oxalate and the presence or absence of oxalate-degrading bacteria in the gut. GI absorption of oxalate has been estimated to be highly variable, with ranges of 2–50% or higher reported, depending on calcium intake and other factors. (105, 106, 111, 112) Gut physiology plays a major role in oxalate absorption, as those with bowel disease or short bowel are prone to malabsorption of calcium, which results in hyperabsorption of oxalate.(40) For these reasons, the control of diet-derived urinary oxalate may remain elusive and may depend as much or more on modulation of other dietary factors and on individual patients' physiology.

Food-derived oxalate precursors. Oxalate biosynthesis from hydroxyproline, an amino acid found in meat and gelatin (82, 83), was discussed above. Other food-derived oxalate precursors may include carbohydrates, specifically, fructose, which may provide carbon skeletons for oxalate synthesis.(112) As ascorbic acid is metabolized to oxalic acid, resulting in an increased biosynthesis of oxalate, it has the potential to increase urinary oxalate excretion. Studies confirm that a high ascorbic acid load, such as is achieved with supplementation, not usually from the recommended intake of fruits and vegetables, is associated with increased urinary oxalate excretion.(113–115) It may be that when supplemental ascorbic acid is ingested in the usual dosages of 200 or more mg per tablet, tissue saturation quickly occurs, leading to substrate for oxalate biosynthesis. In contrast, an appropriate vitamin C intake from fruits and vegetables, consumed throughout the day, may be appropriately handled without overwhelming physiological mechanisms responsible for ascorbic acid metabolism.

Oxalate from dietary supplements. Cranberry juice has been recommended for the treatment of urinary tract infections but has been shown in several studies to increase urinary oxalate excretion.(13, 16, 116) Cranberry tablets were shown in one small study to increase the risk of kidney stone formation by delivering a high oxalate load, which could exceed 300 mg/day if taken per manufacturers' directions, and a subsequent increase in urinary oxalate excretion and calcium oxalate supersaturation.(117) Other concentrated plant extracts may confer similar risk. For example, bilberry extract is a species of the same genus as cranberry (118) and is used by up to 32% of patients with retinitis pigmentosa in one recent study.(119) As bilberry has also been recommended for the treatment of glaucoma and cataracts (120), its use by patients who may be stone formers or potential stone formers could be underestimated. Other plant-derived supplements that are available over-the-counter, such as sorrel, beet extract, and alfalfa, may also confer a high oxalate load that could contribute to excessive urinary oxalate excretion.(121)

PUTATIVE DIETARY EFFECTORS OF LITHOGENESIS: MORE DATA NEEDED

Probiotics. A probiotic is a viable microorganism that exerts a beneficial health effect when, in sufficient concentrations, it reaches the intestine in an active state. Some bacteria degrade oxalate in the GI tract, including *Oxalobacter formigenes* and *Bifidobacterium lactis*, both of which contain the oxalate-degrading enzyme oxalyl-CoA decarboxylase, and certain strains of lactic acid bacteria.(122, 123) Stone formers have been found in some studies to lack colonization with oxalate-degrading bacteria.(124) Fermented milk foods, such as yogurt and kefir, are rich in bacteria and may be helpful in maintaining optimal colonization of appropriate bacterial species in the gastrointestinal tract. Individuals needing supraphysiological dosages of "gut-friendly" bacteria may benefit from food sources of probiotics and over-the-counter supplements of certain bacterial strains. A commercial formulation of *Oxalobacter formigenes* is apparently in the works.(125) Questions about efficacy in stone formers with hyperoxaluria to be answered include determination of the optimal formulation(s) and bacterial species, dosage, length of supplementation, and timing of administration (i.e., with or without regard to meals).

Omega-3 fatty acids. No association between stone risk and total dietary omega-3 fatty acids was found in one large cohort study.(126) However, eicosapentaenoic acid (EPA), a polyunsaturated omega-3 fatty acid, has been associated with decreased stone risk (127–129), possibly by reducing urinary calcium excretion.(129) Fish oil containing marine-derived omega-3 fatty acids have been postulated to reduce inflammation, which may in turn reduce the presence of inflammatory proteins excreted in urine that could contribute to lithogenesis. (127) A study in rats showed reduced renal tubular damage and decreased markers of crystal deposition with administration of EPA.(130)

Vitamin E. Vitamin E is the most potent lipophilic antioxidant in biological membranes. The vitamin E family is comprised of four tocopherols and four tocotrienols: alpha-, beta-, gamma-, and delta-tocopherol and tocotrienol, respectively. Food sources provide all eight compounds of vitamin E; gamma-tocopherol is the most commonly occurring form in the diet whereas alpha-tocopherol is the source most available as an over-the-counter supplement. Gamma-tocopherol protects mostly against nitrogen-based free radicals. Nitrogen free radicals play an important role in diseases associated with chronic inflammation; the renal nitric oxide system has been associated with oxidative stress in a rat model of nephrolithiasis.(131) Vitamin E supplementation in stone formers may prevent oxidative damage to renal epithelial tissue and maximize the inhibitory potential of Tamm-Horsfall glycoprotein.(132, 133) The RDA for vitamin E is 15 mg/day for adult men and women.(37)

Vitamin D. Vitamin D is well known for its role in calcium metabolism. In recent years, vitamin D has also been associated with chemoprevention and prevention of autoimmune diseases. Vitamin D insufficiency has been widely documented.(134, 135) The number of individuals supplementing with vitamin D or undergoing pharmacologic repletion for vitamin D insufficiency is reportedly rising. The AI for vitamin D is suggested by many in both the scientific and medical communities to be too low.(135, 136) It has been suggested that vitamin D metabolism is altered in patients with hypercalciuria (137) and, although conclusive evidence is lacking, that vitamin D supplementation would therefore increase the risk for calcium stone formation in susceptible individuals. An observational study in women showed no increased risk for urinary stones with vitamin D intake.(1) Studies testing for an association in humans between hypercalciuria and vitamin D receptor gene polymorphisms have been inconclusive. (137) Repletion with vitamin D of vitamin D insufficiency in nonstone-forming postmenopausal women did not increase urinary calcium excretion.(138) The role of vitamin D in urolithiasis is unclear. Studies showing the effects on stone risk of vitamin D supplementation in both vitamin D-insufficient and sufficient stone formers are needed. Could it not be possible that vitamin D insufficiency, resulting in parathyroid hormone disregulation, is an unrecognized yet significant contributor to hypercalciuria? The AI for vitamin D is 5 mcg/day for adults 50 years of age and younger, 10 mcg/day for adults 51–70 years, and 15 mcg/day for adults more than 70 years of age.(37)

Herbal supplements. Dietary supplements and various phytotherapeutic concentrates and extracts have historically been alleged to provide lithogenic inhibition. These include various combinations of Chinese herbs (139), *Phyllanthus niruri* (140, 141), *Vediuppu chunnam*, and *Aerva lanata* leaf extract (142), among others. However, appropriately controlled clinical studies in humans that document the mechanisms, efficacy, and side-effects of herbal and other plant-derived formulations after long-term use by stone formers are lacking. The historical use of herbs and other phytochemical agents for preventing lithogenesis has been recently reviewed.(143, 144)

Weight loss. Overweight and obesity are independent risk factors for kidney stone formation and incidence.(64–67) Weight loss to prevent renal disease, including nephrolithiasis, has been recommended.(145) However, prospective studies that confirm a reduced risk or incidence of kidney stones following weight loss are lacking. Does weight loss reverse stone risk and correct risk factors? The answer may vary, depending on the method(s) utilized to achieve weight loss. Modern bariatric surgery, for example, is associated with increased stone risk factors (146–150), as are certain high-protein, low-carbohydrate weight loss diets (e.g., the "Atkins Diet").(151)

APPLICATION OF MEDICAL NUTRITION THERAPY (MNT) TO PATIENTS

Making MNT recommendations to patients with urolithiasis

The efficacy of diet instructions provided to patients by Registered Dietitians for various diseases and conditions is proven.(152–155) Greater adherence by patients to specific lifestyle changes, including diet, is correlated with greater improvements in health that are cost-effective.(156–158) Specific nutrition therapy, adjusted according to a metabolic evaluation, is more effective than nonspecific general nutrition recommendations in secondary stone prevention.(159) Nutrition education should first focus on correcting any myths or misinformation patients have. For example, many calcium stone formers are under the impression that they must avoid dairy and other foods rich in calcium. As this practice could potentially enhance oxalate absorption, depending on the individual's total calcium intake and other dietary factors, this and similar false ideas should be identified and corrected. Second, the nutrition assessment and diagnosis is made. MNT is tailored to the patient based on his/her stone history and composition, urinary risk factors, anthropometric risk factors (e.g., high BMI, excessive body weight), the presence of contributing comorbidities (e.g., bowel disease, gout, metabolic syndrome, premature bone loss), and use of medications with nutrition-related or other interactions that may promote lithogenesis. Table 4.8 provides a brief synopsis of MNT for the various urinary risk factors of stone formers. Third, practical strategies for achieving goals are provided and integrated, when possible, into the patient's usual regimen. Fourth, as monitoring and evaluation is an integral part of the nutrition care process, each patient's learning and understanding of the information provided is measured and assessed during the initial visit and in follow-up consultations. Finally, the intervention and follow-up is documented in the patient's chart and/or otherwise directed to the referring physician.

Although clearly more research is needed on the dietary patterns that promote and inhibit lithogenesis, with therapeutic recommendations derived from appropriately designed experiments that are clinically applied and evaluated, certain dietary patterns and features are suggested from existing studies. Based on the evidence reviewed earlier, there is general support for MNT that addresses the following key concepts:

1   URINE DILUTION – Ample fluids, distributed throughout the day and at bedtime to promote nocturia, are recommended to produce more than 2 L of urine per day.(10–12, 160) While almost all fluids appear protective, low-calorie, nonsweetened beverages should provide the majority of fluid intake.

2   LOW SODIUM CHLORIDE INTAKE – Salt in the form of sodium chloride, which mainly arrives in the diet in processed and preserved foods and not from customary use of the salt shaker, should be limited to ≤10 grams/day, equating to approximately 4,000 mg (174 mEq) sodium. A more vigorous salt restriction can and should be attempted in all patients and may be especially useful for hypercalciuric stone formers, those on thiazide therapy, for cystinuric stone formers, and for anyone in whom excessive bone resorption is suspected, as sodium chloride is implicated in promoting bone loss.(161) A lower sodium chloride intake (approximately 2.6 grams, equivalent to 1,150 mg or 50 mEq sodium) was tested by Borghi et al. in conjunction with other dietary measures. (162) However, 24-h urinary sodium excretion for the low-salt diet, which was protective against calcium oxalate stone formation, averaged 124 mEq over 5 years of follow-up, suggesting that the actual intake of subjects in this group was closer to 2,700 mg of sodium (approximately 6 grams sodium chloride)/day, assuming that the 24-h urinary sodium excretion is 95% reflective of dietary sodium intake. Because such a small percentage of dietary sodium comes from that which is added to foods at the table and during cooking, a detailed diet history should be obtained from each patient and specific salt-reducing strategies developed for each.

3   NORMAL CALCIUM INTAKE, DISTRIBUTED AT MEALS – Calcium intakes per the AI for age and gender should be recommended with the caveat that the calcium be distributed with meals and snacks in order to maximize GI binding of oxalate. This may be generally accomplished by recommending a cup of yogurt or calcium-fortified fruit juice (providing 200–400 mg calcium) with breakfast, and an 8 oz. glass of milk or other calcium-fortified beverage (providing 300 mg calcium) with both lunch and supper. More calcium, a total of 500–600 mg per meal or more, may be required in those with malabsorptive disorders, altered bowel tissue, and when a meal is particularly high in oxalate. Total calcium intake is calculated by the sum of typical daily food sources plus any obtained from dietary supplements.

4   BALANCED FOR PROTEIN – An intake of meat, fish, seafood, and poultry ("flesh foods") that does not exceed 4–6 ozs per day, depending on individual body size, caloric need, and severity of risk factors, is recommended for most individuals. Protein from vegetables need

Table 4.8 Guide to applying Medical Nutrition Therapy to individual stone risk factors.

Stone composition	General concepts
Calcium oxalate	Dilute urine, reduce foods that enhance urinary calcium, obtain adequate calcium to reduce oxalate absorption and maintain calcium balance, enhance intake of foods with inhibitory potential, lose weight if needed, address single risk factors (below)
Calcium phosphate	Dilute urine, reduce foods that enhance urinary calcium, adequate calcium to maintain calcium balance, enhance intake of foods with inhibitory potential, lose weight if needed, address other risk factors as indicated (below)
Uric acid	Dilute urine, reduce dietary uric acid precursors, enhance alkaline load of diet and intake of other foods with inhibitory potential, lose weight if needed, address other risk factors as indicated (below)
Struvite	Dilute urine, may attempt urine acidification with cranberry juice if no history of hyperoxaluria
Cystine	Dilute urine, reduce sodium intake to reduce urinary cystine, may attempt limiting methionine-rich foods in adult patients

Urinary risk factor	Specific recommendations	Example(s) / Special considerations and strategies
Low urine volume - Esp. if high supersaturation	**Increase fluid intake:** Distributed throughout the day, including at bedtime **Include diversity of beverages:** Non-sweetened, low caloric beverages are ideal; most all beverages are protective **Target a goal urine output of >2 L/day**; ≥3 L/day may be optimal	**Distribute fluid intake:** Suggest dividing the day into 3 sub-sections, within which ≥40 ozs. of fluids should be consumed in each **Hot weather, exercise:** Increase fluids to compensate for dermal fluid losses **People in certain professions:** Elementary school teachers and truck drivers are examples of people who may limit fluid intake; strategies to compensate during off-work hours should be provided. Those working in hot environments (e.g., dry cleaners, factories) need more fluids.
Hypercalciuria	**Reduce dietary acid load** **Reduce sodium chloride intake** **Reduce refined carbohydrates** **Reduce caffeine** if excessive **Increase dietary fiber:** May promote GI binding and regulate calcium absorption **Address bone resorption:** If hypercalciuria is from bone, appropriate follow-up and treatment is needed **Adequate calcium intake:** Ensure that dietary + supplemental calcium do not exceed the individual's requirement and that both are taken with foods **Address drug-nutrient interactions:** If a diuretic is prescribed, counsel about drug-nutrient interactions and provide compensatory dietary strategies	**Fruits and vegetables:** Provide dietary fiber, phytate, K^+, and bicarbonate precursors, all of which may reduce calcium excretion. "5-a-day" or more is the goal. **Sodium chloride:** Address hidden sources of sodium chloride, including cheese, processed foods, canned soups & vegetables, convenience foods, luncheon meats, condiments and salad dressings, crackers and other baked goods, bread **Potassium-wasting diuretics:** Certain loop diuretics reduce address hypercalciuria but may cause decreased K^+ excretion, potentially leading to hypocitraturia. Encourage K^+-rich fruits/vegetables daily.
Hyperoxaluria	**Increase calcium intake with meals and snacks:** Focus on calcium-containing foods. Add supplements if needed, titrated against usual dietary intake to meet individual requirements. **Reduce dietary oxalate intake** **Reduce intake of oxalate precursors**	**Fat malabsorption disorders:** In patients with disorders causing malabsorption (e.g., Crohn disease, Celiac disease, cystic fibrosis, inflammatory bowel disease, short bowel), calcium needs are higher than for otherwise healthy adults

(Continued)

Table 4.8   (Continued)

Urinary risk factor	Specific recommendations	Example(s) / Special considerations and strategies
		Dietary oxalate: Focus on major contributors and not a "laundry list" of foods purported to contain oxalate. Suggest simultaneous intake of calcium-containing foods and/or supplement whenever eating high-oxalate foods.
		Oxalate precursors: Limit supplemental ascorbic acid, dietary fructose, gelatin
Hyperuricosuria	**Reduce dietary acid load** to reduce uric acid precipitation	**Fruits and vegetables:** The only food groups providing a dietary alkaline load, ≥5/day is usually required to offset acidic load of typical Western diet
	Reduce meat/fish/poultry intake to reduce uric acid biosynthesis	
	Reduce intake of uric acid precursors: These include alcohol, fructose	**Reducing meat/fish/poultry:** Usually, a combination of reduced portion sizes and reduced frequency of intake throughout the week (e.g., 9 times/wk vs. 14 times/wk) is acceptable. Depending on body size and gender, no more than 4–6 ozs. meat, fish, or poultry/day is recommended.
Hypernatriuria - Esp. if hypercalciuria - Esp. in cystine stone formers	**Reduce Na intake** to <200 mEq (4600 mg)/day – the equivalent of about 2 teaspoons table salt – with eventual goal of a further reduction, to the Adequate Intake (AI) range of 1200-1500 mg/day	**Added salt:** Sodium chloride added to foods at the table and during cooking usually only account for 10–15% of total sodium intake. Limiting the addition of salt is a small but important means to reduce intake.
		Processed foods: Most sodium comes from packaged, convenience, and processed foods. Advise eating fresh and less-processed foods as possible.
		Eating out: Most restaurants, including but not limited to "fast food" restaurants, use more sodium than foods prepared at home. Also, portion sizes of foods ordered out are usually larger, providing more salt. Advise reducing frequency of eating out or taking out foods.
		High salt foods: A few foods are notoriously rich in sodium chloride and should be limited. These include salted meats (sausage, bacon, ham, etc.), most cheese and cottage cheese, salty snacks (pretzels, chips, crackers, etc.), certain condiments (soy sauce, some salad dressings, etc.), and luncheon meats that are not sliced fresh from the carcass.
Hyperphosphaturia - Esp. if CaPhos stone former	**Reduce intake** to ≤700 mg/day, consistent with the RDA for adult men and women	**Reducing phosphorus:** As it is widely distributed in foods, especially protein foods, a combination of reduced portion sizes of meat, fish, poultry, dairy (if excessive), and beans is recommended. May also recommend reduced frequency of intake throughout the week.
Hypocitraturia	**Reduce acid load of diet** to enhance urinary citrate excretion	**Fruits and vegetables:** The only food groups providing a dietary alkaline load, ≥5/day is usually required to offset acidic load of typical Western diet
	Increase intake of fruits and vegetables rich in K⁺ and organic acids, which are bicarbonate precursors	**Distribute intake throughout the day:** Suggest eating at least one fruit or vegetable with each meal plus as between-meal snacks

(Continued)

Table 4.8 (Continued)

Urinary risk factor	Specific recommendations	Example(s) / Special considerations and strategies
		Double up on portions: Suggest doubling up on vegetable portions, especially non-starchy vegetables to maintain appropriate kcal intake, if frequency of intake throughout the day is a problem
		Suggest using 4 ozs. lemon or lime juice daily, distributed in water or other beverages: Some studies show a modest increase in urinary citrate with use of concentrated forms of these fruit juices
Hypomagnesiuria	**Reduce dietary acid load** to increase urine pH	**Increase intake of magnesium-rich foods:** Generally, these are whole grains, beans, seeds, nuts, and leafy greens; refer to Table 4.4
	Address Mg malabsorption from chronic diarrhea, vomiting, and other medical problems	
Acid urine	**Reduce dietary acid load** to increase urine pH	**Fruits and vegetables:** The only food groups providing a dietary alkaline load, ≥5/day is usually required to offset acidic load of typical Western diet
	Address bicarbonaturia from diarrhea, vomiting, wasting, and other medical problems	**Other high acid foods:** Cheese and eggs are also high acid foods and should be limited. Grains are slightly acidic; dairy is nearly neutral; dietary fat is neutral
	Address need for weight loss, if overweight	

not be restricted. Most studies (73, 76, 79, 162), but not all (163), are clear about the utility of a dietary protein content that is neither deficient nor excessive. A diversity of protein sources should be encouraged, including those from vegetables, dairy, and nondairy animal/fowl/marine sources.

5   STONE INHIBITORS – Ample fruits and vegetables, meeting or exceeding 5 servings (about 3 cups) or more per day, depending on individual caloric need, are recommended.(60, 79, 164) Fruits and vegetables provide a dietary alkaline load, potassium, magnesium, fiber, phytate, citric acid, and antioxidants, all of which inhibit stone formation by various mechanisms.

6   WEIGHT NEUTRAL DIET – As body weight and other parameters associated with body habitus appear to have a profound influence on kidney stone risk (64–71), diets that promote weight loss or weight maintenance are highly recommended. If necessary, overweight patients should receive appropriate referrals to a Registered Dietitian or other specialized professional for weight loss counseling and support. Community weight loss programs may also be suggested. A sensible weight loss or weight maintenance diet is generally balanced for macronutrients, low in saturated fat as compared with mono- and polyunsaturated fats, adequate for micronutrients, rich in plant foods and fiber, and low in refined carbohydrates and fructose.

7   SUPPLEMENTS – The use of all dietary supplements by patients should be queried and documented. Supraphysiological dosages of any micronutrient should be endorsed cautiously and individually, if at all. Supplemental ascorbic acid, i.e., beyond that which is obtained in a diet rich in fruits and vegetables, for example, should be avoided by calcium oxalate stone formers. Herbal and other plant-derived concentrates may confer an appreciable oxalate load and should be limited until their influence on urinary oxalate excretion is known. Calcium supplements, if they are not timed with meals and snacks, provide little GI oxalate–binding capacity.

8   INDIVIDUALIZATION AND ADJUSTMENT OF MNT – As with pharmacologic and other therapies, the effects of MNT and any barriers to compliance with recommendations should be evaluated and adjusted as needed, during follow-up and according to patients' individual risk factors and disease progression.

Obstacles to applying MNT

The "one diet for all" approach. There is no one stone diet to fit all stone formers. Patients with hypertension are not told that they all need the same antihypertensive medication. Rather, various medications at varying dosages are attempted with appropriate clinical and biochemical monitoring with adjustments made as needed. In the same way, no "one size fits all" approach should be taken with stone formers as even multiple patients who form the same type of stones have variable risk factors. Yet, patients are often told to go on "the stone diet." While occasionally this advice may be followed with the recommendation to see a dietitian, often times, little or no explanation of why and how dietary changes will affect stone risk is provided. Written handouts may be handed to the patient, but without adequate explanation and individualization, they fail to target the patient's individual risk factors and leave the impression that the patient must comply with all of the recommendations, which may include unnecessary avoidance of foods from many food groups. "What's left for me to eat?" patients often ask. Targeted MNT should be offered to all willing patients with recurrent stones. General guidelines are useful; however, MNT is most useful when targeted to the individual patient's risk factors.(159) Table 4.8 provides a list of lithogenic risk factors and specific nutrition recommendations.

The "low oxalate diet." Only a minority of calcium oxalate stone formers have hyperoxaluria, and no randomized-controlled studies to date have shown that a restriction of foods high in oxalate results in reduced stone risk factors or reduced stone formation. Thus, the traditional "low oxalate diet," advised to all calcium oxalate stone-forming patients with or without hyperoxaluria, and without also emphasizing the importance of adequate calcium intakes for optimum GI binding of oxalate, has questionable clinical value. Indeed, only a few foods among the many that contain oxalate have been associated with an increase in urinary oxalate excretion. These are: spinach, nuts, tea, chocolate, beets, rhubarb, strawberries, and wheat bran.(108) Of these, the most clinically relevant foods to limit are those that patients eat on a regular basis. Calcium oxalate stone-forming patients are frequently told to avoid "all green leafy vegetables" and other foods analyzed by various laboratory methods that were found to be high in oxalate. If their intake of vegetables and other high-oxalate foods is already low, this advice is meaningless to patients. Lists of foods reportedly high in oxalate abound on the Internet and from other sources and frequently include foods that are not actually high in oxalate (e.g., cola beverages) or foods that are high in oxalate on a gram for gram basis but not in terms of what is commonly consumed (e.g., black pepper). As patients are told to increase their fruit and vegetable intake, they may be understandably confused by what they perceive as conflicting and unnecessarily restrictive dietary advice. Although it makes sense to limit the intake of the few notoriously high-oxalate foods, achieving an adequate calcium intake that is distributed at all meals is paramount in reducing urinary oxalate excretion. The role of dietary oxalate precursors, e.g., fructose (112) and hydroxyproline (82, 83), needs further elucidation. In the meantime, excessive fructose intake could lead to weight gain and obesity in susceptible individuals so should be limited.

Diet vs. medication. Patients are frequently told that they can try dietary changes instead of or prior to initiating pharmacologic therapy but that diet alone "doesn't usually work." It appears to be a common belief among health-care practitioners that "patients don't comply with dietary recommendations," yet there are few data to either support or reject this notion. For many people, nutrition therapy does work, but the efficacy of nutrition recommendations may wane as the disease progresses and/or as lithogenic risk factors change without concomitant modifications to the therapeutic regimen or if the therapy is not given in an understandable way. Moreover, patients whose health-care providers deliver dietary recommendations in a disdainful way may lack the conviction that it is an effective strategy to be attempted in earnest. Usually, neither diet nor medication is a successful therapy in isolation. In most cases, both strategies may and should be employed. For example, the efficacy of hydrochlorothiazide and other diuretics may only be optimized when the patient also maintains a low sodium chloride intake and an ample potassium intake to offset the hypokalemic potential of the diuretic.

QUESTIONS AND FUTURE IMPLICATIONS FOR MNT FOR UROLITHIASIS

If a balance between nutrient needs and control of urinary stone risk factors cannot be achieved, then concurrent medication therapy is needed to assist in reducing risk factors and improving overall health outcomes. MNT, as with pharmacologic therapy or physical therapy, is a self-management therapy. Education, support, and follow-up are required to assist the patient to make lifestyle changes essential to successful nutrition therapy. Diets for other conditions (e.g., low saturated fat, low salt, high polyunsaturated fats for metabolic syndrome; DASH diet for hypertension) may be useful. The Mediterranean diet, a balanced diet rich in polyunsaturated and monounsaturated fats as well as fiber, fruits, and vegetables, may be useful. The Weight Watchers diet and similar group education and support programs may be useful for weight loss and maintenance. These dietary patterns have the advantage of having been studied in multiple cohorts, and their influence on risk factors for other diseases, many of which are shared by stone formers, is known. Additionally, data have been acquired with respect to patient education on and adherence to these diets, something which is relatively understudied in stone disease. The following are some questions that should be considered in further evaluating the role and efficacy of nutrition therapy to prevent urolithiasis:

- What is the role of gender, age, and body size on specific dietary effectors of stone disease?
- Do patients comply with, adhere to, and understand nutrition recommendations to prevent kidney stones?
- What are patients' obstacles and barriers to compliance; and how may these be overcome?
- What is the average length of time for MNT to take effect? What is its durability?
- Do patients who are medically managed, especially with nutrition therapy, have a higher health-related quality of life?
- Are there specific nutrients or dietary factors that can prevent or promote renal epithelial injury and/or crystal retention?
- Is expression of urinary macromolecules influenced by dietary factors?

REFERENCES

1. Taylor EN, Stampfer MJ, Curhan GC. Dietary factors and the risk of incident kidney stones in men: new insights after 14 years of follow-up. J Am Soc Nephrol 2004; 15: 3225–32.
2. Taylor EN, Curhan GC. Diet and fluid prescription in stone disease. Kidney Int 2006; 70: 835–9.
3. Siener R. Impact of dietary habits on stone incidence. Urol Res 2006; 34: 131–3.
4. Siener R, Hesse A. Recent advances in nutritional research on urolithiasis. World J Urol 2005; 23: 304–8.
5. Smith RE, Patrick S, Michael P, Hager M. Medical nutrition therapy: the core of ADA's advocacy efforts (part 1). J Am Diet Assoc 2005; 105: 825–34.
6. Hess B, Mauron H, Ackermann D, Jaeger P. Effects of a 'common sense diet' on urinary composition and supersaturation in patients with idiopathic calcium urolithiasis. Eur Urol 1999; 36: 136–43.
7. Siener R, Glatz S, Nicolay C, Hesse A. Prospective study on the efficacy of a selective treatment and risk factors for relapse in recurrent calcium oxalate stone patients. Eur Urol 2003; 44: 467–74.
8. Siener R, Schade N, Nicolay C, von Unruh GE, Hesse A. The efficacy of dietary intervention on urinary risk factors for stone formation in recurrent calcium oxalate stone patients. J Urol 2005; 173: 1601–5.
9. Parks JH, Asplin JR, Coe FL. Patient adherence to long-term medical treatment of kidney stones. J Urol 2001; 166: 2057–60.
10. Pak CYC, Sakhaee K, Crowther C, Brinkley L. Evidence justifying a high fluid intake in treatment of nephrolithiasis. Ann Intern Med 1980; 93: 36–9.
11. Curhan GC, Willett WC, Rimm EB, Spiegelman D, Stampfer MJ. Prospective study of beverage use and the risk of kidney stones. Am J Epidemiol 1996; 143: 240–7.
12. Curhan GC, Willett WC, Speizer FE, Stampfer MJ. Beverage use and risk for kidney stones in women. Ann Intern Med 1998; 126: 534–40.
13. Gettman MT, Ogan K, Brinkley LJ et al. Effect of cranberry juice consumption on urinary stone risk factors. J Urol 2005; 174: 590–4.
14. Goldfarb DS, Asplin JR. Effect of grapefruit juice on urinary lithogenicity. J Urol 2001; 166: 263–7.
15. Hönow R, Laube N, Schneider A, Kessler T, Hesse A. Influence of grapefruit-, orange- and apple-juice consumption on urinary variables and risk of crystallization. Br J Nutr 2003; 90: 295–300.
16. Kessler T, Jansen B, Hesse A. Effect of blackcurrant-, cranberry- and plum juice consumption on risk factors associated with kidney stone formation. Eur J Clin Nutr 2002; 56: 1020–3.
17. Wabner CL, Pak CY. Effect of orange juice consumption on urinary stone risk factors. J Urol 1993; 149: 1405–8.
18. Choi JW, Ford ES, Gao X, Choi HK. Sugar-sweetened soft drinks, diet soft drinks, and serum uric acid level: the third national health and nutrition examination survey. Arthritis Rheum 2008; 59: 109–16.

19. Choi HK, Curhan G. Soft drinks, fructose consumption, and the risk of gout in men: prospective cohort study. BMJ 2008; 336: 309–12.

20. Gao X, Qi L, Qiao N et al. Intake of added sugar and sugar-sweetened drinks and serum uric acid concentration in U.S. men and women. Hypertension 2007; 50: 306–12.

21. Taylor EN, Curhan GC. Fructose consumption and the risk of kidney stones. Kidney Int 2008; 73: 207–12.

22. Shuster J, Finlayson B, Scheaffer RL et al. Primary liquid intake and urinary stone disease. J Chronic Dis 1985; 38: 907–14.

23. Heaney RP. Effects of caffeine on bone and the calcium economy. Food Chem Toxicol 2002; 40: 1263–70.

24. Massey LK, Sutton RAL. Acute caffeine effects on urine composition and calcium kidney stone risk in calcium stone formers. J Urol 2004; 172: 555–8.

25. Choi HK, Curhan G. Beer, liquor, and wine consumption and serum uric acid level: the third national health and nutrition examination survey. Arthritis Rheum 2004; 51: 1023–9.

26. Zechner O, Pfluger H, Scheiber V. Idiopathic uric acid lithiasis: epidemiologic and metabolic aspects. J Urol 1982; 128: 1219–23.

27. Penniston KL, Steele TH, Nakada SY. Lemonade therapy increases urinary citrate and urine volumes in patients with recurrent calcium oxalate stone formation. Urology 2007; 70: 856–60.

28. Seltzer MA, Low RD, McDonald M, Shami GS, Stoller ML. Dietary manipulation with lemonade to treat hypocitraturic calcium nephrolithiasis. J Urol 1996; 156: 907–9.

29. Kang DE, Sur RL, Haleblian GE et al. Long-term lemonade based dietary manipulation in patients with hypocitraturic nephrolithiasis. J Urol 2007; 144: 1358–62.

30. Koff SG, Paquette EL, Cullen J et al. Comparison between lemonade and potassium citrate and impact on urine pH and 24-hour urine parameters in patients with kidney stone formation. Urology 2007; 69: 1013–6.

31. Odvina CV. Comparative value of orange juice vs. lemonade in reducing stone-forming risk. Clin J Am Soc Nephrol 2006; 1: 1269–74.

32. Grossmann W. The current urinary stone wave in center Europe. Br J Urol 1938; 10: 46–54.

33. Zarembski PM, Hodgkinson A. Some factors influencing the urinary excretion of oxalic acid in man. Clin Chim Acta 1969; 25: 1–10.

34. Curhan GC, Willett WC, Rimm EB et al. A prospective study of dietary calcium and other nutrients and the risk of symptomatic kidney stones. N Engl J Med 1993; 328: 833–8.

35. Curhan GC, Willett WC, Speizer FE, Spiegelman D, Stampfer MJ. Comparison of dietary calcium with supplemental calcium and other nutrients as factors affecting the risk for kidney stones in women. Ann Intern Med 1997; 126: 497–504.

36. von Unruh GE, Voss S, Sauerbruch T, Hesse A. Dependence of oxalate absorption on the daily calcium intake. J Am Soc Nephrol 2004; 15: 1567–73.

37. Food and Nutrition Board, Institute of Medicine. Dietary reference intakes: applications in dietary assessment. Washington, DC: National Academies Press; 2000. Available at http://www.iom.edu/CMS/3788/4574.aspx, accessed 05/05/2008.

38. Heilberg IP. Update on dietary recommendations. Nephrol Dial Transplant 2000; 15: 117–23.

39. McCarron DA, Heaney RP. Estimated healthcare savings associated with adequate dairy food intake. Am J Hypertens 2004; 17: 88–97.

40. Worcester EM. Stones from bowel disease. Endocrinol Metal Clin North Am 2002; 31: 979–99.

41. Barilla DE, Notz C, Kennedy D, Pak CY. Renal oxalate excretion following oral oxalate loads in patients with ileal disease and with renal and absorptive hypercalciurias. Am J Med 1978; l64: 579–585.

42. Stauffer JQ. Hyperoxaluria and intestinal disease: the role of steatorrhea and dietary calcium in regulating intestinal oxalate absorption. Digest Dis 1977; 22: 921–8.

43. Pak CYC. Physiological basis for absorptive and renal hypercalciurias. Am J Physiol 1979; 237: F415–F423.

44. Stitchantrakul W, Sopassathit W, Prapaipanich S, Domrongkitchaiporn S. Effects of calcium supplements on the risk of renal stone formation in a population with low oxalate intake. Southeast Asian J Trop Med Public Health 2004; 35: 1028–33.

45. Domrongkitchaiporn S, Sopassathit W, Stitchantrakul W et al. Schedule of taking calcium supplement and the risk of nephrolithiasis. Kidney Int 2004; 65: 1835–41.

46. Sakhaee K, Poindexter JR, Griffith CS, Pak CY. Stone forming risk of calcium citrate supplementation in healthy postmenopausal women. J Urol 2004; 172: 958–61.

47. Pierratos A, Dharamsi N, Carr LK et al. Higher urinary potassium is associated with reduced stone growth after shock wave lithotripsy. J Urol 2000; 164: 1486–9.

48. Volpe SL. Serving on the Institute of Medicine's dietary reference intake panel for electrolytes and water. J Am Diet Assoc 2004; 104: 1885–7.

49. artini LA, Cuppari L, Cunha MA, Schor N, Heilberg IP. Potassium and sodium intake and excretion in calcium stone forming patients. J Ren Nutr 1998; 8: 127–31.

50. Ford ES, Mokdad AH. Dietary magnesium intake in a national sample of U.S. adults. J Nutr 2003; 133: 2879–82.
51. Cochat P, Liutkus A, Fargue S et al. Primary hyperoxaluria type 1: still challenging! Pediatr Nephrol 2006; 21: 1075–81.
52. Turnlund JR, Betschart AA, Liebman M, Kretsch MJ, Sauberlich HE. Vitamin B-6 depletion followed by repletion with animal- or plant-source diets and calcium and magnesium metabolism in young women. Am J Clin Nutr 1992; 56: 905–10.
53. Curhan GC, Willett WC, Rimm EB, Stampfer MJ. A prospective study of the intake of vitamins C and B6, and the risk of kidney stones in men. J Urol 1996; 155: 1847–51.
54. Curhan GC, Willett WC, Speizer FE, Stampfer MJ. Intake of vitamins B6 and C and the risk of kidney stones in women. J Am Soc Nephrol 1999; 10: 840–5.
55. Silva CD, D'Cruz DP. Pyridoxine toxicity courtesy of your local health food store. Ann Rheum Dis 2006; 65: 1666–7.
56. Greiner R, Konietzny U, Jany KD. Phytate - an undesirable constituent of plant-based foods? J für Ernährungsmed 2006; 8: 18–28.
57. Grases F, Isern B, Sanchis P et al. Phytate acts as an inhibitor in formation of renal calculi. Front Biosci 2007; 12: 2580–7.
58. Grases F, March JG, Prieto RM et al. Urinary phytate in calcium oxalate stone formers and healthy people – dietary effects on phytate excretion. Scand J Urol Nephrol 2000; 34: 162–4.
59. Curhan GC, Willett WC, Knight EL, Stampfer MJ. Dietary factors and the risk of incident kidney stones in younger women: nurses' health study II. Arch Intern Med 2004; 164: 885–91.
60. Meschi T, Maggiore U, Fiaccadori E et al. The effect of fruits and vegetables on urinary stone risk factors. Kidney Int 2004; 66: 2402–10.
61. Jahnen A, Heynck H, Gertz B, Glassen A, Hesse A. Dietary fiber: the effectiveness of a high bran intake in reducing renal calcium excretion. Urol Res 1992; 20: 3–8.
62. Al Zahrani H, Norman RW, Thompson C, Weerasinghe S. The dietary habits of idiopathic calcium stone-formers and normal control subjects. BJU Int 2000; 85: 616–20.
63. Hirvonen T, Pietinen P, Virtanen M, Albanes D, Virtamo J. Nutrient intake and use of beverages and the risk of kidney stones among male smokers. Am J Epidemiol 1999; 150: 187–94.
64. Curhan GC, Willett WC, Rimm EB, Speizer FE, Stampfer MJ. Body size and risk of kidney stones. J Am Soc Nephrol 1998; 9: 1645–52.
65. Taylor EN, Stampfer MJ, Curhan GC. Obesity, weight gain, and the risk of kidney stones. JAMA 2005; 293: 455–62.
66. Taylor EN, Curhan GC. Body size and 24-hour urine composition. Am J Kidney Dis 2006; 48: 905–15.
67. Siener R, Glatz S, Nicolay C, Hesse A. The role of overweight and obesity in calcium oxalate stone formation. Obes Res 2004; 12: 106–13.
68. Ekeruo WO, Tan YH, Young MD et al. Metabolic risk factors and the impact of medical therapy on the management of nephrolithiasis in obese patients. J Urol 2004; 172: 159–63.
69. Lemann J Jr, Pleuss JA, Worcester EM et al. Urinary oxalate excretion increases with body size and decreases with increasing dietary calcium intake among healthy adults. Kidney Int 1996; 49: 200–8.
70. Powell CR, Stoller ML, Schwartz BF et al. Impact of body weight on urinary electrolytes in urinary stone formers. Urology 2000; 55: 825–30.
71. Maalouf NM, Sakhaee K, Parks JH et al. Association of urinary pH with body weight in nephrolithiasis. Kidney Int 2004; 65: 1422–5.
72. Caudarella R, Vescini F, Buffa A, Stefoni S. Citrate and mineral metabolism: kidney stones and bone disease. Front Biosci 2003; 8: s1084–106.
73. Breslau NA, Brinkley L, Hill KD, Pak CY. Relationship of animal protein-rich diet to kidney stone formation and calcium metabolism. J Clin Endocrinol Metab 1988; 66: 140–6.
74. Coe FL, Moran E, Kavalich AG. The contribution of dietary purine over-consumption to hyperuricosuria in calcium oxalate stone formers. J Chron Dis 1976; 29: 793–800.
75. Robertson WG, Heyburn PJ, Peacock M, Hanes FA, Swaminathan R. The effect of high animal protein intake on the risk of calcium stone-formation in the urinary tract. Clin Sci 1979; 57: 285–8.
76. Giannini S, Nobile M, Sartori L et al. Acute effects of moderate protein restriction in patients with idiopathic hypercalciuria and calcium nephrolithiasis. Am J Clin Nutr 1999; 69: 267–71.
77. Barzel US, Massey LK. Excess dietary protein can adversely affect bone. J Nutr 1998; 128: 1051–3.
78. Remer T, Manz F. Potential renal acid load of foods and its influence on urine pH. J Am Diet Assoc 1995; 95: 791–7.
79. Siener R, Hesse A. The effect of a vegetarian and different omnivorous diets on urinary risk factors for uric acid stone formation. Eur J Nutr 2003; 42: 332–7.
80. Choi HK, Liu SM, Curhan GC. Intake of purine-rich foods, protein, and dairy products and relationship to serum levels of uric acid: the third national health and nutrition examination survey. Arthritis Rheum 2005; 52: 283–9.

81. Choi HK, Atkinson K, Karlson EW, Willett W, Curhan G. Purine-rich foods, dairy and protein intake, and the risk of gout in men. N Engl J Med 2004; 350: 1093–103.
82. Nguyen QV, Kalin A, Drouve U, Casez JP, Jaeger P. Sensitivity to meat protein intake and hyperoxaluria in idiopathic calcium stone formers. Kidney Int 2001; 59: 2272–81.
83. Knight J, Jiang J, Assimos DG, Holmes RP. Hydroxyproline ingestion and urinary oxalate and glycolate excretion. Kidney Int 2006; 70: 1929–34.
84. Naya Y, Ito H, Masai M, Yamaguchi K. Association of dietary fatty acids with urinary oxalate excretion in calcium oxalate stone-formers in their fourth decade. BJU Int 2002; 89: 842–6.
85. Porena M, Guiggi P, Micheli C. Prevention of stone disease. Urol Int 2007; 79: 37–46.
86. Lemann J Jr, Piering WF, Lennon E. Possible role of carbohydrate-induced calciuria in calcium oxalate kidney-stone formation. N Engl J Med 1969; 280: 232–7.
87. Lemann J Jr, Adams ND, Gray RW. Urinary calcium excretion in human beings. N Engl J Med 1979; 30: 535–41.
88. Centers for Disease Control and Prevention (CDC): Trends in intake of energy and macronutrients: United States, 1971-2000. MMWR Morb Mortal Wkly rep 2004; 53: 80–2.
89. Raskin P, Stevenson MRM, Barilla DE, Pak CY. The hypercalciuria of diabetes mellitus: its amelioration with insulin. Clin Endocrinol 1978; 9: 329–35.
90. Griffith HM, O'Shea B, Kevany JP, McCormick JS. A control study of dietary factors in renal stone formation. Br J Urol 1981; 53: 416–20.
91. Hsu TC, Chen J, Huang HS, Wang CJ. Association of changes in the pattern of urinary calculi in Taiwanese with diet habit change between 1956 and 1999. J Formos Med Assoc 2002; 101: 5–10.
92. Baggio B, Gambaro G, Zambon S et al. Anomalous phospholipids n-6 polyunsaturated fatty acid composition in idiopathic calcium nephrolithiasis. J Am Soc Nephrol 1996; 7: 613–20.
93. Messa P, Londero D, Massarino F et al. Abnormal arachidonic acid content of red blood cell membranes and main lithogenic factors in stone formers. Nephrol Dial Transplant 2000; 15: 1388–93.
94. Naya Y, Ito H, Masai M, Yamaguchi K. Effect of dietary intake on urinary oxalate excretion in calcium oxalate stone formers in their forties. Eur Urol 2000; 37: 140–4.
95. Institute of Medicine, Food and Nutrition Board: Dietary reference intakes for water, potassium, sodium, chloride, and sulfate. Washington, DC: National Academy Press; 2004: 269-423.
96. Loria CM, Obarzanek E, Ernst ND. Choose and prepare foods with less salt: dietary advice for all Americans. J Nutr 2001; 131: 536S–551S.
97. Mattes RD, Donnelly D. Relative contributions of dietary sodium sources. J Am Coll Nutr 1991; 10: 383–93.
98. Harrington M, Cashman KD. High salt intake appears to increase bone resorption in postmenopausal women but high potassium intake ameliorates this adverse effect. Nutr Rev 2003; 61: 179–83.
99. Sakhaee K, Harvey JA, Padalino PK, Whitson P, Pak CY. The potential role of salt abuse on the risk for kidney stone formation. J Urol 1993; 150: 310–2.
100. Pak CY. Citrate and renal calculi: new insights and future directions. Am J Kidney Dis 1991; 17: 420–5.
101. Devine A, Criddle RA, Dick IM, Kerr DA, Prince RL. A longitudinal study of the effect of sodium and calcium intakes on regional bone density in postmenopausal women. Am J Clin Nutr 1995; 62: 740–5.
102. Loghman-Adham M. Adaptation to changes in dietary phosphorus intake in health and in renal failure. J Lab Clin Med 1997; 129: 176–88.
103. Roberts DH, Knox FG. Renal phosphate handling and calcium nephrolithiasis: role of dietary phosphate and phosphate leak. Semin Nephrol 1990; 10: 24–30.
104. de OG Mendonca C, Martini LA, Baxmann AC et al. Effects of an oxalate load on urinary oxalate excretion in calcium stone formers. J Ren Nutr 2003; 13: 39–46.
105. Holmes RP, Kennedy M. Estimation of the oxalate content of foods and daily oxalate intake. Kidney Int 2000; 57: 1662–7.
106. Holmes RP, Goodman HO, Assimos DG. Contribution of dietary oxalate to urinary oxalate excretion. Kidney Int 2001; 59: 270–6.
107. Massey LK, Palmer RG, Horner HT. Oxalate content of soybean seeds (Glycine max: Leguminosae), soyfoods, and other edible legumes. J Agric Food Chem 2001; 49: 4262–6.
108. Massey LK, Roman-Smith H, Sutton RA. Effect of dietary oxalate and calcium on urinary oxalate and risk of calcium oxalate kidney stones. J Am Diet Assoc 1993; 93: 901–6.
109. Siener R, Hönow R, Voss S, Seidler A, Hesse A. Oxalate content of cereals and cereal products. J Agric Food Chem 2006; 54: 3008–11.
110. Taylor EN, Curhan GC. Oxalate intake and the risk for nephrolithiasis. J Am Soc Nephrol 2007; 18: 2198–04.
111. Holmes RP, Knight J, Assimos DG. Origin of urinary oxalate. CP900, Renal Stone Disease, 1st Annual International Urolithiasis Research Symposium, edited by AP Evan, JE Lingeman, and JC Williams, 2007.
112. Rofe AM, James HM, Bais R, Conyers RA. Hepatic oxalate production: the role of hydroxypyruvate. Biochem Med Metab Biol 1986; 36: 141–50.

113. Baxmann AC, de OG Mendonca C, Heilberg IP. Effect of vitamin C supplements on urinary oxalate and pH in calcium stone-forming patients. Kidney Int 2003; 63: 1066–71.

114. Massey LK, Liebman M, Kynast-Gales SA. Ascorbate increases human oxaluria and kidney stone risk. J Nutr 2005; 135: 1673–7.

115. Traxer O, Huet B, Poindexter J, Pak CY, Pearle MS. Effect of ascorbic acid consumption on urinary stone risk factors. J Urol 2003; 170: 397–401.

116. McHarg T, Rodgers A, Charlton K. Influence of cranberry juice on the urinary risk factors for calcium oxalate kidney stone formation. BJU Int 2003; 92: 765–8.

117. Terris MK, Issa MM, Tacker JR. Dietary supplementation with cranberry concentrate tablets may increase the risk of nephrolithiasis. Urology 2001; 57: 26–9.

118. USDA, ARS, National Genetic Resources Program. Germplasm Resources Information Network - (GRIN) [Online Database]. National Germplasm Resources Laboratory, Beltsville, Maryland. URL: http://www.ars-grin.gov/cgi-bin/npgs/html/splist.pl?12610. Accessed May 28, 2008.

119. Kiser AK, Dagnelie G. Reported effects of non-traditional treatments and complementary and alternative medicine by retinitis pigmentosa patients. Clin Exp Optom 2008; 91: 166–76.

120. Head K. Natural therapies for ocular disorders part two: cataracts and glaucoma. Altern Med Rev 2001; 6: 141–66.

121. Blowey DL. Nephrotoxicity of over-the-counter analgesics, natural medicines, and illicit drugs. Adolesc Med 2005; 16: 31–43.

122. Hoppe B, von Unruh G, Laube N, Hesse A, Sidhu H. Oxalate degrading bacteria: new treatment option for patients with primary and secondary hyperoxaluria? Urol Res 2005; 33: 372–5.

123. Lieske JC, Goldfarb DS, De Simone C, Regnier C. Use of a probiotic to decrease enteric hyperoxaluria. Kidney Int 2005; 68: 1244–9.

124. Troxel SA, Dishu H, Kaul P, Low RK. Intestinal Oxalobacter formigenes colonization in calcium oxalate stone formers and its relation to urinary oxalate. J Endourol 2003; 17: 173–6.

125. Hoppe B, Beck B, Gatter N et al. Oxalobacter formigenes: a potential tool for the treatment of primary hyperoxaluria type 1. Kidney Int 2006; 70: 1305–11.

126. Taylor EN, Stampfer MJ, Curhan GC. Fatty acid intake and incident nephrolithiasis. Am J Kidney Dis 2005; 45: 267–74.

127. Buck AC, Davies RL, Harrison T. The protective role of eicosapentaenoic acid (EPA) in the pathogenesis of nephrolithiasis. J Urol 1991; 146: 188–94.

128. Rothwell PJ, Green R, Blacklock NJ, Kavanagh JP. Does fish oil benefit stone formers? J Urol 1993; 150: 1391–4.

129. Yasui T, Tanaka H, Fujita K, Kguchi M, Kohri K. Effects of eicosapentaenoic acid on urinary calcium excretion in calcium stone formers. Eur Urol 2001; 39: 580–5.

130. Lenin M, Thiagarajan A, Nagaraj M, Varalakshmi P. Attenuation of oxalate-induced nephrotoxicity by eicosapentaenoate-lipoate (EPA-LA) derivative in experimental rat model. Prostaglandins Leukot Essent Fatty Acids 2001; 65: 265–70.

131. Huang HS, Ma MC, Chen CF, Chen J. Changes in nitric oxide production in the rat kidney due to CaOx nephrolithiasis. Neurourol Urodyn 2006; 25: 252–8.

132. Sumitra K, Pragasam V, Sakthivel R, Kalaiselvi P, Varalakshmi P. Beneficial effect of vitamin E supplementation on the biochemical and kinetic properties of Tamm-Horsfall glycoprotein in hypertensive and hyperoxaluric patients. Nephrol Dial Transplant 2005; 27: 1407–15.

133. Thamilselvan S, Menon M. Vitamin E therapy prevents hyperoxaluria-induced calcium oxalate crystal deposition in the kidney by improving renal tissue antioxidant status. BJU Int 2005; 96: 117–26.

134. Holick MF, Chen TC. Vitamin D deficiency: a worldwide problem with health consequences. Am J Clin Nutr 2008; 87: 1080S–1086S.

135. Vieth R, Fraser D. Vitamin D insufficiency: no recommended dietary allowance exists for this nutrient. CMAJ 2002; 166: 1541–2.

136. Maalouf J, Nabulsi M, Vieth R et al. Short-term and long-term safety of weekly high-dose vitamin D3 supplementation in school children. J Clin Endocrinol Metab 2008; 93: 2693–701.

137. Vezzoli G, Soldati L, Gambaro G. Update on primary hypercalciuria from a genetic perspective. J Urol 2008; 179: 1676–82.

138. Hansen KE, Jones AN, Lindstrom MJ et al. Vitamin D insufficiency: disease or no disease? J Bone Miner Res 2008; 23(7): 1052–60.

139. Gohel MD, Wong SP. Chinese herbal medicines and their efficacy in treating renal stones. Urol Res 2006; 34: 365–72.

140. Micali S, Sighinolfi MC, Celia A et al. Can Phyllanthus niruri affect the efficacy of extracorporeal shock wave lithotripsy for renal stones? A randomized, prospective, long-term study. J Urol 2006; 176: 1020–22.

141. Nishiura JL, Campos AH, Boim MA, Heilberg IP, Schor N. Phyllanthus niruri normalizes elevated urinary calcium levels in calcium stone forming (CSF) patients. Urol Res 2004; 32: 362–6.

142. Selvam R, Kalaiselvi P, Govindaraj A et al Effect of A. lanata leaf extract and vediuppu chunnam on the urinary risk factors of calcium oxalate urolithiasis during experimental hyperoxaluria. Pharmacol Res 2001; 43: 89–93.

143. Gurocak S, Kupeli B. Consumption of historical and current phytotherapeutic agents for urolithiasis: a critical review. J Urol 2006; 176: 450–5.

144. Pardalidis N, Tsiamis C, Diamantis A, Andriopoulos N, Sofikitis N. Methods of lithotripsy in ancient Greece and Byzantium. J Urol 2007; 178: 1182–3.

145. Rutkowski P, Klassen A, Sebekova K, Bahner U, Heidland A. Renal disease in obesity: the need for greater attention. J Ren Nutr 2006; 16: 216–23.

146. Nelson WK, Houghton SG, Milliner DS, Lieske JC, Sarr MG. Enteric hyperoxaluria, nephrolithiasis, and oxalate nephropathy: potentially serious and unappreciated complications of Roux-en-Y gastric bypass. Surg Obes Relat Dis 2005; 1: 481–5.

147. Durrani O, Morrisroe S, Jackman S, Averch T. Analysis of stone disease in morbidly obese patients undergoing gastric bypass surgery. J Endourol 2006; 20: 749–52.

148. Asplin JR, Coe FL. Hyperoxaluria in kidney stone formers treated with modern bariatric surgery. J Urol 2007; 177: 565–9.

149. Sinha MK, Collazo-Clavell ML, Rule A et al. Hyperoxaluric nephrolithiasis is a complication of Roux-en-Y gastric bypass surgery. Kidney Int 2007; 72: 100–7.

150. Duffey BG, Pedro RN, Makhlouf A et al. Roux-en-Y gastric bypass is associated with early increased risk factors for development of calcium oxalate nephrolithiasis. J Am Coll Surg 2008; 206: 1145–53.

151. Reddy ST, Wang CY, Sakhaee K, Brinkley L, Pak CY. Effect of low-carbohydrate high-protein diets on acid-base balance, stone-forming propensity, and calcium metabolism. Am J Kidney Dis 2002; 40: 265–74.

152. Rhodes KS, Weintraub MS, Biesemeier CK, Rubenfire M. The lipid management nutrition outcomes project: perspectives from a national experience in protocol implementation and nutrition outcomes tracking. J Am Diet Assoc 2008; 108: 332–9.

153. Raatz SK, Wimmer JK, Kwong CA, Sibley SD. Intensive diet instruction by registered dietitians improves weight-loss success. J Am Diet Assoc 2008; 108: 110–3.

154. Lin PH, Appel LJ, Funk K et al. The PREMIER intervention helps participants follow the dietary approaches to stop hypertension dietary pattern and the current dietary reference intakes recommendations. J Am Diet Assoc 2007; 107: 1541–51.

155. Henkin Y, Shai I, Zuk R et al. Dietary treatment of hypercholesterolemia: do dietitians do it better? A randomized, controlled trial. Am J Med 2000; 109: 549–55.

156. Fappa E, Yannakoulia M, Pitsavos C et al. Lifestyle intervention in the management of metabolic syndrome: could we improve adherence issues? Nutrition 2008; 24: 286–91.

157. Daubenmier JJ, Weidner G, Sumner MD et al. The contribution of changes in diet, exercise, and stress management to changes in coronary risk in women and men in the multisite cardiac lifestyle intervention program. Ann Behav Med 2007; 33: 57–68.

158. Pronk NP, Goodman MJ, O'Connor PJ, Martinson BC. Relationship between modifiable health risks and short-term health care charges. JAMA 1999; 282: 2235–9.

159. Kocvara R, Plasgura P, Petrik A et al. A prospective study of nonmedical prophylaxis after a first kidney stone. BJU Int 1999; 84: 393–8.

160. Borghi L, Meschi T, Amato F et al. Urinary volume, water and recurrence in idiopathic calcium nephrolithiasis: a 5-year randomized prospective study. J Urol 1996; 155: 839–43.

161. Borghi L, Schianchi T, Meschi T et al. Comparison of two diets for the prevention of recurrent stones in idiopathic hypercalciuria. N Engl J Med 2002; 346: 77–83.

162. Devine A, Criddle RA, Dick IM, Kerr DA, Prince RL. A longitudinal study of the effect of sodium and calcium intakes on regional bone density in postmenopausal women. Am J Clin Nutr 1995; 62: 740–5.

163. Hiatt RA, Ettinger B, Caan B et al. Randomized controlled trial of a low animal protein, high fiber diet in the prevention of recurrent calcium oxalate kidney stones. Am J Epidemiol 1996; 144: 25–33.

164. Robertson WG, Peacock M, Marshall DH. Prevalence of urinary stone disease in vegetarians. Eur Urol 1982; 8: 334–9.

165. Choi HK, Curhan G. Coffee, tea, and caffeine consumption and serum uric acid level: the third national health and nutrition examination survey. Arthritis Rheum 2007; 57: 816–21.

166. Choi HK, Willett W, Curhan G. Coffee consumption and risk of incident gout in men: a prospective study. Arthritis Rheum 2007; 56: 2049–55.

167. Goldfarb DS, Fischer ME, Keich Y, Goldberg J. A twin study of genetic and dietary influences on nephrolithiasis: a report from the Vietnam Era Twin (VET) Registry. Kidney Int 2005; 67: 1053–61.

168. Grases F, Costa-Bauza A, Prieto RM. Renal lithiasis and nutrition. Nutrition J 2006; 5: 23–9.

169. Joung H, Nam G, Yoon S et al. Bioavailable zinc intake of Korean adults in relation to the phytate content of Korean foods. J Food Comp Analysis 2004; 17: 713–24.

5 | The role of imaging in the management of urolithiasis

Gyan Pareek

INTRODUCTION

Radiographic studies are integral for the management of urolithiasis. Ideally, these studies should provide optimal assessment of urinary tract anatomy and detailed stone characterization. Various imaging modalities are utilized during the management of urolithiasis such as intravenous urography (IVU), ultrasound (US), noncontrast computed tomography (NCCT), and magnetic resonance urography (MRU). Of these, NCCT has evolved to become the imaging modality of choice for the assessment of patients with suspected urinary tract stones. Besides its superior speed and accuracy in comparison to other radiologic tests, NCCT can also provide alternative diagnosis in patients without stones. As a first-line assessment tool for patients presenting with acute renal colic, NCCT has proven to be more effective for diagnosing urinary stones than IVU, ultrasound, and MRU.(1) This chapter will summarize the various imaging modalities employed for the diagnosis and management of urolithiasis. Special emphasis will be placed on NCCT, the first-line imaging modality for the management of urinary stones. Specific attention to current literature providing scientific evidence on the role of NCCT as a prognostic tool will be a primary focus. The goal of the chapter is to provide the reader with an evidence-based algorithmic approach for the radiographic work-up and management of urolithiasis.

IMAGING MODALITIES FOR DIAGNOSIS

NCCT

NCCT provides rapid assessment of stone size, shape, number, and location. Many studies have assessed the utility value of NCCT and have concluded a greater than 95% sensitivity and specificity for its assessment of urinary calculi.(2) As previously mentioned, the NCCT has proven to be superior to IVU and ultrasound.(3, 4, 5)

Evidence demonstrates that NCCT provides additional detail such as stone location, density, and other secondary signs of urolithiasis. Clinical details of value include the degree of hydronephrosis, assessment of perinephric and periureteral tissue as well as the detailed radiographic assessment of other urological and nonurological organ systems. One study assessed the secondary diagnosis found by NCCT and found that 14% of patients who underwent NCCT for the evaluation of stone disease were found to have another diagnosis requiring treatment.(6) Associated signs of renal enlargement, perinephric or periureteral inflammation or "stranding," and distension of the collecting system or ureter are especially important parameters emphasized by NCCT. These findings have proven to be sensitive indicators of the degree of ureteral obstruction. Additionally, renal parenchyma thickness (RPT) may be evaluated, allowing relative comparison of the health of the kidneys (Figure 5.1). Additional information from a NCCT includes the density assessment of stones, measured in Hounsfield units (HU). Clinically, these measurements may be used to distinguish cystine and uric acid stones from calcium-bearing stones (see section: *NCCT for Prognosis*). Additional, rare pathology may be diagnosed by NCCT, such as abdominal aortic aneurysms and cholelithiasis. NCCT also is a valuable tool for stone size assessment although the estimated sizes of renal calculi determined using NCCT vary slightly from those obtained with KUB radiography (see section *NCCT for Prognosis*).

Of note, NCCT is generally more expensive than IVU and ultrasound, but the increased cost is certainly balanced by more definitive, faster diagnosis. The cost of NCCT is reported

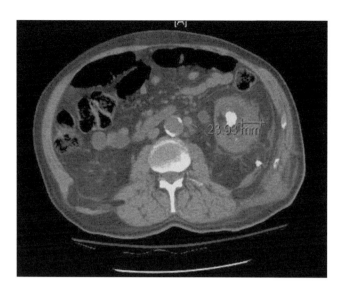

Figure 5.1 Renal parenchyma thickness (RPT) (arrows) allows for an easy, useful measurement to assess relative kidney health.

as $600 to $800 compared with $400 for IVU, varying from institution to institution and by accounting methods.

Plain-film Radiography

Plain-film radiography of the kidneys, ureters, and bladder (KUB) may be sufficient to document the size and location of radiopaque urinary calculi.

Calcium oxalate and calcium phosphate stones, due to their calcium content, are easiest to detect by radiography. Uric acid stones are less radio opaque and stones composed mainly of cystine or magnesium ammonium phosphate (MAP), may be difficult, if not impossible, to detect on plain-film radiographs. Overlying stool or bowel gas may obscure radio opaque calculi, and identification of ureteral stones overlying the bony pelvis or transverse processes of vertebrae may be difficult. On the contrary, false positives on a KUB are common. Radiopacities, such as calcified mesenteric lymph nodes, gallstones, stool, and phleboliths (calcified pelvic veins), may be misread as stones.

Although 90% of urinary calculi have historically been considered to be radiopaque, the sensitivity and specificity of KUB radiography alone remain poor (sensitivity: 45–59%; specificity: 71–77%).(7)

KUB radiographs are useful in the initial evaluation of patients with known stone disease and in following the course of patients with known radiopaque stones.

IVU

Until the advent of NCCT, IVU was considered the gold standard for the diagnosis of urolithiasis. Currently, IVU has a limited role in management. IVU provides useful information about the stone size, location, and radiodensity. Calyceal anatomy, degree of obstruction, as well as the contralateral renal unit may also be assessed with accuracy. IVU is widely available, and its interpretation is well standardized. Additionally, IVU allows for ureteral calculi to be easily distinguished from nonurologic radiopacities. The accuracy of IVU can be maximized with proper bowel preparation, and the adverse renal effects of contrast media may be minimized by ensuring that the patient is well hydrated. Preparatory steps require time and often cannot be accomplished when a patient presents in an emergency situation. Compared with abdominal ultrasonography and KUB radiography, IVU has greater sensitivity (64–87%) and specificity (92–94%) for the detection of renal calculi.(7)

Contrast is necessary for performing IVU. The nephrotoxic effects of contrast are well documented from the IVU literature and are briefly discussed in order to allow the reader to clinically deal with situations where contrast use may be in question. Serum creatinine levels must always be measured before contrast media are administered. At our institution a creatinine level greater then 1.5 mg per dL (130 μmol per L) is generally used as a cutoff value for contrast administration. The risks and benefits of using contrast media above this creatinine level must be carefully weighed, particularly in patients with diabetes mellitus, cardiovascular disease, or other systemic disorders. Certain steps can be taken to minimize the risks of contrast reaction and include adequate hydration, minimizing the amount of contrast material that is infused and maximizing the time interval between consecutive contrast studies. The role of nonionic contrast media continues to evolve. Use of these materials may decrease reactions associated with contrast injections including, nausea, flushing, and bradycardia. Fatal metabolic acidosis after radiologic procedures using intravenous contrast media in patients with diabetes with preexisting renal failure and who were taking metformin (Glucophage) has been reported.(8) Basic mechanism of this interaction involves impairment of renal metformin excretion by contrast media-induced nephrotoxicity that results in elevated serum metformin levels.(8) Current recommendation from the United States FDA is to discontinue metformin at the time of or before a procedure using contrast material and to withhold the drug for 48 hours after the procedure. Metformin therapy is reinstituted only after renal function has been reevaluated and found to be normal.

Ultrasound

Currently, ultrasound has a limited use in the diagnosis of urolithiasis.

Ultrasonography is a readily available technique and is quickly performed with a high sensitivity in detecting renal calculi. Ultrasound sensitivity in detecting lower urinary stones is poor, being virtually blind to ureteral stones (sensitivity: 19 percent).(9) Since the latter group is likely to represent most of the patients presenting with symptomatic renal calculi, the routine use of ultrasound in patents presenting with acute renal colic is limited. Interestingly, if a ureteral stone is visualized by ultrasound, the finding is reliable with a reported specificity of 97%.(9)

Although the role for diagnosis is limited, ultrasound may play a vital role for management and follow-up for patients with urolithiasis. Ultrasound is highly sensitive to hydronephrosis, which may be a manifestation of ureteral obstruction. Although it is limited in defining the level or nature of obstruction, it is useful in assessing renal anatomy and in defining any other disease processes which may be mimicking renal colic.

Additionally, abdominal ultrasonography is the preferred imaging modality for the evaluation of gynecologic pain, which is more common than urolithiasis in women of childbearing age. Patients in the pediatric age group as well as those patients with a history of nonradio opaque stones (uric acid) may also be managed radiographically by ultrasound.

At our institution, ultrasound is used routinely during follow-up and as part of the preventive care protocol for the prevention of urolithiasis (see section *Imaging for Surveillance*).

MRU

Magnetic resonance urography (MRU) has a minimal role in the diagnosis and management of urolithiasis. MRU provides an alternative to NCCT in certain clinical settings, including pediatric and pregnant patients. MRU provides superb depiction of the urinary tract and has been shown to have accuracy in stone diagnosis of 92.8 %.(10) The current role of MRU is evolving and not considered standard of care.

NCCT FOR PROGNOSIS

Size

Stone measurements on NCCT vs. other radiographic modalities have been shown to be significantly different. Studies have revealed that NCCT may underestimate stone size by 12%.(11) Others have shown an overestimation.(12) As summarized by Parsons et al. CT and plain film differ minimally in their measurements in the transverse and longitudinal axes, but NCCT overestimates dimensions in the cephalo-caudal dimension.(13) In a review by Potretzke and Monga, accurate assessment of stone size should be approached with caution. The authors concluded that one should be cautious and not treat a small stone too conservatively if assessed on NCCT if a high level of clinical suspicion is present.(14) It is apparent that the accurate assessment of stone size is one of the key parameters to guide therapy, whether conservative or endourolgic intervention. As revealed by Wang et al. along with stone density on NCCT, size and morphology are powerful predictors of clinical outcome.(15)

Table 5.1   HU of Urinary Stones.

Composition	Avg. % Composition	No. of Stones	Avg. Size (mm)	HU ± SD
Brushite	75%	4	10.0	1123 ± 254
Apatite	60%	9	15.6	865 ± 341
100–80% CaOMH	83%	15	7.3	857 ± 243
<80–60% CaOMH	66%	16	9.0	718 ± 311
<60–50% CaOMH	53%	8	8.0	667 ± 293
CaODH	66%	9	6.0	524 ± 266
Cystine	100%	2	7.5	550 ± 74
Uric Acid	100%	11	14.9	338 ± 159

Composition

Investigators have demonstrated that the HU density of stones obtained on NCCT may be used to predict stone composition.(16, 17) Others have suggested that the pre-SWL HU determination on NCCT may help predict stone fragility before SWL.(18) Additionally, recent unpublished data at our institution has correlated HU to the various calcium stone subtypes. In this latter study, we evaluated patients undergoing endourologic management for urinary stones and attempted to determine whether HU on NCCT could predict the subtype composition of the various calcium stones. Indeed, the preliminary data from these findings revealed that certain subtypes may be predicted by HU measurement on NCCT (Table 5.1).

Interestingly, the ability to assess stone characteristics and predict fragility is not a new phenomenon. Chaussy and Fuchs suggested that stones are less likely to break if their radiodensity is greater than that of the spine.(19) Others have studied opacity as a determinant of stone fragility and found that highly opaque stone are less fragile.(20) As mentioned previously, recent reviews have reported on the value of the attenuation value of calculi measured in HU as a predictor of stone composition, fragility, and stone-free status following SWL.(17, 18) Although these measures may provide more insight pre-operatively for the urologist, the precise meaning of this data in the management of stone disease remains controversial.

Recent studies have also suggested that HU calculations on NCCT bone window settings may be able to determine the internal structure of a stone, possibly deciphering multiple stone components due to variations in internal structure. Specifically, in the setting of a patient with a ureteral stent or nephrostomy tube in place, the bone windows setting may be used to allow visual distinction between the stent/tube and the calculus. Additionally, further distinction can be attained by measuring the HU value of the stent/tube which tend to exceed 1,600 HU, while most stones are <1,600 HU in attenuation.(21) However, an important observation is that the viewing window does not alter the HU in CT scans.(22)

The collimation size of the CT scanner and the size of the stone may affect the HU of the stone on NCCT. In an *in vitro* study, Saw et al. demonstrated that stone composition may be separated by the absolute HU on CT scan, but that the ability to distinguish the various compositions decreases as the collimation size increases. These findings correlate with stone size, a parameter which may affect the absolute HU measurement.(23) Williams et al. showed that the volume-averaging effects on attenuation in helical CT scans could be partially corrected as long as collimation width did not excessively exceed the diameter of the structure.(24) If the size of the calculus is smaller than the collimation size, the attenuation of the stone will be subject to larger partial-volume inaccuracy than in the case of a larger stone.(23) Thus, a smaller collimation size combined with a larger stone will allow the HU measurement to approach the "true HU attenuation value" which will lead to the ability to separate urinary stones by stone composition.

Previous *in vivo* studies correlating HU values to stone composition have demonstrated that calcium oxalate stones or pure calcium stones may be distinguished from uric acid stones (Table 5.2). (16, 17, 25–27) Motley et al. studied 87 calcium stones which had a mean HU of 440±262 and 7 uric acid stones which had a mean HU of 270±134 at a 5 mm collimation but the average stone size varied from 1 to 19 mm.(16) Nakada et. al. found the *in vivo* HU values for 82 calcium oxalate stones to be 652±490 with a mean size of 5.3±3.9 mm and 17 uric acid stones to be 344±152 with a mean size of 6.8±4.5 mm using 3 and 5 mm collimation.(17) Furthermore, Hounsfield unit density (HUD) has been shown to differentiate calcium from uric acid stones. (16, 17, 26) Nakada et al. showed that using an attenuation-to-size ratio cutoff of 80 HU/mm,

Table 5.2 *In Vivo* Studies Using Helical CT Scan to Differentiate Stone Composition.

Study	Collimation (mm)	Stone Size Range (mm)	Results[†]
Motley et al.(11)	5	1–19	UA from CaOx and CaPO4
Nakada et al.(12)	3-5	1–28	UA from CaOx
Pareek et al.(10)	5	5–10	UA from CaOx and CaPO4
Demirel & Suma(13)	5	NR	UA from CaOx; Overlap between UA, STV, CaOx*

† Composition separation based on absolute HU measurement
* Statistically significant difference between groups, but overlap in absolute HU
NR: Not Reported, UA: Uric Acid, CaOx: Calcium Oxalate, CaPO4: Calcium Phosphate, STV: Struvite

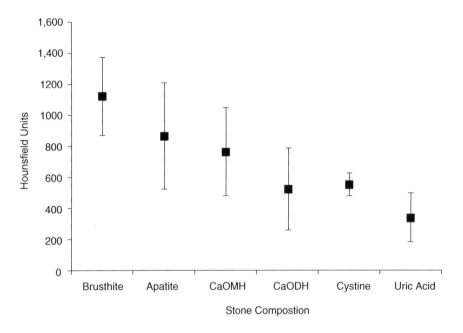

Figure 5.2 Hounsfield Unit measurements based on stone composition.

the negative predictive value that a stone would be predominantly calcium oxalate was 99%. Figure 5.2 summarizes the contemporary series studying HUD and stone composition.

Thus, stone size and collimation are important variables that affect HU measurement both *in vivo* and *in vitro*. HU measurement of urinary stones on NCCT demonstrates a significant difference between calcium and uric acid stones. Furthermore, early evidence suggests that HUD may help differentiate calcium stone subtypes, specifically CaOMH (hard stones) and CaODH. The only conclusion that can be formulated is that the information may be helpful in deciding the best management modality for each individual stone. Multi-institutional randomized trials are required to study the HU attenuation values of urinary stones by taking into account various stone sizes at a fixed collimation.

Lower Pole Anatomy

The management of lower pole stones (LPSs) differs from stones in other renal or ureteral areas (Chapters 11–13). Certain criteria on NCCT for LPS must be considered before treatment recommendations.

Previously, we have reported the value of body mass index (BMI), Hounsfield unit density (HU), and skin-to-stone distance (SSD) for LPS.(27) The analysis studied patients with a single lower pole renal stones between 5 and 15 mm and the data revealed that SSD calculated on pre-treatment NCCT provides a simple, easily reproducible, and readily available quantitative measurement (Figure 5.3). The logistic regression analysis fit for SSD, HU, and BMI revealed SSD

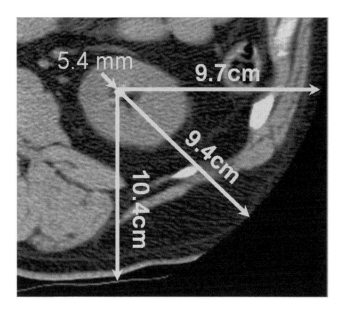

Figure 5.3 Skin-to-stone distance (SSD) calculation computed tomography. The average of the 3 calculations is used in SWL management protocols.

to be a significant predictor of SF rates. The data showed that patients who failed SWL had an SSD greater or equal to 10 cm. Specifically, 85% of the RS patients had a measured SSD greater than 10 cm. Of the SF patients only 6 of 30 (20%) had a SSD greater than 10 cm. We postulate that the focal distance of the shockwave generated by the lithotripter becomes increasingly less effective as the SSD approaches the maximum focal distance from the shockwave initiation point (F1) to the stone (F2). The DoliS lithotripter used in the study had a pressure field measured F1 to F2 distance of 14cm. We believe this may be an overestimation of the optimal F1 to F2 distance required for treatment success. We theorize that the F1 to F2 distance described on a lithotripsy unit represents a clinically insignificant value and that each lithotripter should be studied to determine its optimal treatment distance. Whether this finding holds true across a wider range of lithotripters remains to be determined by larger randomized multi-institutional trials. Therapeutic considerations emerge from these findings. Lower pole renal stones with a SSD of greater than 10 cm may be more amenable to endourological treatment such as ureteroscopy or PCNL.

The prognostic value of NCCT is in assessing the location, size, HU, and SSD of stones. Figures 5.4 and 5.5 provide an algorithmic approach to the radiograhic management of urolithiasis.(28) Certainly, all the evidence is based on retrospective data, but until the literature provides more randomized controlled data, treatment decisions will be based on the current literature.

Imaging for Surveillance

There are no surveillance protocols for the management of patients followed conservatively by surveillance or those managed by endourological management. Certainly, repeated computed tomography examinations are not warranted and would expose the patient to mega doses of radiation. At our institution, after the initial diagnosis is established by NCCT, treatment recommendations are made depending on conservative or interventional management.

Conservative Management

We employ a nonradiation approach to patients managed conservatively. Outpatient ultrasound is utilized as a primary tool management for patients on preventive care protocol. Plain-film radiography is only utilized for patients following SWL as these patients have had pretreatment radiographs for comparison. Ultrasound is utilized semiannually or annually depending on the patient-specific surveillance protocol.

Radiation Exposure

An estimated 60–80 million computed tomography examinations are performed in the U.S. annually.(29) Radiation exposure is of great concern and knowledge of the amounts of radiation exposure during NCCT and other radiographic modalities should be a part of every

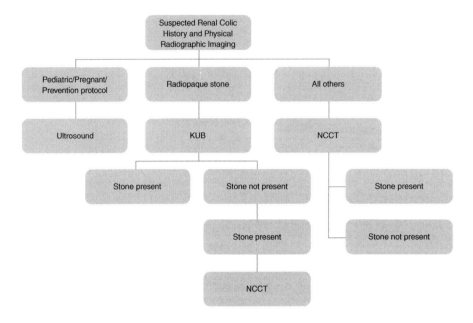

Figure 5.4 Algorithm for radiographic management of patients presenting with acute renal colic.

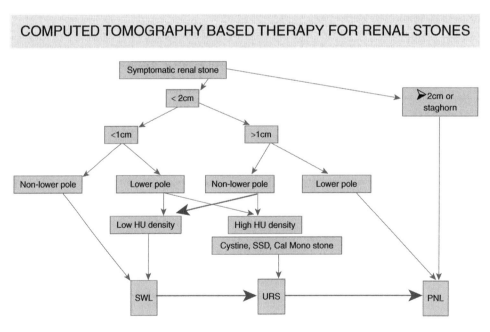

Figure 5.5 Evidence-based algorithm for radiographic management of patients diagnosed with renal urolithiasis (Reproduced with permission34).

clinician's armamentarium. In general, standard NCCT protocols use approximately 180 mAs of radiation. The effects of radiation exposure at these levels in the long term are unknown, but certainly limiting exposure is of the utmost importance.

Imaging in Pregnancy

Abdominal ultrasonography is the gold standard radiographic modality during the initial work-up of renal colic in pregnancy. It offers an easy, cost-effective methodology without exposing the mother or fetus to radiation. As outlined earlier the sensitivity of ultrasound as compared to NCCT is poor, with reported sensitivity ranging from 34 to 86%.(30)

Radiation exposure to the fetus during pregnancy precludes NCCT as a radiographic modality in pregnant women presenting with acute renal colic. The threshold for induction of developmental defects, birth defects, or miscarriages is 20,000 mrads during organogenesis and 50000 mrads during the second and third trimesters.(31) Interestingly, recent review revealed that 95% of academic institutions utilized NCCT during pregnancy if the benefits are thought to outweigh the risks.(32) The estimated radiation dose to the fetus is reported to be approximately 1,600 rads.(33)

In certain instances, IVU may be utilized for the diagnosis of urolithiasis in pregnancy. The high radiation exposure to the mother and fetus is of concern and therefore a limited 1-shot protocol should be utilized with a radiograph taken 10 minutes after contrast injection.

As mentioned earlier, the future may have a role for MRU. Spencer et al. reported that MRU was a very powerful modality in the investigation of hydronephrosis during pregnancy. Calculi on MRU are represented by filling defects, in which there is an absence of signal on a T2-weighted image distal to the obstruction, along with other obstructive signs such as hydronephrosis and hydroureter.(33)

SUMMARY

Imaging is of paramount importance for the appropriate management of urolithiasis. NCCT is the current radiographic modality of choice for diagnosis, prognosis, and treatment of urolithiasis. Future directions will focus on the ideal radiographic modality, one which will limit radiation exposure to the patient while providing fine anatomical and stone detail. Additionally, the ideal tool for surveillance of stones managed nonsurgically will continue to be the focus. Newer 4-dimensional ultrasounds and fused ultrasound/MRI machines are on the horizon and may provide superior diagnostic capabilities to NCCT. Certainly, for the near future NCCT will remain the standard of care and diagnostic modality of choice in patients with urolithiasis.

REFERENCES

1. Miller N, Lingeman J. Management of kidney stones. BMJ 2007; 334: 468–72.
2. Heidenreich A, Desgrandschamps F, Terrier F. Modern approach of diagnosis and management of acute flank pain: review of all imaging modalities. Eur Urol 2002; 41: 351–62.
3. Ulusan S, Koc Z, Tokmak N. Accuracy of sonography for detecting renal stone comparison with CT. J Clin Ultrasound 2007; 35: 256–61.
4. Palmer JS, Donaher ER, O'Riordan MA, Dell KM. Diagnosis of pediatric urolithiasis: role of ultrasound and computerized tomography. J Urol 2005; 174: 1413–6.
5. Liu W, Esler S, Kenny B et al. Low-dose non-enhanced helical CT of renal colic: assessment of ureteric stone detection and measurement of effective dose equivalent. Radiology 2000; 215: 51–4.
6. Hoppe H, Studer R, Kessler T et al. Alternate or additional findings to stone disease on unenhanced computerized tomography for acute flank pain can impact management. J Urol 2006; 175: 1725–30.
7. Sameh WM. Value of intravenous urography before shockwave lithotripsy in the treatment of renal calculi: a randomized study. J Endourol 2007; 21: 574–7.
8. Jain V, Sharma D, Prabhakar H, Dash HH. Metformin-associated lactic acidosis following contrast-induced nephrotoxicity. Eur J Anaesthesiol. 2008 Feb; 25(2): 166–7.
9. Pepe R, Motta L, Pennisi M, Aragona F. Functional evaluation of the urinary tract by color-Doppler ultrasonography (CDU) in 100 patients with renal colic. Eur J Radiol 2005; 53: 131–5.
10. Jung P, Brauers A, Nolte-Ernsting C et al. Magnetic resonance urography enhanced by gadolinium and diuretics: a comparison with conventional urography in diagnosing the cause of ureteric obstruction. BJU Int 2000; 86: 960–5.
11. Dundee P, Bouchier-Hayes D, Haxhimolla H et al. Renal tract calculi: comparison of stone size on plain radiography and noncontrast spiral CT scan. J Endourol 2006; 20: 1005–9.
12. Tisdale BE, Siemens DR, Lysack J et al. Correlation of CT scan vs. plain radiography for measuring urinary stone dimensions. Can J Urol 2007; 14: 3489–92.
13. Parsons J, Lancini V, Shetye K et al. Urinary stone size: comparison of abdominal plain radiography and non contrast CT measurements. J Endourol 2003; 17: 725–8.

14. Potretzke A, Monga M. Imaging modalities for urolithiasis: Impact on Management. Current Opinion Urol 2008; 18: 199–204.
15. Wang LJ, Wong YC, Chuang CK et al. Predictions of outcomes of renal stones after extracorporeal shock wave lithotripsy from stone characteristics determined by unenhanced helical computed tomography: a multivariate analysis. [see comment]. Eur J Radiol 2005; 15: 2238–43.
16. Motley G, Dalrymple N, Keesling C et al. Hounsfield unit density in the determination of urinary stone composition. Urology 2001; 58: 170–3
17. Nakada SY, Hoff DG, Attai S et al. Determination of stone composition by noncontrast spiral computed tomography in the clinical setting. Urology 2000; 55: 816–9.
18. Pareek G, Armenakas NA, Fracchia JA. Hounsfield units on computerized tomography predict stone-free rates after extracorporeal shock wave lithotripsy. J Urol 2003; 169: 1679–81.
19. Chaussy CG, Fuchs GJ. Extracorporeal shockwave lithotripsy. Monogr Urol 1987; 4: 80.
20. Yankovski SZ, Yankovski JA. Obesity. N Engl J Med 2002; 346: 591–602.
21. Tanrikut C, Sahani D, Dretler SP. Distinguishing stent from stone: use of bone windows. Urology 2004; 63: 823–6.
22. Williams JC: Viewing windows do not alter Hounsfield units in CT scans. Urol Res 2005; 33: 481–2.
23. Saw KC, McAteer JA, Monga AG et al. Helical CT of urinary stones: effect of stone composition, stone size, and scan collimation. AJR Am J Roentgenol 2000; 175: 329–32
24. Williams JC, Saw KC, Monga AG et al. Correction of helical CT attenuation values with wide beam collimation: in vitro test with urinary stones. Acad Radiol 2001; 8: 478–3.
25. Demirel A, Suma S. The efficacy of non-contrast helical computed tomography in the prediction of urinary stone composition in vivo. J Int Med Res 2003; 31: 1–5.
26. Williams JC, Paterson RF, Kopecky KK et al. High resolution detection of internal structure of renal stones by helical computerized tomography. J Urol 2001; 167: 322–6.
27. Pareek G, Hedican SP, Lee FT et al. Shock wave lithotripsy success determined by skin-to-stone distance on computed tomography. Urology 2005; 66: 941–4.
28. Semelka R, Armao D, Elias J, Huda W. Imaging strategies to reduce the risk of radiation in CT studies, including selective substitution with MRI. J Magn Reson Imaging 2007; 25: 900–9.
29. Mitterberger M, Pinggera G, Maier E et al. Value of 3-dimensional transrectal/ transvaginal sonography in diagnosis of distal ureteral calculi. J Ultrasound Med 2007; 26: 19–27.
30. Brent RL. Utilization of developmental basic science principles in the evaluation of reproductive risks from pre and postconception environmental radiation exposures. Teratology 1999; 59: 182–204.
31. Jaffe TA, Miller CM, Merkle EM. Practice patterns in imaging of the pregnant patient with abdominal pain: a survey of academic centers. AJR Am J Roentgenol 2007; 189: 1128–34.
32. Lazarus E, Mayo-Smith W, Mainiero M, Spencer P. CT in the evaluation of nontraumatic abdominal pain in pregnant women. Radiology 2007; 244: 784–90.
33. Regan F, Kuszyk B, Bohlman M, Jackson S. Acute ureteric calculus obstruction: unenhanced spiral CT vs. HASTE MR urography and abdominal radiograph. Br J Radiol 2005; 78: 506–11.

6 | Evaluation and management of the patient with acute renal colic

Bhavin N Patel, Corey M Passman, and Dean G Assimos

INTRODUCTION

Patients with acute colic due to renal or ureteral stones need to be promptly evaluated so that the diagnosis can be established and treatment instituted. The components of this evaluation process include history, physical examination, laboratory studies, imaging, and symptom management. Herein, we review these various steps.

History and Physical Examination

The patient's presenting complaints need to be initially chronicled and characterized. Pertinent information includes the onset, duration, intensity, and location of the pain along with associated symptoms and signs including the presence of chills, fever, malaise, nausea, emesis, gross hematuria, and lower urinary tract symptoms. Prior stone events, stone compositions, and treatments need to be elicited. Medical history is obtained as various maladies may impact stone formation.(1) These include bowel disease, gout, diabetes mellitus, hyperparathyroidism, cystic fibrosis, sarcoidosis, immobilization, recurrent urinary tract infections, distal renal tubular acidosis, cystinuria, primary hyperoxaluria, and neurogenic bladder.(1) Previous stone analyses may aid in the identification of some of these conditions.(2, 3) Prior surgical procedures are recorded. The drugs or supplements (calcium and ascorbic acid) which the patient is taking should be documented as these drugs or their metabolites may promote stone formation.(4) A comprehensive review of systems is elicited. Dietary history including fluid, sodium, animal protein, dairy product, oxalate, fructose, and citrus fruit consumption is obtained.(5, 6) Family history is also relevant as stone disease can have a polygenic or monogenic pattern.(7)

A focused physical examination is conducted. The components include vital signs, general appearance, mentation, and cardiac, pulmonary, abdominal and flank exams. Genital examination is performed selectively.

Laboratory Studies

Urinalysis is obtained in all cases as important information may be garnered. Bacteruria may be present especially in those with signs of sepsis. pH is an important parameter in those with uric acid, calcium phosphate, cystine and struvite stones. Specific gravity is reflective of the patient's state of hydration. Urine culture testing is obtained in those with bacteruria or signs of sepsis.

Certain blood tests are obtained including serum electrolytes, BUN, creatinine, and calcium. These tests reflect the patient's overall renal function and may suggest primary hyperparathyroidism and renal tubular acidosis.(8–10) A complete blood count and blood cultures are obtained if there are signs of sepsis.

Imaging

Noncontrast computed tomography (CT) of the abdomen and pelvis is the most sensitive, specific, and accurate imaging technique for detecting stones in the urinary tract. The performance in all three of these metrics approaches 100 %.(11–13) It is the preferred imaging approach in the majority for patients with acute flank pain. There are a number of advantages of this technology including superior accuracy, sensitivity and specificity, no intravenous contrast requirement, rapid performance, and its ability to detect other causes of flank/abdominal pain.(14) These features decrease time in the emergency room as compared to evaluation with intravenous pyelography, thus reducing indirect costs.(15)

A multidetector row CT scanner is currently utilized in the majority of institutions. It permits an analysis of a large volume of data with near isotopic resolution in all three planes. This permits high-quality multiplanar reconstruction including longitudinal display of the urinary tract which requires thin section data acquisition. The utilization of overlapping 3 mm sections permits detection of stones as compared to thicker sections where calculi less than 3 mm may be missed.(16)

The diagnosis of a ureteral stone can be rapidly made if the stone is visible within the lumen of the ureter. However, when not, a search for secondary signs associated with ureteral stones is undertaken to corroborate this diagnosis.(17) These include peri-renal stranding and fluid, peri-ureteral edema, hydronephrosis, proximal ureteral dilation, ipsilateral renal enlargement, tissue rim sign, and decreased renal density. Extremely small stones and those composed of protease inhibitors such as indinavir may not be detected with this technology.(18)

Many patients with ureteral stones will be given a chance to pass their stones spontaneously. The anatomic position of the stone will need to be monitored to assess for distal migration. This is typically done with follow-up KUB X-rays. There are some limitations of the CT-generated scout film. Ege and associates reported that the sensitivity of the scout CT was 40 % as compared to 52 % for KUB; mean stone size 3.9 mm. This improved for stones greater than 5 mm where it was 66% for the CT scout and 87.5% for abdominal radiography. (19) Therefore, if the stone is not detected on the scout CT, a KUB X-ray should be obtained at the same time as this may aid in follow-up. The measurements of stone size on KUB X-ray correlate fairly well with those generated from CT. Katz and colleagues reported that the transverse diameters and longitudinal dimensions were similar. However, the mean anterior-posterior dimension measured on the CT was significantly greater than the transverse dimensions assessed on CT and KUB.(20)

Other useful stone information can be garnered from the CT scan. The attenuation coefficient may identify stone composition. For example, uric acid stones which have a low attenuation value can be distinguished from other stones.(21) In addition, this parameter may predict response to shock-wave lithotripsy (SWL).(22) The skin-to-stone distance for those with renal stones may also influence SWL results.(23) Relationships with peri-renal structures are also defined with CT which may be important for percutaneous nephrolithotomy (PNL).

Radiation exposure is a potential problem with CT especially for children or those previously subjected to multiple prior imaging studies utilizing ionizing radiation. The estimated cancer risks for CT imaging have recently been chronicled.(24, 25) The utilization of low-dose CT for evaluation of stone patients has recently been described.(26–29) The amount of radiation for such studies is equivalent to that of a KUB X-ray.(30) Stone size and patient size may influence the sensitivity of this study. Poletti and associates reported a sensitivity of 86 % for detecting ureteral stones less than 3 mm when BMI is less than 30 and 0% when it is greater. This discrepancy was less for larger ureteral stones where it was 100% for stones greater than 3 mm in size in subjects with a BMI less than 30 and 67% when it was greater. Similar findings were demonstrated for detection of renal stones using this approach.(26)

Other imaging may be considered if either CT is not available or ionizing radiation needs to be avoided or limited. Intravenous pyelography (IVP) may be employed if CT is not available. The reported sensitivities (64–97%), and specificities (92–94%) are inferior to those of CT.(11–13) It requires intravenous contrast administration placing the patient at risk for allergic reactions and contrast-induced nephropathy. It should not be undertaken in the majority of those with renal insufficiency or a contrast allergy. This study consumes more time especially if high-grade obstruction is present as delayed imaging may be necessary. However, an advantage is that it provides information about renal function, ureteral and renal anatomy all of which may influence choice and timing of treatment. Although IVP is reported to be more sensitive than ultrasound alone, the combination of ultrasonography with a KUB X-ray improves sensitivity.(13, 31) The latter can be further increased with the utilization of newer ultrasound technology such as harmonic imaging ultrasonography.(32) Therefore, this approach may be preferable to IVP as it is less burdensome and risky. Utilization of Doppler ultrasonography may provide useful information as resistive indices may be measured and ureteral jets may be seen; both of which may infer the degree of renal obstruction.(33–35) Renal ultrasonography is also commonly used in the follow-up of patients who are attempting to spontaneously pass a stone as it monitors for the presence of obstruction. Nuclear renography may be used if high-grade renal obstruction is suspected as this may influence the timing and nature of treatment.

The typical isotopes utilized are [99m]technetium diethylenetriamine-pentaacetic acid (DTPA), or [99m]technetium mercaptoacetylglycine 3 (MAG3). (36, 37) These studies provide excellent delineation of quantitative and differential renal function. Magnetic resonance urography (MRU) has been used in an attempt to identify ureteral or renal stones.(38, 39) The major advantage is that it does not involve ionizing radiation and thus may benefit certain groups such as pregnant women or children. Two MRU approaches have been utilized. T-2 weighted techniques are rapid and do not require the administration of gadolinium chelates. However, it has limited sensitivity.(39) The other approach is T-1 imaging with the administration of gadolinium which has greater sensitivity.(39) However, these studies consume more time, and frequently require the administration of furosemide. In addition, gadolinium chelates should not be administered in patients who are pregnant or have renal insufficiency or failure.(40) The detection of calculi is based on the presence of a filling defect and therefore is not specific. Tumor, blood clot, and other soft tissue lesions may have similar appearance.

A special imaging approach is required for the pregnant patient as ionizing radiation may impact fetal development and also increase risk of future malignancy. Ultrasonography is the preferred initial evaluation.(41) If the diagnosis cannot be confirmed with this technique, limited IVP or T-2 MRU are considerations.(41) The utilization of low-dose CT has been used in this setting and reported to be highly sensitive and specific.(42) Further evaluation of this imaging approach for pregnant women is needed. It is anticipated that it may supplant limited IVP and perhaps T-2 MRU.

MANAGEMENT OF PAIN, NAUSEA, AND EMESIS

Intense and debilitating pain is often the presenting manifestation of a stone patient. The pain may be located in the flank, abdomen, or genital area. Nonsteroidal anti-inflammatory agents (NSAIDs) and opioid analgesics are the most commonly used medications for the acute management of patients with renal colic.

NSAIDs directly inhibit the synthesis of prostaglandins, thereby decreasing activation of pain receptors. They also reduce renal blood flow resulting in decreased urine output which conceptually abrogates pain.(43) In addition, *in vitro* experiments have demonstrated a reduction in ureteral contractility with NSAIDs which could also attenuate pain.(44, 45) They can be given intravenously, orally, or by suppository. These agents are inexpensive and generally well tolerated. Side effects include gastrointestinal disturbances, qualitative platelet dysfunction, and renal functional impairment. Therefore, they should not be utilized in those afflicted with peptic ulcer disease/gastritis, renal insufficiency, or pregnancy. There are many NSAIDs available for utilization including ibuprofen, naproxen, diclofenac, indomethacin, celecoxib, and ketorolac. An advantage of ketorolac is that it can be administered via several routes including oral, intravenous, and intramuscular. All of the aforementioned agents except celecoxib are nonselective cyclooxygenase(COX) inhibitors while celecoxib is a COX-2 inhibitor which limits the risk of gastrointestinal side effects. While there are no reported studies of the utilization of this agent for renal colic, it is anticipated that it would be as effective as another COX-2 inhibitor, rofecoxib, which has been demonstrated to attenuate renal colic.(46) The latter agent was taken off the market because of cardiovascular risks.

Opioid analgesics are extremely effective for the treatment of renal colic. They can be administered via the aforementioned routes in addition to transdermal application. The administration of narcotics needs to be tailored to the patient as responses may differ. Side effects are common and may include nausea, emesis, constipation, drowsiness, respiratory depression, and hypotension. Intravenous administration is preferred because of rapid onset and the ability to titrate the dose based on the patients response. Morphine is the most common parenteral narcotic used for management of acute renal colic.

There have been multiple trials comparing opioid analgesia to NSAIDs for renal colic.(47, 48) The majority of these studies demonstrate that opioids provide faster pain control but both agents provide similar pain relief 20–30 minutes after administration. A significantly higher percentage of patients are able to resume usual activities at 60 minutes and be discharged from the emergency room sooner after NSAID administration compared to opioid analgesic administration. Fewer patients need break through narcotic therapy when initially given an NSAID as compared to those receiving narcotic monotherapy.(49) Side effects are also less common with NSAID therapy. Combined therapy may be the best alternative as the administration of a parenteral NSAID and an opioid analgesic is superior to either agent alone for acute pain management. In addition, a smaller amount of narcotics are required with combination therapy.(50)

Other measures have been used to treat patients with renal colic. These include the administration of antispasmodics, atypical or synthetic opioid analgesics (tramadol, butorphanol), transcutaneous electrical nerve stimulation, acupuncture, regional nerve block, local warming, nitrites, calcium channel blockers, and α-1 blockers. The latter agents have also been demonstrated to facilitate stone passage.(51–60) The role of hydration in pain management and stone passage was recently evaluated. There is no difference in pain score or rate of spontaneous stone passage with forced hydration compared to minimal hydration.(61)

Approximately one-third of patients with renal colic have nausea or emesis.(62) In addition, some experience these problems after being administered opioid analgesics. The dopamine receptor antagonist, promethazine (phenergan), is commonly prescribed in this setting. It can be administered intravenously, intramuscularly, via suppository, or orally as an elixir or tablet. Another agent utilized is the serotonin 5-HT$_3$ receptor antagonist, ondansetron (zofran) which may be given intravenously, intramuscularly, or by tablet. Other anti-emetic agents may be used. A critical analysis of these agents for the treatment of nausea and emesis in those suffering from renal colic has not been performed.

Medical Expulsive Therapy

Patients with ureteral stones are candidate for Medical expulsive therapy (MET), the administration of drugs to facilitate stone passage obviating the need for surgical interventions. MET is an option for patients who have a reasonable chance of spontaneous stone passage, controllable pain, adequate renal function, and no evidence of sepsis. The basis for MET is that a ureteral stone decreases ureteral peristaltic activity and increases the amplitude of ureteral contractions.(63) Relaxation of the ureter in the area of a stone is thought to promote stone passage.(64) Calcium channel blockers and α-1 blockers reduce ureteral activity and thus have been used for MET.(65, 66)

The most common medications used for MET are α-1 blockers, calcium channel blockers, and corticosteroids. Two meta-analytic studies have assessed the effectiveness of the aforementioned agents. Hollingsworth and colleagues reported that MET with the administration of a α-1 blocker or a calcium channel blocker had a 65% greater likelihood of spontaneous stone passage as compared to those not receiving such therapy. They reported that the pooled risk ratios and 95% confidence intervals for calcium channel blockers and α-1 blockers were 1.9 (1.51–2.4) and 1.54 (1.29–1.85). They also noted that the concomitant administration of steroids had marginal benefit.(67) Preminger and associates reported that the calcium channel blocker nifedipine had a 9% increase in stone passage as compared to controls, a difference which was not statistically significant. They also noted that patients with ureteral stones receiving α-1 blockers had a 29% better chance of stone passage than controls, a statistically significant difference. This group of investigators recommended that presently α-1 blockers are the preferred agents for MET.(68) Additional benefits of MET is a reduction in the intensity of pain and analgesic requirements, fewer episodes of colic and quicker stone passage.(69, 70)

Tamsulosin has been the most common α-1 blocker used in MET trials. However, the utilization of other α-1 blockers including terazosin and doxazosin has been demonstrated to be equally effective.(71) Side effects of α-1 blocker therapy include dizziness, nasal congestion, ejaculatory disturbances, and hypotension. Patients who are to undergo cataract surgery should inform their ophthalmologist that they are taking an α-1 blocker as there is a risk of floppy iris syndrome.(72) Patients should be informed of the off label utilization of α-1 blockers in this setting.

Acute Intervention

Septic patients with ureteral stones or obstructing renal stones need urgent drainage of the involved renal unit(s). This can be accomplished with placement of a ureteral stent or percutaneous nephrostomy tube. A randomized prospective study demonstrated that both approaches were equally effective.(73) Patients who have uncontrollable colic or who have high-grade renal obstruction with a threat of permanent renal damage may need urgent stent or percutaneous nephrostomy tube placement, or definitive stone removal. The latter is usually accomplished with a ureteroscopic approach as SWL may not be readily available. However, if it is available, several groups have achieved reasonable results with urgent/emergent SWL.(74–76)

REFERENCES

1. Matlaga BR, Assimos DG. Urologic manifestations of nonurologic disease urolithiasis. Urol Clin North Am 2003; 30(1): 91–9.
2. Pak CY, Poindexter JR, Adams-Huet B et al. Predictive value of kidney stone composition in the detection of metabolic abnormalities. Am J Med 2003; 115(1): 26–32.
3. Kourambas J, Aslan P, Teh CL et al. Role of stone analysis in metabolic evaluation and medical treatment of nephrolithiasis. J Endourol 2001; 15(2): 181–6.
4. Matlaga BR, Shah OD, Assimos DG. Drug-induced urinary calculi. Rev Urol 2003; 5(4): 227–31.
5. Assimos DG, Holmes RP. Role of diet in the therapy of urolithiasis. Urol Clin North Am 2000; 27(2): 255–68.
6. Taylor EN, Curhan GC. Fructose consumption and the risk of kidney stones. Kidney Int 2008; 73(2): 207–12.
7. Goodman HO, Holmes RP, Assimos DG. Genetic factors in calcium oxalate stone disease. J Urol 1995; 153(2): 301–7.
8. Derrick FC Jr. Renal calculi in association with hyperparathyroidism: a changing entity. J Urol 1982; 127(2): 226.
9. Jabbour N, Corvilain J, Fuss M, Kinnaert P, Van Geertruyden J. The natural history of renal stone disease after parathyroidectomy for primary hyperparathyroidism. Surg Gynecol Obstet 1991; 172(1): 25–8.
10. Mollerup CL, Lindewald H. Renal stones and primary hyperparathyroidism: natural history of renal stone disease after successful parathyroidectomy. World J Surg 1999; 23(2): 173–5.
11. Miller OF, Rineer SK, Reichard SR et al. Prospective comparison of unenhanced spiral computed tomography and intravenous urogram in the evaluation of acute flank pain. Urology 1998; 52(6): 982–7.
12. Niall O, Russell J, MacGregor R et al. A comparison of noncontrast computerized tomography with excretory urography in the assessment of acute flank pain. J Urol 1999; 161(2): 534–7.
13. Yilmaz S, Sindel T, Arslan G et al. Renal colic: comparison of spiral CT, US and IVU in the detection of ureteral calculi. Eur Radiol 1998; 8(2): 212–7.
14. Chen MY, Zagoria RJ, Saunders HS, Dyer RB. Trends in the use of unenhanced helical CT for acute urinary colic. AJR Am J Roentgenol 1999; 173(6): 1447–50.
15. Pfister SA, Deckart A, Laschke S et al. Unenhanced helical computed tomography vs. intravenous urography in patients with acute flank pain: accuracy and economic impact in a randomized prospective trial. Eur Radiol 2003; 13(11): 2513–20.
16. Memarsadeghi M, Heinz-Peer G, Helbich TH et al. Unenhanced multi-detector row CT in patients suspected of having urinary stone disease: effect of section width on diagnosis. Radiology 2005; 235(2): 530–6.
17. Katz DS, Lane MJ, Sommer FG. Unenhanced helical CT of ureteral stones: incidence of associated urinary tract findings. AJR Am J Roentgenol 1996; 166(6): 1319–22.
18. Sundaram CP, Saltzman B. Urolithiasis associated with protease inhibitors. J Endourol 1999; 13(4): 309–12.
19. Ege G, Akman H, Kuzucu K, Yildiz S. Can computed tomography scout radiography replace plain film in the evaluation of patients with acute urinary tract colic? Acta Radiol 2004; 45(4): 469–73.
20. Katz D, McGahan JP, Gerscovich EO, Troxel SA, Low RK. Correlation of ureteral stone measurements by CT and plain film radiography: utility of the KUB. J Endourol 2003; 17(10): 847–50.
21. Nakada SY, Hoff DG, Attai S et al. Determination of stone composition by noncontrast spiral computed tomography in the clinical setting. Urology 2000; 55(6): 816–9.
22. Perks AE, Gotto G, Teichman JM. Shock wave lithotripsy correlates with stone density on preoperative computerized tomography. J Urol 2007; 178: 912–5.
23. Pareek G, Hedican SP, Lee FT Jr et al. Shock wave lithotripsy success determined by skin-to-stone distance on computed tomography. Urology 2005; 66(5): 941–4.
24. Brody AS, Donald P. Frush MD et al. Radiation risk to children from computed tomography. Pediatrics 2007; 120(3): 677–82.
25. Brenner DJ, Hall EJ. Computed tomography--an increasing source of radiation exposure. N Engl J Med 2007; 357(22): 2277–84.
26. Poletti PA, Platon A, Rutschmann OT et al. Low-dose vs. standard-dose CT protocol in patients with clinically suspected renal colic. AJR Am J Roentgenol 2007; 188(4): 927–33.
27. Kalra MK, Maher MM, D'Souza RV et al. Detection of urinary tract stones at low-radiation-dose CT with z-axis automatic tube current modulation: phantom and clinical studies. Radiology 2005; 235(2): 523–9.
28. Heneghan JP, McGuire KA, Leder RA et al. Helical CT for nephrolithiasis and ureterolithiasis: comparison of conventional and reduced radiation-dose techniques. Radiology 2003; 229(2): 575–80.
29. Meagher T, Sukumar VP, Collingwood J et al. Low dose computed tomography in suspected acute renal colic. Clin Radiol 2001; 56(11): 873–6.

30. Kluner C, Hein PA, Gralla O et al. Does ultra-low-dose CT with a radiation dose equivalent to that of KUB suffice to detect renal and ureteral calculi? J Comput Assist Tomogr 2006; 30(1): 44–50.

31. Unal D, Yeni E, Karaoglanoglu M et al. Can conventional examinations contribute to the diagnostic power of unenhanced helical computed tomography in urolithiasis? Urol Int 2003; 70(1): 31–5.

32. Mitterberger M, Pinggera GM, Pallwein L et al. Plain abdominal radiography with transabdominal native tissue harmonic imaging ultrasonography vs. unenhanced computed tomography in renal colic. BJU Int 2007; 100(4): 887–90.

33. Pepe P, Motta L, Pennisi M, Aragona F. Functional evaluation of the urinary tract by color-Doppler ultrasonography (CDU) in 100 patients with renal colic. Eur J Radiol 2005; 53(1): 131–5.

34. Opdenakker L, Oyen R, Vervloessem I et al. Acute obstruction of the renal collecting system: the intrarenal resistive index is a useful yet time-dependent parameter for diagnosis. Eur Radiol 1998; 8(8): 1429–32.

35. Akcar N, Ozkan IR, Adapinar B, Kaya T. Doppler sonography in the diagnosis of urinary tract obstruction by stone. J Clin Ultrasound 2004; 32(6): 286–93.

36. Sfakianakis GN, Cohen DJ, Braunstein RH et al. MAG3-F0 scintigraphy in decision making for emergency intervention in renal colic after helical CT positive for a urolith. J Nucl Med 2000; 41(11): 1813–22.

37. Lorberboym M, Kapustin Z, Elias S, Nikolov G, Katz R. The role of renal scintigraphy and unenhanced helical computerized tomography in patients with ureterolithiasis. Eur J Nucl Med 2000; 27(4): 441–6.

38. Sudah M, Vanninen RL, Partanen K et al. Patients with acute flank pain: comparison of MR urography with unenhanced helical CT. Radiology 2002; 223(1): 98–105.

39. Sudah M, Vanninen R, Partanen K et al. MR urography in evaluation of acute flank pain: T2-weighted sequences and gadolinium-enhanced three-dimensional FLASH compared with urography. Fast low-angle shot. AJR Am J Roentgenol 2001; 176(1): 105–12.

40. Saxena SK, Sharma M, Patel M, Oreopoulos D. Nephrogenic systemic fibrosis: an emerging entity. Int Urol Nephrol 2008; 40(3): 715–24.

41. Cormier CM, Canzoneri BJ, Lewis DF et al. Urolithiasis in pregnancy: current diagnosis, treatment, and pregnancy complications. Obstet Gynecol Surv 2006; 61(11): 733–41.

42. White WM, Zite NB, Gash J et al. Low-dose computed tomography for the evaluation of flank pain in the pregnant population. J Endourol 2007; 21(11): 1255–60.

43. Caron N, El Hajjam A, Declèves AE et al. Changes in renal haemodynamics induced by indomethacin in the rat involve cytochrome P450 arachidonic acid-dependent epoxygenases. Clin Exp Pharmacol Physiol 2004; 31(10): 68–90.

44. Brough RJ Lancashire MJ, Prince JR et al. The effect of diclofenac (voltarol) and pethidine on ureteric peristalsis and the isotope renogram. Eur J Nucl Med 1998; 25(11): 1520–3.

45. Nakada SY, Jerde TJ, Bjorling DE, Saban R. Selective cyclooxygenase-2 inhibitors reduce ureteral contraction in vitro: a better alternative for renal colic? J Urol 2000; 163(2): 607–12.

46. Engeler DS, Ackermann DK, Osterwalder JJ, Keel A, Schmid HP. A double-blind, placebo controlled comparison of the morphine sparing effect of oral rofecoxib and diclofenac for acute renal colic. J Urol 2005; 174(3): 933–6.

47. Sandhu DP, Iacovou JW, Fletcher MS et al. A comparison of intramuscular ketorolac and pethidine in the alleviation of renal colic. Br J Urol 1994; 74(6): 690–3.

48. Holdgate A, Pollock T. Systematic review of the relative efficacy of non-steroidal anti-inflammatory drugs and opioids in the treatment of acute renal colic. BMJ 2004; 328(7453): 1401.

49. Wood VM, Christenson JM, Innes GD, Lesperance M, McKnight D. The NARC (Nonsteroidal Anti-inflammatory in Renal Colic) Trial. Single-dose intravenous ketorolac vs. titrated intravenous meperidine in acute renal colic: a randomized clinical trial. CJEM 2000; 2(2): 83–9.

50. Safdar B, Degutis LC, Landry K et al. Intravenous morphine plus ketorolac is superior to either drug alone for treatment of acute renal colic. Ann Emerg Med 2006; 48(2): 173–81.

51. Mora B, Giorni E, Dobrovits M et al. Transcutaneous electrical nerve stimulation: an effective treatment for pain caused by renal colic in emergency care. J Urol 2006; 175(5): 1737–41.

52. Nikiforov S, Cronin AJ, Murray WB, Hall VE. Subcutaneous paravertebral block for renal colic. Anesthesiology 2001; 94(3): 531–2.

53. Morita T, Wada I, Saeki H, Tsuchida S, Weiss RM. Ureteral urine transport: changes in bolus volume, peristaltic frequency, intraluminal pressure and volume of flow resulting from autonomic drugs. J Urol 1987; 137(1): 132–5.

54. Caravati EM, Runge JW, Bossart PJ et al. Nifedipine for the relief of renal colic: a double-blind, placebo-controlled clinical trial. Ann Emerg Med 1989; 18(4): 352–4.

55. Dellabella M, Milanese G, Muzzonigro G. Efficacy of tamsulosin in the medical management of juxtavesical ureteral stones. J Urol 2003; 170: 2202–5.

56. Lee YH, Lee WC, Chen MT et al. Acupuncture in the treatment of renal colic. J Urol 1992; 147(1): 16–8.

57. Hussain Z, Inman RD, Elves AW et al. Use of glyceryl trinitrate patches in patients with ureteral stones: a randomized, double-blind, placebo-controlled study. Urology 2001; 58(4): 521–5.

58. Henry H 2nd, Nordan J, Tomlin EM. Comparison of butorphanol tartrate and meperidine in moderate to severe renal colic. Urology 1987; 29(3): 339–45.

59. Mortelmans LJ, Desruelles D, Baert JA, Hente KR, Tailly GG. Use of tramadol drip in controlling renal colic pain. J Endourol 2006; 20(12): 1010–5.

60. Kober A, Dobrovits M, Djavan B et al. Local active warming: an effective treatment for pain, anxiety and nausea caused by renal colic. J Urol 2003; 170(3): 741–4.

61. Springhart WP, Marguet CG, Sur RL et al. Forced vs. minimal intravenous hydration in the management of acute renal colic: a randomized trial. J Endourol 2006; 20(10): 713–6.

62. Cupisti A, Pasquali E, Lusso S et al. Renal colic in Pisa emergency department: epidemiology, diagnostics and treatment patterns. Intern Emerg Med 2008; 3(3): 241–4.

63. Laird JM, Roza C, Cervero F. Effects of artificial calculosis on rat ureter motility: peripheral contribution to the pain of ureteric colic. Am J Physiol 1997; 272: R1409–16.

64. Sivula A, Lehtonen T. Spontaneous passage of artificial concretions applied in the rabbit ureter. Scand J Urol Nephrol 1967; 1(3): 259–63.

65. Maggi CA, Giuliani S. A pharmacological analysis of calcium channels involved in phasic and tonic responses of the guinea-pig ureter to high potassium. J Auton Pharmacol 1995; 15(1): 55–64.

66. Morita T, Wada I, Suzuki T, Tsuchida S. Characterization of alpha-adrenoceptor subtypes involved in regulation of ureteral fluid transport. Tohoku J Exp Med 1987; 152(2): 111–8.

67. Hollingsworth JM, Rogers MA, Kaufman SR et al. Medical therapy to facilitate urinary stone passage: a meta-analysis. Lancet 2006; 368(9542): 1171–9.

68. Preminger GM, Tiselius HG, Assimos DG et al. Guideline for the management of ureteral calculi. Eur Urol 2007; 52(6): 1610–31.

69. Porpiglia F, Destefanis P, Fiori C, Fontana D. Effectiveness of nifedipine and deflazacort in the management of distal ureter stones. Urology 2000; 56(4): 579–82.

70. Resim S, Ekerbicer H, Ciftci A. Effect of tamsulosin on the number and intensity of ureteral colic in patients with lower ureteral calculus. Int J Urol 2005; 12(7): 615–20.

71. Yilmaz E, Batislam E, Basar MM et al. The comparison and efficacy of 3 different alpha1-adrenergic blockers for distal ureteral stones. J Urol 2005; 173(6): 2010–2.

72. Chang DF, Osher RH, Wang L, Koch DD. Prospective multicenter evaluation of cataract surgery in patients taking tamsulosin (Flomax). Ophthalmology 2007; 114(5): 957–64.

73. Pearle MS, Pierce HL, Miller GL et al. Optimal method of urgent decompression of the collecting system for obstruction and infection due to ureteral calculi. J Urol 1998; 160(4): 1260–4.

74. Sighinolfi MC, Micali S, De Stefani S et al. Noninvasive management of obstructing ureteral stones using electromagnetic extracorporeal shock wave lithotripsy. Surg Endosc 2008; 22(5): 1339–41.

75. Tombal B, Mawlawi H, Feyaerts A et al. Prospective randomized evaluation of emergency extracorporeal shock wave lithotripsy (ESWL) on the short-time outcome of symptomatic ureteral stones. Eur Urol 2005; 47(6): 855–9.

76. Tligui M, El Khadime MR, Tchala K et al. Emergency extracorporeal shock wave lithotripsy (ESWL) for obstructing ureteral stones. Eur Urol 2003; 43(5): 552–5.

7 | Pathophysiology and management of calcium stones

Elaine M Worcester

NATURAL HISTORY OF CALCIUM STONES

Most kidney stones in the industrialized world are composed primarily of calcium salts, in both adults and children. For example, among 2011 patients seen in the Kidney Stone clinic at the University of Chicago who have had a stone analysis, 76% formed stones composed mainly of calcium oxalate, in either the monohydrate (whewhellite) or dihydrate (weddellite) form, and 12% stones that were mainly calcium phosphate (as either hydroxyapatite or brushite). Most stones contain a mixture of both salts, bound together by a macromolecular matrix. The distribution of calcium phosphate as a component of analyzed stones from idiopathic calcium stone formers in our clinic is shown in **Figure 7.1**. Phosphate-containing stones are relatively more common among women (1), although overall, stone disease is more common in men.

After passage of a first idiopathic calcium stone, recurrence is the rule, although it may be delayed. Untreated first-time calcium stone formers have been found to have a 27% chance of recurrence by 5 years (2), 50% by 8–9 years (3), and about 75% by 20 years.(3) However, in those who have already had a recurrence, future stone formation becomes more likely; treatment trials in recurrent calcium stone formers demonstrated new stone formation in about 43–48% of patients in the placebo arm by 3 years.(4–6) Accurate prediction of relapse is difficult with current diagnostic tools, although increasing levels of hypercalciuria (2, 7) and of urine pH (8), as well as increasing number of prior stone events (9) and younger age at first stone (8, 9) have been associated with a tendency to recurrence. Those patients with stones in the setting of systemic disease are likely to recur at higher rates than those with idiopathic stones.

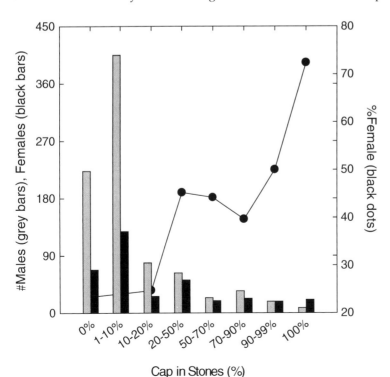

Figure 7.1 Numbers of stones and sex distribution with increasing percent of calcium phosphate (CaP) in stones. The majority of stones formed by both males (grey bars) and females (black bars) were composed primarily of calcium oxalate. However, as percent CaP in stones rose, percent female (black circles connected by line) increased. At CaP% above 90, females predominated. (From ref. 1).

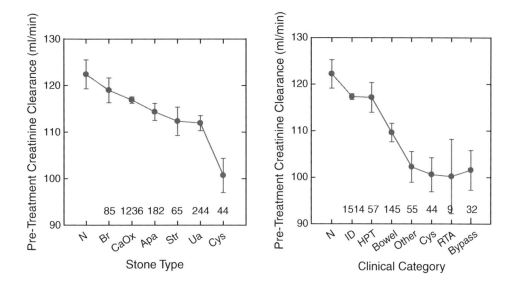

Figure 7.2 Pretreatment creatinine clearances by stone type or clinical category, adjusted for age, weight, and gender, shown as means ± SEM. Patients are from the University of Chicago Kidney Stone Program. Numbers represent patients in each category; overall, 1856 stone formers, 153 normal subjects. N, normal; BR, brushite; CaOx, calcium oxalate; Apa, apatite; Str, struvite; Ua, uric acid; Cys, cystine; ID, idiopathic; HPT, hyperparathyroid; Bowel, bowel disease with or without surgery; Other, rare diseases such as sarcoidosis, drug stones, eating disorders; RTA, renal tubular acidosis; Bypass, obesity bypass. (From ref 10).

Stone formation may be associated with systemic complications, such as hypertension and chronic kidney disease.(10–13) Patients with stones caused by systemic disorders such as distal renal tubular acidosis or enteric hyperoxaluria have a particularly high risk of decreased creatinine clearance (**Figure 7.2**). Causative factors probably include the renal damage from extensive nephrocalcinosis and tubule obstruction, coupled with repeated episodes of obstruction and need for surgical procedures for stone removal, with attendant risk of infection. It is likely that prevention of recurrent stone episodes would be beneficial to prevent further deterioration of renal function, but this is not yet proven.

PHYSICAL CHEMISTRY AND HISTOPATHOLOGY OF CALCIUM STONES

Supersaturation

Effective treatment of stones relies on an understanding of the underlying causes. The fundamental requirement for stone formation is that urine must be supersaturated with respect to the relevant stone mineral; that is, the concentration of the mineral phase exceeds its solubility. Supersaturation may be produced when excretion rates of minerals are high or when urine volume is low, as both situations will raise urine mineral concentrations. The concentrations of the active, ionic form of the minerals may also be modified by substances such as citrate or magnesium that form soluble complexes with calcium or oxalate, respectively, and thereby alter the level of supersaturation. In the case of calcium phosphate, urine pH is another important determinant of solubility. Therefore, simple determination of solute excretion is often not a perfect reflection of urinary supersaturation with respect to calcium salts. Computer algorithms are available to calculate the prevailing levels of supersaturation in a urine sample (14), and usually express the degree of supersaturation as a ratio of the urinary concentration to the known solubility of the given mineral phase. Levels above 1 denote supersaturation and the greater the degree of supersaturation, the higher the risk of crystal formation and stones. Studies of stone formers show that urinary supersaturation correlates with the type of stones that form in a given patient (15), and treatment to lower supersaturation is effective in preventing recurrent stones.

As would be predicted, the level of urinary supersaturation with respect to calcium oxalate increases directly with urine calcium excretion, and inversely with urine volume (**Figure 7.3**).

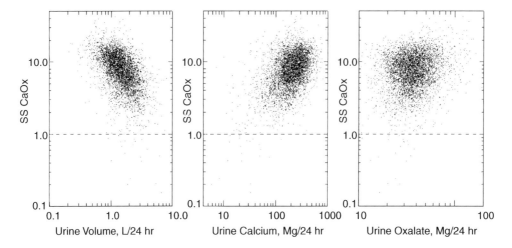

Figure 7.3 Determinants of urine calcium oxalate (CaOx) supersaturation (SS). Calcium oxalate SS, y-axes of each panel, varies strongly with urine volume (left panel), modestly with urine calcium excretion (middle panel), but very little with urine oxalate excretion (right panel). Each point is a single 24-hour urine sample from a patient with nephrolithiasis or normal subject. (From ref 37).

It should be clear from this figure that both calcium and volume are graded risk factors. Data from population studies confirm that risk of stone formation rises directly with urine calcium excretion, with no observable risk threshold over the range of normal values.(16) Urine oxalate excretion may be somewhat higher in idiopathic calcium stone formers than in nonstone formers, but the effect of urine oxalate excretion on supersaturation is more modest than that of calcium and water excretion over the range found in idiopathic stone formers.

Supersaturation with respect to calcium phosphate has a similar relation to volume and calcium excretion as calcium oxalate, except that supersaturation values are distributed above and below 1. In addition to solute concentrations, urine pH is an important determinant of calcium phosphate solubility. Urinary phosphate is a buffer of excreted protons; at low urine pH, phosphate exists in the di-hydrogen form, which does not interact with calcium ion. Higher urine pH leads to increased abundance of urinary mono-hydrogen phosphate (pKa about 6.7), which forms insoluble complexes with calcium, as brushite, which may transform to apatite. More alkaline urine pH (persistently > 6.2) is almost invariably found in patients with greater amounts of calcium phosphate in their stones.(1)

Inhibitors of Crystallization

Since **Figure 7.3** includes data from both normal subjects and stone formers, it is apparent that urine in nonstone formers is almost always supersaturated with respect to calcium oxalate (and sometimes calcium phosphate), indicating that supersaturation, while necessary, is not sufficient to produce stones. Urine of stone formers is usually more supersaturated than that of nonstone formers, which raises the risk of crystal formation. In addition, urine contains inhibitors of crystallization, which can retard nucleation, growth and aggregation of crystals in urine (17); in fact, it is the presence of these substances in urine that allows metastable supersaturation to exist at all. Both small molecules such as citrate and pyrophosphate, and a number of macromolecules, have been shown to possess inhibitory properties *in vitro*. Experimental studies have demonstrated some abnormalities of inhibition in the urine of stone formers compared to that of nonstone formers (18), as well as abnormalities in the excretion pattern of inhibitory proteins (19), suggesting that mechanisms that normally protect against crystallization in the kidney are defective in certain stone formers. The role these molecules play in stone formation is still poorly understood, and is not yet a target for preventive treatment of stones, with the exception of citrate therapy, which will be discussed below.

Histopathology of the Renal Papilla in Stone Formers

Recent studies show that all calcium stone formers studied so far have deposits of calcium phosphate in their renal medulla, but there are different patterns of mineral deposition in the tissue of stone formers who make calcium oxalate and calcium phosphate stones. Although supersaturation is the driving force in all cases, the differing location of crystal deposition suggests that there is more than one mechanism by which crystallization can occur in the kidney.

Idiopathic calcium oxalate stone formers have interstitial apatite deposits, called Randall's plaque, and the amount of plaque found in the papilla correlates directly with urine calcium excretion, and inversely with urine volume (20), that is, with the major determinants of supersaturation. Calcium oxalate stones usually grow attached to these sites of plaque.(21) By contrast, the kidneys of idiopathic stone formers who make calcium phosphate stones composed of brushite have only modest amounts of interstitial apatite, but the inner medullary collecting ducts are filled with crystal deposits composed of apatite, and ducts may be quite dilated, with plugs of crystal protruding from the mouths of the ducts of Bellini.(22) Other phosphate stone formers, such as those with distal renal tubular acidosis (23) or primary hyperparathyroidism (24), share the finding of inner medullary tubule plugs of apatite, with variable amounts of interstitial plaque. In these patients, stones were seldom found attached to plaque, implying a different mechanism by which stone formation was initiated.

Overall, these studies show that there are several different patterns of mineral deposition in medullary tissue, but calcium phosphate is the mineral found in all cases. In patients with severe hyperoxaluria, the intratubular phosphate deposits may also contain small amounts of calcium oxalate.(25) When intra-tubular crystals are found, interstitial scarring is also apparent, suggesting that this route to stone formation may also result in eventual tissue damage. The histopathology of stone formers is described in more detail in Chapter 2.

DIAGNOSISTIC EVALUATION OF CALCIUM STONE FORMERS

Recurrent stone formation is associated with the potential for renal injury, and stone passage or surgical treatment to remove stones is costly in time lost from work and in use of medical resources.(26) Since preventive therapy significantly reduces recurrence rates, it is worthwhile to evaluate patients for underlying causes of stone formation, to guide appropriate treatment. Laboratory evaluation should be done as an outpatient, after the acute stone passage event has resolved, when patients are eating their normal diet. Medications that affect mineral metabolism, such as diuretics, vitamins or mineral supplements, should be stopped for several days before the laboratory studies.

Identification of the type of stone is important to guide evaluation. Any stone material passed should be analyzed by X-ray crystallography or infrared spectroscopy; there are many commercial labs that provide this service. In the absence of a stone analysis, a urinalysis may be helpful to identify crystals, but will often be unrevealing. When there is no evidence to the contrary, it is reasonable to presume that the stone is calcium containing, but pains should be taken to try to analyze any future stones passed or removed to confirm this. A single urine sample to rule out cystinuria with a cyanide- nitroprusside test is advisable.

Determine whether the patient is a single or recurrent stone former. History of prior stone episodes should be taken, including surgical treatments required. X-rays, especially noncontrast CT scans, can define the location, size, and number of stones remaining in the kidneys; coronal sections are particularly helpful. A patient with several stones on X-ray is already a recurrent stone former. A baseline X-ray also allows one to judge the success of treatment by the yardstick of new stone formation or growth of old stones.

Rule out systemic diseases or anatomical abnormalities that increase risk of recurrence or renal damage. For patients with a single episode of calcium stone, or if stone type is unknown, initial evaluation should rule out systemic disorders such as hyperparathyroidism, distal renal tubular acidosis, or hyperoxaluria (**Table 7.1**), by taking a history focused on family history of stones, suggesting a genetic disorder, and on co-existing problems that may indicate a systemic disease causing or aggravating the patient's stones. Important data include onset of stones in childhood or adolescence; a history of inflammatory bowel disease, bowel resection, or bariatric surgery, which may result in enteric hyperoxaluria or volume depletion; nontraumatic bone fractures, which may indicate a disease affecting calcium conservation; or unusual dietary patterns or use of large amounts of calcium supplements. Frequent or recurrent urinary tract infections should also be noted, as well as any history of other kidney or urologic abnormalities such

Table 7.1 Causes of Calcium Stone Formation.

HYPERCALCIURIA

 Hypercalciuria with normocalcemia
  Idiopathic hypercalciuria (commonest)
  Granulomatous diseases (sarcoid, etc.) (rare)
 Hypercalciuria with hypercalcemia
  Primary hyperparathyroidism
  Granulomatous diseases (sarcoid)
  Vitamin D excess
  Malignancy
  Hyperthyroidism
 Hypercalciuria with normocalcemia and metabolic acidosis
  Distal renal tubular acidosis

HYPOCITRATURIA

  Secondary to metabolic acidosis (including protein load)
  Secondary to hypokalemia
  Idiopathic

HYPEROXALURIA

 Dietary hyperoxaluria
  Low calcium diet
  Excess vitamin C
 Enteric hyperoxaluria
  Small bowel resection
  Bariatric surgery
  Fat malabsorption from any cause
 Primary hyperoxaluria – Type 1, Type 2

HYPERURICOSURIA

  High purine diet
  Myeloproliferative disorder

PERSISTENT LOW URINE VOLUME

  Diarrheal states

as single kidney, uretero-pelvic junction obstruction, horseshoe kidney or medullary sponge kidney. Laboratory screening should include a serum panel including calcium, creatinine, bicarbonate, and potassium. Elevated serum calcium suggests primary hyperparathyroidism, but granulomatous diseases should also be considered. Decreased serum bicarbonate should raise the possibility of distal renal tubular acidosis, particularly if accompanied by low serum potassium.

 Conservative therapy with increased fluids is indicated for patients with a single probable calcium stone and without systemic illness.

 For patients with recurrent idiopathic stones, or with systemic disease that makes recurrence likely, preventive treatment is indicated and relies on measures that decrease supersaturation. The correct treatment for a given patient will depend on the assessment of their specific risk factors, and will usually include a combination of fluids, dietary advice, and medications. 24-hour urines should be collected at least twice before starting therapy to assess for factors leading to supersaturation. Several commercial labs offer urine testing for stone formers which is cost effective and includes the analytes shown in **Table 7.2** as well as calculated supersaturation for CaOx, CaP, and uric acid. Increased solute concentrations correlate with supersaturation, but it is difficult to accurately estimate supersaturation without a computer algorithm, particularly when solubilities are pH dependent. Normal ranges for urine solute excretion are suggested in **Table 7.2**, however there is a great deal of overlap between stone formers and nonstone formers, and these values should be thought of as continuous risk factors. After treatment has been prescribed, another 24-hour urine should be collected in 4–8 weeks to evaluate the results. Successful therapy should decrease supersaturation into the normal or low-normal range; in practice, lower is better.

Table 7.2   24-hour urine stone chemistries.

Analyte	Units	Normal Values (non-stone formers)
VOLUME		> 1.5 L/day
pH		5.8–6.2
CALCIUM	mg/day	<250 (F), <300 (M), < 4 mg/kg or <140mg/g creat (both sexes)
OXALATE	mg/day	30–50
CITRATE	mg/day	>550 (F), >450 (M)
URIC ACID	mg/day	<750 (F), < 800 (M)
PHOSPHATE	mg/day	500–1500
MAGNESIUM	mg/day	50–150
SULFATE	mmol/day	20–80
AMMONIA	mmol/day	15–60
SODIUM	mmol/day	50–150
POTASSIUM	mmol/day	20–100
CREATININE	mg/day	15–19 mg/kg (F), 20–24 mg/kg (M)
SS CAOX		6–10
SS CAP		0.5–2
SS URIC ACID		0–1

F, female; M, male; creat, creatinine; GFR, glomerular filtration rate.
Values from University of Chicago Stone Clinic.

PATHOPHYSIOLOGY AND TREATMENT OF CALCIUM STONES

Genetics and Environment

Nephrolithiasis resembles diseases such as diabetes and hypertension, which result from the interplay between genetic predisposition and environmental triggers such as diet.(27) There are rare monogenic disorders that are associated with formation of calcium stones, usually because they cause hypercalciuria or hyperoxaluria (**Table 7.3**). Idiopathic hypercalciuria (IH), which is far more common, appears to have a familial association as well (28), and is found in about 50% of first degree relatives of hypercalciuric stone formers (29) but it is a complex trait, polygenic, and the genes that contribute to it are presently under study.(30)

Environment, especially diet, can modify solute and fluid excretion, which may promote supersaturation and stone formation; the increased incidence of kidney stones in the industrialized countries in the past century probably reflects the intersection of genetic risk and dietary factors. High salt intake is accompanied by increased urine calcium excretion; in healthy subjects the urine calcium increases about 0.6 mmol/day for each 100 mmol/day increment in sodium excretion.(31) Patients with IH have higher calcium excretion at any given sodium excretion, compared to normals (32), and decreasing salt intake can decrease calcium excretion. Sugar (or rapidly metabolized carbohydrate) intake can also increase urine calcium excretion. (33) Likewise, very high protein intakes will increase calcium excretion, in part because of the acid production that occurs as the sulfated amino acids are metabolized. On the other hand, in large epidemiologic studies, higher dietary calcium intake, 800–1000 mg/day, has been found to be protective, compared to low-calcium diets.(34) The impact of diet on stone formation is discussed at greater length in Chapter 4.

Idiopathic Hypercalciuria

Metabolic abnormalities associated with calcium stones are shown in **Table 7.1**. Of these, IH is the most common, being found in 30–60% of adult stone formers.(35) The normal ranges for urine calcium are shown in **Table 7.2**; IH is defined as calcium excretion above these levels. Patients with IH have normal serum calcium, normal or slightly low serum phosphorus, and no overt evidence of bone disease, although subtle bone defects may be present; known causes of hypercalciuria such as primary hyperparathyroidism, sarcoidosis, Cushing's syndrome, cancer, excess vitamin D intake, hyperthyroidism, glucocorticoid use, Paget's disease, or renal tubular acidosis are absent. As noted above, IH has a genetic basis, but expression is influenced by environmental factors, notably diet.

Table 7.3 Monogenic disorders of nephrocalcinosis and calcium stone formation.

Disease	Inheritance	Gene/Gene product	Function	Stones	NC	Phenotype
Dent's disease	X-linked	CLCN5/ClC-5	Endosomal Cl channel	+	+	Hypercalciuria, LMW proteinuria, CRF
Bartter syndrome Type I	AR	SLC12A1/NKCC2	Na-K-2Cl co-transporter		+	Hypercalciuria, hypokalemic alkalosis
Bartter syndrome Type II	AR	KCNJ1/ROMK	K channel		+	Hypercalciuria, hypokalemic alkalosis
Bartter syndrome Type III	AR	CLCNKB/ClC-Kb	Basolateral Cl channel	+	+	Hypercalciuria, hypokalemic alkalosis
Bartter syndrome Type V	AD	CASR/CaSR (severe gain of function)	Calcium sensing receptor	+	+	Hypercalciuria, hypokalemic alkalosis, CRF, hypocalcemia
AD Hypocalcemic hypercalciuria	AD	CASR/CaSR (gain of function)	Calcium sensing receptor		+	Hypercalciuria, CRF, hypocalcemia
Familial hypomagnesemia with hypercalciuria	AR	PCLN1/Paracellin 1	Tight junction protein	+	+	Hypercalciuria, hypermagnesuria, CRF, hypomagnesemia
Hereditary hypophosphatemic rickets with hypercalciuria	AR	SLC34A3/NaPi-IIc	Sodium-phosphate co-transporter	rare	rare	Hypercalciuria, hypophosphatemia, rickets
AD distal renal tubular acidosis	AD	SLC4A1/AE1	Cl-bicarbonate exchanger	+	+	Hypercalciuria, hypokalemia, osteomalacia,
AR distal RTA with hearing loss	AR	ATP6V1B1/B1 subunit of vacuolar H-ATPase	Proton secretion	+	+	Hypercalciuria, hypokalemia, rickets
AR distal RTA	AR	ATP6V0A4/A4 subunit of vacuolar H-ATPase	Proton secretion	+	+	Hypercalciuria, hypokalemia, rickets
Primary hyperoxaluria Type I	AR	AGXT/alanine glyoxylate aminotransferase	Converts glyoxalate to glycine	+		Hyperoxaluria, CRF
Primary hyperoxaluria Type II	AR	GRHPR/Glyoxylate reductase	Converts glyoxylate to glycolate	+		Hyperoxaluria, CRF

NC, nephrocalcinosis; LMW, low molecular weight; CRF, chronic renal failure; AR, autosomal recessive; AD, autosomal dominant; RTA, renal tubular acidosis; aa, amino acid.

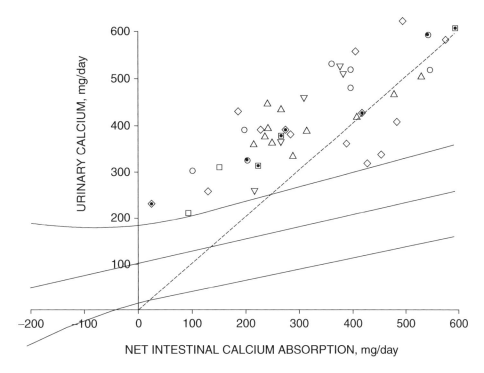

Figure 7.4   Balance studies in subjects with idiopathic hypercalciuria (IH) and controls. In each of 42 metabolic balance studies (studies from different laboratories are denoted by different symbols) IH subjects excrete more calcium (y axis) for their level of net GI calcium absorption (x axis) than did 203 normal subjects represented by the 95% confidence limits (solid lines). In most subjects calcium excretion equaled or exceeded absorption, as shown by the dotted line of identity. (From ref. 36).

IH involves accelerated calcium transport in gut, kidney, and bone, to varying extents. Increased gut absorption of calcium is a feature noted in essentially all patients with IH. Studies that have compared intestinal calcium absorption in patients with IH to that in normal subjects find consistently increased calcium uptake in IH (36, 37) at all levels of calcium intake (38), reflecting an increase in active calcium transport by the intestine. One potential mechanism for increased absorption may be the higher levels of serum calcitriol found in patients with IH compared to normal subjects in many studies.(36, 37) Calcitriol upregulates expression of calcium transport proteins in the intestine, including the apical calcium channel, TRPV6 (39), and calcium absorption is directly related to calcitriol levels. Serum calcium and PTH levels have generally been reported as normal or slightly low in IH.(40)

Careful balance studies show that urine calcium excretion rises in normal subjects as net intestinal calcium absorption (calculated as [diet calcium-fecal calcium]) increases (**Figure 7.4,** solid lines). However, in the same studies, patients with IH excrete more calcium than normal subjects at any level of net calcium absorption (36), and in many cases excrete more calcium than they have absorbed, meaning that some of the urine calcium must be derived from bone, especially at lower levels of calcium intake. This finding implies that IH involves abnormal renal calcium conservation in addition to increased intestinal absorption of calcium.

The cause of the increased urine calcium excretion appears to be decreased renal tubular calcium reabsorption. Although increased gut calcium absorption led to a rise in serum calcium (and therefore the filtered load of calcium at the glomerulus) in studies using single high-calcium foods or calcium alone (41), in studies done using a diet composed of ordinary food containing about 1200 mg calcium, neither ultrafiltrable calcium nor filtered load of calcium differed between the normal subjects and those with IH.(42) Urine calcium excretion was significantly higher after meals in IH subjects, and fractional reabsorption was lower, meaning that the increased calcium absorbed with meals in IH is excreted into the urine mainly via decreased tubule reabsorption. However, PTH levels did not differ between normal subjects and those with IH, nor did urine sodium excretion, as would be expected on this controlled diet. Studies using lithium as a marker for proximal tubule function show that proximal tubule sodium and calcium reabsorption is decreased in patients with IH (43); the increased sodium that reaches the distal nephron is completely reabsorbed, but the extra calcium is not. A second defect in calcium reabsorption may also exist in the distal nephron. The underlying mechanism for such defects remains to be explained.

The fact that patients with IH are prone to go into negative calcium balance, as shown in **Figure 7.4**, also implies that they are at risk of bone mineral loss. Recent studies have confirmed that bone mineral density is often decreased in patients with IH (44), and there is an increased risk of fracture, as well, particularly vertebral fracture.(45, 46) Abnormalities of bone histomorphometry have been demonstrated, which include increased resorption, low bone formation, and a mineralization defect.(47, 48) Abnormal bone formation may contribute to increased urine calcium in patients with IH, and can lead to decreased bone mineralization particularly in the setting of low calcium intake.

Treatment

Treatment trials for patients with calcium stones are shown in **Table 7.4**. Many of the subjects in these trials had IH, sometimes combined with other mild metabolic abnormalities; some had normal levels of calcium excretion, but still responded well to treatment. A randomized trial of fluid intake in patients who had formed a single stone showed a significant decrease in recurrent stones in patients who significantly increased their fluid intake and urine output.(2) Urine volume at the baseline visit was just over 1 L in both groups, but rose to over 2 L in the fluid group and remained there, while the control group had an unchanged urine volume. In the group with greater fluid intake, mean urine saturations for calcium oxalate, brushite, and uric acid all fell significantly, compared to the control group. Patients who relapsed (in either group) had higher baseline calcium excretion than those who did not. Water is the beverage of choice, but other fluids need not be restricted; only grapefruit juice and apple juice have been associated with increased risk of stones in large epidemiologic studies.(49)

Epidemiologic studies have also suggested that higher calcium intake is protective against stone formation, and that high protein and salt intake are associated with increased risk of stones.(34) A controlled trial done in Italy tested whether a diet that had a normal amount of calcium (30 mmol/day) but was restricted in salt (100mmol) and animal protein (52 gm/day) would be superior to a low-calcium diet in preventing relapse in patients with recurrent calcium stones (50) (**Table 7.4**). Both groups were instructed to avoid oxalate rich foods, and were encouraged to increase fluid intake. The men on the higher calcium diet had significantly fewer recurrent stones by five years than those on low calcium diet; both groups had a fall in calcium oxalate supersaturation, but the decrease was significantly greater in the normal calcium group, who also had a significant fall in urine oxalate excretion. In a second trial of a low protein – normal calcium diet, the control group actually had fewer stones than the subjects on the low protein diet, however the diet was not sodium restricted, and urine calcium and oxalate excretions did not appear to fall; supersaturations were not reported.(51) Overall, the trial by Borghi, et al. validates the potential for success with dietary intervention, but emphasizes the need for close supervision and adequate follow-up, which may not be practical for many patients. The DASH-sodium diet (52), which has been shown to lower blood pressure, provides a dietary pattern that matches important features of the diet used by Borghi, and may be useful for dietary counseling.

For many patients with idiopathic recurrent calcium stones, thiazide diuretics are the optimal treatment (**Table 7.4**). Three trials validate their ability to lower urine calcium excretion and calcium oxalate supersaturation, and decrease stone relapse. Trials of less than three years duration have failed to show significance, but all trials lasting at least three years showed efficacy of thiazide to prevent recurrence. The patients in these studies were a mixture of hypercalciuric and normocalciuric stone formers, so the ability of thiazide to decrease urine calcium oxalate supersaturation may be of benefit to those patients without marked increases in urine calcium, as well as those with hypercalciuria. A balance study suggests that thiazide treatment leads to positive calcium balance, as the decrease in urine calcium exceeds the fall in gut calcium absorption that also occurs (53); this would be predicted to be beneficial for bone mineralization. Common side effects of thiazide are a fall in serum potassium, which may require supplementation. A sodium restricted diet will improve response to the medication.

Table 7.4 Treatment trials for prevention of idiopathic calcium stones in adults.

Treatment	Dose	Population studied	Study Duration	Comparison	Recurrence (%)		Quality of Evidence
					Treated	Control	
First Calcium Stone (+/- hypercalciuria, mild hyperoxaluria, hypocitraturia, hyperuricosuria)							
Fluid[a]	Increase fluid intake to keep urine volume > 2 liters/day	CaOx SF (n=199) (M/F=134/65)	5 years	High fluid intake vs. usual intake	12	27	RC (p=0.008)
Recurrent Calcium Stones (+/- hypercalciuria, mild hyperoxaluria, hypocitraturia, hyperuricosuria)							
Diet[b]	Ca 1200 mg/d Na 50 mmol/d Protein 52 gm/d	HC CaOx SF (n=120) (M=120)	5 years	Study diet vs. 400 mg Ca diet	20	38	RC (p=0.04)
Chlorthalidone[c]	25 or 50 mg/day	CaOx SF (n=73) (M/F=63/10)	3 years	Drug vs. placebo	14	46	RCD (p<0.05)
HCTZ[d]	25 mg bid	CaSF (n=50) (M/F=38/12)	3 years	Drug vs. placebo	20	48	RCD (p=0.04)
Indapamide[e] (+/- allopurinol)	2.5 mg/day	HC CaOx SF (n=75) (M/F=59/16)	3 years	Drug vs. placebo	15	43	RCD (p<0.02)
K citrate[f]	20 meq tid	Hypocit Ca SF (n=57) (M/F=25/32)	3 years	Drug vs. placebo	28	80	RCD (p<0.001)
K-Mg citrate[g]	21 meq tid	CaOx SF (n=64) (M/F=50/14)	3 years	Drug vs. placebo	13	64	RCD (RR 0.16)
Na-K citrate[h]	Dose adjusted to keep urine pH 7-7.2	CaOx SF (n=50) (M/F=31/19)	3 years	Drug vs. no Rx	69	73	RC (p=0.65)
Recurrent Calcium Stones (hyperuricosuric, normocalciuric)							
Allopurinol[i]	100 mg tid	CaOx SF (n=72)	39 mo	Drug vs. placebo	31	58	RCD (p<0.05)

Patients are idiopathic calcium stone formers. In all trials, patients with systemic disease, such as hyperparathyroidism, bowel disease, renal tubular acidosis etc. were excluded. CaOx, calcium oxalate; SF, stone former; M, male; F, female; RC, randomized controlled; RCD, randomized controlled double blind; HCTZ, hydrochlorothiazide; HC, hypercalciuric; Ca, calcium; Hypocit, hypocitraturic; RR, relative risk.
a, ref. 2; b, ref. 50; c, ref. 5; d, ref. 6; e, ref. 4; f, ref. 61; g, ref. 62; h, ref. 63; i, ref. 82;

Primary Hyperparathyroidism

Kidney stones occur in approximately 20% of patients with primary hyperparathyroidism (54), and they account for an estimated 5% of all calcium stone formers. In 85% to 95% of cases a single parathyroid adenoma is the cause, while four gland hyperplasia is found in 5–15% of cases, often as part of an inherited syndrome such as multiple endocrine adenomatosis. Parathyroid cancer is rare, found in less than 1% of cases of primary hyperparathyroidism. Elevated PTH levels in serum enhance renal tubule calcium reabsorption and stimulate increased production of calcitriol, which increases gut calcium absorption. Hypercalciuria results from an increased filtered load of calcium, and from the effect of hypercalcemia on the calcium sensing receptor in the kidney to increase calcium excretion. Fractional excretion of calcium is higher than in normal subjects or idiopathic stone formers, despite the increased PTH level.(55)

Serum calcium levels are elevated, but the elevation may be mild; in 105 stone formers diagnosed with hyperparathyroidism in our program the mean serum calcium was 10.81±0.03 mg/dl, compared with 9.54±0.01 in idiopathic stone formers (**Figure 7.5**).(55) Decreased serum phosphate is also found, consistent with the effect of PTH to decrease renal tubular phosphate reabsorption. Serum PTH levels may be elevated, but are not always above the upper limit of normal; however, failure of PTH to be completely suppressed by hypercalcemia strongly suggests hyperparathyroidism. Diagnosis may require repeated measurement of serum calcium and PTH to confirm that they are abnormal, and these should preferably be done fasting to ensure consistency. Urine calcium excretion may be quite elevated compared to idiopathic stone formers or nonstone formers (**Figure 7.5**), and urine supersaturation with respect to both calcium oxalate and calcium phosphate are quite high as a result. Stones may contain both calcium oxalate and calcium phosphate, and renal papillary histology shares features with both idiopathic calcium stone formers (Randall's plaque) and brushite stone formers (plugs of apatite crystals filling inner medullary collecting ducts).(24)

Definitive treatment for stone disease in primary hyperparathyroidism is surgical removal of the enlarged gland(s), preferably by a surgeon experienced in parathyroidectomy. Preoperative localization of parathyroid glands may be done, using radionuclide scans or sometimes ultrasound, CT, or MRI, but it is not clear that such studies improve surgical outcome. Post-operatively, serum calcium and phosphate correct, and urine calcium falls markedly, although it may remain somewhat high (**Figure 7.5**); supersaturation for both calcium oxalate and calcium phosphate also decreases markedly. Stone recurrence and need for urologic procedures drops markedly.(55, 56)

Granulomatous Diseases

Sarcoid, and perhaps other granulomatous diseases, may be complicated by hypercalcemia and hypercalciuria, which may occur in up to 20 and 50% of cases, respectively.(57) The cause is increased calcitriol production in macrophages in the granulomas, which is not under control of PTH. The elevated serum calcitriol levels lead to increased calcium absorption in the GI tract, and suppression of PTH. Both kidney stones and nephrocalcinosis may occur. Treatment may require steroids, but suppression of calcitriol production can be achieved with the use of hydroxychloroquine or ketoconazole, which are inhibitors of the 1-alpha-hydroxylase enzyme.(58)

Hypocitraturia

Citrate is a tricarboxylic organic anion found in urine that can inhibit stone formation by forming soluble complexes with urinary calcium, thus lowering the calcium ion available for binding with oxalate or phosphate. In addition, citrate is a direct inhibitor of calcium crystallization. Low urine citrate, which is found in up to 60% of stone formers (59), is therefore a risk factor for stone formation.

Citrate is filtered at the glomerulus, and reabsorbed in the proximal tubule, and urinary citrate represents the filtered citrate that escaped reabsorption.(60) Control of proximal tubule citrate uptake is not fully understood, but acid–base balance appears to be the most important determinant of urinary citrate excretion (**Table 7.1**). Urine citrate excretion is enhanced by alkalosis and decreased by acidosis. However, frank acidosis, such as in patients with distal renal tubular acidosis, is rare among stone formers; a more common cause may be the acid load imposed by high protein diet. Gastrointestinal loss of bicarbonate with diarrhea will also lead

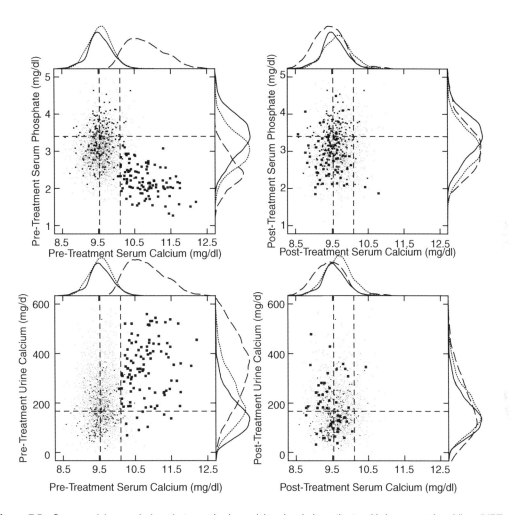

Figure 7.5 Serum calcium and phosphate, and urine calcium levels in patients with hyperparathyroidism (HPT, large symbols), normal subjects (N, small circles), and routine stone formers (SF, cloud of tiny points). Pre-treatment (left panels), serum calcium (x axis of all panels) in HPT was > 10 (females) or 10.1 (males). Non-parametric density distributions (shown at upper and right borders of the figures) show the difference in calcium levels in HPT (dashed lines) compared with N (solid lines) and SF (dotted lines). Serum phosphorus (y axis, upper left panel) decreased with increasing serum calcium in HPT, density distributions shown at right side. Urine calcium (y axis, lower left panel) was higher in HPT than in SF. Post-treatment (right panels) values for calcium, phosphorus and urine calcium in HPT overlapped with SF and NS, with a few exceptions. The mean value and upper limit of normal for serum calcium are depicted by dashed vertical lines on each panel; normal mean values for serum phosphate (upper panels) and urine calcium (lower panels) are shown as horizontal dashed lines. (From ref. 56).

to low urine citrate. Hypokalemia is another common cause of hypocitraturia, and acts via an effect to decrease intracellular pH, which leads to increased uptake of citrate from the glomerular filtrate. Many patients with calcium kidney stones have hypocitraturia with no apparent cause, however, and are currently considered to have idiopathic hypocitraturia.

Treatment

Patients with hypocitraturia can be treated with oral alkali in order to increase urinary citrate excretion (**Table 7.4**); the form of alkali that has been used successfully in treatment trials is potassium citrate or potassium-magnesium citrate.(61, 62) The oral citrate is metabolized to bicarbonate, and the alkali load leads to an increase in urine citrate excretion. In the two trials using a form of potassium citrate, stone recurrences dropped compared to the placebo group; the trial using sodium citrate did not show reduced stone recurrence.(63) Benefit was not limited to patients with hypocitraturia; the ability to lower calcium oxalate supersaturation and augment crystal inhibition may be beneficial to many patients with calcium oxalate stones. Urine pH rises, which may increase calcium phosphate supersaturation, however, and patients should be monitored to avoid excessively high urine pH. In patients treated with thiazide, the resulting hypokalemia may cause hypocitraturia, and use of potassium citrate to raise serum potassium may also correct the hypocitraturia, and enhance the therapeutic effect of thiazide.(64)

Hyperoxaluria

Oxalate is an end-product of glyoxalate, amino acid, and ascorbic acid metabolism produced in the liver. Dietary oxalate also contributes to the daily oxalate load; ordinarily about 10% of ingested oxalate is absorbed. Normally, about half of urinary oxalate is derived from the diet and half from endogenous production (65), and hyperoxaluria can result from an increase in either production or absorption. The recent appreciation that a significant amount of oxalate is secreted into the gut raises the possibility that decreased secretion might also lead to hyperoxaluria (66), but this has not yet been shown in humans.

Dietary hyperoxaluria

Mild dietary hyperoxaluria is common in patients with idiopathic kidney stones, and may be seen if patients adopt a low-calcium diet, which will result in an increase in oxalate absorption from the gut (67); diets unusually high in protein or oxalate may also increase oxalate excretion. Another factor that may affect net oxalate absorption is the presence in the gut of bacteria that can metabolize oxalate, such as *Oxalobacter formigenes*. Stone formers have been found to be colonized with this bacteria at a significantly lower rate than controls (68), although urine oxalate levels did not correlate with the presence or absence of the bacteria. Two short-term studies using pharmacologic preparations of oxalate-degrading bacteria to lower oxalate absorption and thereby urine oxalate have had divergent results (69, 70); no longer term studies have been done as yet. Although there are no trials specifically of low-oxalate diet for idiopathic calcium stone formers, patients with higher oxalate excretion should be advised to avoid oxalate rich foods such as spinach, nuts, potatoes, chocolate, or rhubarb.(71)

Enteric hyperoxaluria

Intestinal oxalate absorption may be significantly increased in the presence of fat malabsorption, which occurs in the setting of small bowel and pancreatico-biliary disease, provided that the colon is present and receiving small bowel effluent (72); examples include ileal resection or bypass. The mechanism of increased absorption is thought to involve binding of diet calcium by free fatty acids in the gut, allowing increased absorption of free oxalate, and possibly altered colonic permeability. Stool losses of fluid and alkali, in addition to the increased oxalate excretion, lead to high levels of supersaturation with respect to calcium oxalate and uric acid in the urine. Patients undergoing modern forms of bariatric surgery also appear to have an increase in urine oxalate excretion (73) and stone formation.

There are no treatment trials of stone prevention in these patients, but urine oxalate may be decreased by diets reduced in fat and oxalate.(72) Use of dietary calcium or calcium supplements taken with meals to bind oxalate may also be helpful; if hypercalciuria occurs, thiazide diuretics may be used to lower urine calcium excretion. Cholestyramine, a bile acid-binding resin, has also been used to bind oxalate in some patients. Sevelamer, a cationic phosphate binder, was tested in patients with enteric hyperoxaluria; urine oxalate levels and urine calcium oxalate supersaturation did not fall significantly, although urine phosphate did.(74) Alkali and fluid supplementation is also beneficial, if tolerated. Monitoring of outcome with 24-hour urines is important to tailor treatment.

Primary hyperoxaluria

Type 1 (PH1) and type 2 (PH2) primary hyperoxaluria arise from rare autosomal recessive genetic disorders of oxalate synthesis.(75, 76) PH1, the most common, is caused by deficiency of a liver-specific enzyme, alanine:glyoxylate aminotransferase (AGT) which leads to impaired glyoxylate metabolism in the peroxisomes of hepatocytes. In 35% of cases, the enzyme is present but mistargeted to the mitochondria, where it is inactive. In remaining cases, the enzyme may be either absent, or nonfunctional. The end result is an increase in synthesis and excretion of oxalate; urine oxalate excretion is 100–300 mg/day, and urine glycolate may also be elevated.

The clinical manifestations include kidney stones, nephrocalcinosis, and renal failure; symptoms usually begin in childhood, often by age 5. Diagnosis should also be suspected in patients with elevated urine oxalate excretion in the absence of bowel disease, or patients with stones and renal failure. Diagnosis depends on metabolic workup and liver biopsy or genetic testing when appropriate.(77, 78)

High doses of pyridoxine, which is a cofactor for the enzyme, lower oxalate production and excretion in some patients, largely those with the targeting error, and can result in long-term clinical stability. Treatment should also include high fluid intake, as in all stone formers. In addition, neutral orthophosphate has been used with success.(79) In those with persistent hyperoxaluria and end-organ damage, definitive treatment is liver-kidney transplantation which supplies a functional enzyme.

PH2, which accounts for about 20% of cases of primary hyperoxaluria, results from deficiency of the enzymes glyoxylate reductase and hydroxypyruvate reductase, caused by the lack of a single cytosolic protein with multiple enzyme activities. The clinical manifestations are similar to PH1, but the course seems to be milder, with less renal failure. An international registry exists for patients with primary hyperoxaluria, to improve the diagnosis and treatment of patients with these rare disorders.(80)

Hyperuricosuria

Elevated urinary uric acid (>800 mg/day in men, > 750 mg/day in women) may be seen in calcium oxalate stone formers.(81) That the elevated uric acid may be causally related to the stone formation is suggested by a placebo-controlled trial using allopurinol to decrease uric acid synthesis and excretion in a group of calcium oxalate stone formers (**Table 7.4**).(82) Over three years, stone recurrence was significantly lower in the group that took allopurinol. The most common cause for the elevated uric acid excretion is a high protein intake, suggesting that modest restriction would also be effective, and potentially safer than allopurinol. The physicochemical mechanism of increased calcium oxalate stone formation is not certain, but uric acid can decrease the solubility of calcium oxalate in solution, so-called "salting out", and this may be the cause.

CALCIUM PHOSPHATE STONES WITH AND WITHOUT DISTAL RENAL TUBULAR ACIDOSIS

Stones composed predominantly of calcium phosphate are less common than calcium oxalate stones (**Figure 7.1**), but they deserve a special mention. The pathological studies described earlier show that the presence of a significant amount of calcium phosphate in stones, as either apatite or brushite, correlates with plugging of inner medullary collecting ducts with apatite crystals, and variable amounts of interstitial scarring, so that formation of such stones seems particularly clinically undesirable. It is worrisome that formation of calcium phosphate stones has been increasing over the past three decades in both sexes.(1) As discussed earlier, formation of calcium phosphate stones correlates with the presence of calcium phosphate supersaturation in urine, which is largely due to an increased urine pH (**Figure 7.6**). Although some patients suffer from abnormalities of urine acidification such as distal renal tubular acidosis, most patients have no systemic disorder, and the higher urine pH is not associated with a defect in proton excretion. We have noted that formation of calcium phosphate stones is strongly associated with an increased number of extracorporeal shock-wave lithotripsy treatments.(1) However, although comparison of patients who converted from calcium oxalate to calcium phosphate stone formation with those who did not convert confirms that those who convert have had a larger number of lithotripsy treatments (83), it does not provide evidence that the lithotripsy itself is clearly responsible for the higher pH. Rather, high pH appears to be present even when patients were still forming calcium oxalate stones, in those destined to convert. Likewise, there was no more use of citrate therapy in those who converted compared to those who did not. However, unlike the other patients, converters had a rise in urine pH on citrate without a rise in citrate concentration, which may have placed them at increased risk for calcium phosphate crystallization. In patients being treated with citrate, it is prudent to monitor the level of urine pH and supersaturation with calcium phosphate, to avoid increasing the risk for calcium phosphate stones. The reason for the rise in phosphate stone formation in recent years is still

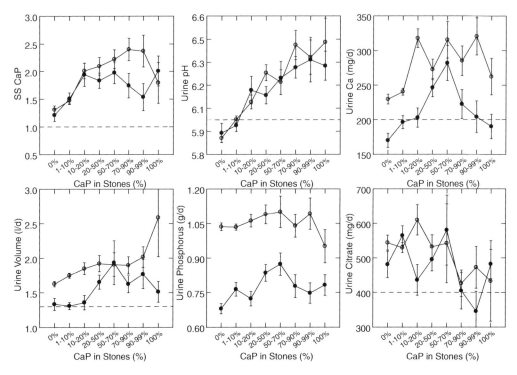

Figure 7.6 Urine stone risk factors with increasing stone CaP%. CaP supersaturation (SS) (y axis) rose with the percent of CaP in stones (x axis) (upper left panel) in men (gray circles) and women (black circles). Urine pH rose with CaP%, which would increase CaP SS (upper middle panel). Urine calcium rose initially, but then plataued in men and fell in women as CaP% increased (upper right panel). Urine volumes were higher at high CaP% values in both sexes (lower left panel). Urine phosphorus excretion (lower middle panel) was variable across CaP%, but higher in men. Urine citrate excretion was lowest at high CaP% values, (lower right panel) but values overlapped, and no significant trend is present. Values are mean ± SEM (From ref. 1).

unsettled, and the link with lithotripsy is provocative, but still unexplained. Also unexplained is the persistently higher urine pH in this group of patients.

Although most calcium phosphate stone formers do not have systemic acidosis, patients with distal renal tubular acidosis (type 1 RTA) have a persistent abnormality in proton secretion and urinary acidification that leads to systemic acidosis. The defect may be inherited (**Table 7.3**) or acquired; acquired RTA may be secondary to autoimmune disease (Sjogren's syndrome, lupus), hypergammaglobulinemic disorders, or idiopathic.(84) In addition to persistently alkaline urine, low urine citrate and hypercalciuria are commonly found, and increase the risk of both stones and nephrocalcinosis.(84, 85) Bone disease and growth retardation are common in pediatric patients. Treatment with potassium citrate can correct acidosis and decrease hypercalciuria, but careful follow-up is needed to ensure that urinary supersaturation with respect to calcium phosphate falls; persistent hypercalciuria should be treated as for idiopathic hypercalciuria when acidosis has been corrected.

REFERENCES

1. Parks JH, Worcester EM, Coe FL et al. Clinical implications of abundant calcium phosphate in routinely analyzed kidney stones. Kidney Int 2004; 66: 777–85.
2. Borghi L, Meschi T, Amato F et al. Urinary volume, water and recurrences of idiopathic calcium nephrolithiasis: a 5-year randomized prospective study. J Urol 1996; 155: 839–43.
3. Sutherland JW, Parks JH, Coe FL. Recurrence after a single renal stone in a community practice. Miner Electrolyte Metab 1985; 11: 267–9.
4. Borghi L, Meschi T, Guerra A, Novarini A. Randomized prospective study of a nonthiazide diuretic, indapamide, in preventing calcium stone recurrences. J Cardiovasc Pharmacol 1993; 22(Suppl 6): S78–S86.

5. Ettinger B, Citron JT, Livermore B, Dolman LI. Chlorthalidone reduces calcium oxalate calculous recurrence but magnesium hydroxide does not. J Urol 1988; 139: 679–84.

6. Laerum E, Larsen S. Thiazide Prophylaxis of Urolithiasis: a double-blind study in general practice. Acta Med Scand 1984; 215: 383–9.

7. Strauss AL, Coe FL, Deutsch L, Parks JH. Factors that predict relapse of calcium nephrolithiasis during treatment: a prospective study. Am J Med 1982; 72: 17–24.

8. Trinchieri A, Ostini F, Nespoli R et al. A prospective study of recurrence rate and risk factors for recurrence after a first renal stone. J Urol 1999; 162 (1): 27–30.

9. Parks JH, Coe FL. An increasing number of calcium oxalate stone events worsens treatment outcome. Kidney Int 1994; 45: 1722–30.

10. Worcester EM, Parks JH, Evan AP, Coe FL. Renal function in patients with nephrolithiasis. J Urol 2006; 176: 600–3.

11. Gillen DL, Worcester EM, Coe FL. Decreased renal function among adults with a history of nephrolithiasis: a study of NHANES III. Kidney Int 2005; 67: 685–90.

12. Gillen DL, Coe FL, Worcester EM. Nephrolithiasis and increased blood pressure among females with high body mass index. Am J Kidney Dis 2005; 46: 263–9.

13. Madore F, Stampfer MJ, Rimm EB, Curhan GC. Nephrolithiasis and risk of hypertension. Am J Hypertens 1998; 11: 46–53.

14. Werness PG, Brown CM, Smith LH, Finlayson B. Equil 2: a basic computer program for the calculation of urinary saturation. J Urol 1985; 134: 1242–4.

15. Asplin J, Parks J, Lingeman J et al. Supersaturation and stone composition in a network of dispersed treatment sites. J Urol 1998; 159: 1821–5.

16. Curhan GC, Willett WC, Speizer FE, Stampfer MJ. Twenty-four-hour urine chemistries and the risk of kidney stones among women and men. Kidney Int 2001; 59: 2290–8.

17. Kumar V, Lieske JC. Protein regulation of intrarenal crystallization. Curr Opin Nephrol Hypertens 2006; 15: 374–80.

18. Asplin JR, Parks JH, Chen MS et al. Reduced crystallization inhibition by urine from men with nephrolithiasis. Kidney Int 1999; 56: 1505–16.

19. Bergsland KJ, Kelly JK, Coe BJ, Coe FL. Urine protein markers distinguish stone-forming from non-stone-forming relatives of calcium stone formers. Am J Physiol Renal Physiol 2006; 291: F530–F536.

20. Kuo RL, Lingeman JE, Evan AP et al. Urine calcium and volume predict coverage of renal papilla by Randall's plaque. Kidney Int 2003; 64: 2150–4.

21. Matlaga BR, Williams JC Jr, Kim SC et al. Endoscopic evidence of calculus attachment to Randall's plaque. J Urol 2006; 175: 1720–4.

22. Evan AP, Lingeman JE, Coe FL et al. Crystal-associated nephropathy in patients with brushite nephrolithiasis. Kidney Int 2005; 67: 576–91.

23. Evan AP, Lingeman J, Coe F et al. Renal histopathology of stone-forming patients with distal renal tubular acidosis. Kidney Int 2007; 71: 795–801.

24. Evan AP, Lingeman JE, Coe FL et al. Histopathology and surgical anatomy of patients with primary hyperparathyroidism and calcium phosphate stones. Kidney Int 2008; 74: 223–9.

25. Evan AP, Coe FL, Gillen D et al. Renal intratubular crystals and hyaluronan staining occur in stone formers with bypass surgery but not with idiopathic calcium oxalate stones. Anat Rec (Hoboken) 2008; 291: 325–34.

26. Saigal CS, Joyce G, Timilsina AR. Urologic diseases in america project: Direct and indirect costs of nephrolithiasis in an employed population:opportunity for disease management? Kidney Int 2005; 68: 1808–14.

27. Gambaro G, Vezzoli G, Casari G et al. Genetics of hypercalciuria and calcium nephrolithiasis: From the rare monogenic to the common polygenic forms. Am J Kidney Dis 2004; 33: 963–86.

28. Goldfarb DS, Fischer ME, Keich Y, Goldberg J. A twin study of genetic and dietary influences on nephrolithiasis: a report from the Vietnam Era Twin (VET) registry. Kidney Int 2005; 67: 1053–61.

29. Coe FL, Parks JH, Moore ES. Familial idiopathic hypercalciuria. N Engl J Med 1979; 300: 337–40.

30. Vezzoli G, Soldati L, Gambaro G. Update on primary hypercalciuria from a genetic perspective. J Urol 2008; 179: 1676–82.

31. Lemann J Jr. Pathogenesis of idiopathic hypercalciuria and nephrolithiasis, chap. 32, in Disorders of bone and mineral metabolism, 1st ed., edited by Coe FL, Favus MJ, New York, Raven Press, 1992: 685–706.

32. Lemann J Jr, Worcester EM, Gray RW. Hypercalciuria and stones. [Review]. Am J Kidney Dis 1991; 17: 386–91.

33. Lemann J Jr, Piering WF, Lennon EJ. Possible role of carbohydrate-induced calciuria in calcium oxalate kidney-stone formation. N Engl J Med 1969; 280: 232–7.

34. Curhan GC, Willett WC, Rimm EB, Stampfer MJ. A Prospective study of dietary calcium and other nutrients and the risk of symptomatic kidney stones. N Engl J Med 1993; 328: 833–8.

35. Worcester EM, Coe FL. New insights into the pathogenesis of idiopathic hypercalciuria. Semin Nephrol 2008; 28: 120–32.

36. Coe FL, Favus MJ, Asplin JR. Nephrolithiasis, chap. 39, in The Kidney, 7th ed., edited by Brenner BM, Rector FCJr, Philadelphia, Elsevier, 2004: 1819–66.

37. Coe FL, Parks JH, Evan AP, Worcester E. Pathogenesis and treatment of nephrolithiasis, chap. 68, in Seldin and Giebisch's The Kidney, edited by Alpern R, Hebert S Elsevier, Inc., 2007: 1945–77.

38. Lemann J Jr. Idiopathic hypercalciuria, chap. 30, in Disorders of bone and mineral metabolism, 2nd ed., edited by Coe FL, Favus M Lippincott, 2002: 673–97.

39. Hoenderop JGJ, Nilius B, Bindels RJM. Calcium absorption across epithelia. Physiol Rev 2005; 85: 373–422.

40. Monk RD, Bushinsky DA. Pathogenesis of idiopathic hypercalciuria, chap. 32, in Kidney stones: Medical and surgical management, edited by Coe FL, Favus MJ, Pak CYC et al. Lippincott-Raven, 1996: 759–72.

41. Schwille PO, Rumenapf G, Schmidtler JKR. Fasting and post calcium load serum calcium, parathyroid hormone, calcitonin, in male idiopathic calcium urolithiasis. Exp Clin Endocrinol 1987; 90: 71–5.

42. Worcester EM, Gillen DL, Evan AP et al. Evidence that postprandial reduction of renal calcium reabsorption mediates hypercalciuria of patients with calcium nephrolithiasis. Am J Physiol Renal Physiol 2007; 292: F66–F75.

43. Worcester E, Coe FL, Evan AP et al. Evidence for increased postprandial distal nephron calcium delivery in hypercalciuric stone forming patients. Am J Physiol Renal Physiol epubm 2008; 295: F1286–F1294.

44. Bataille P, Achard JM, Fournier A et al. Diet, Vitamin D and vertebral mineral density in hypercalciuric calcium stone formers. Kidney Int 1991; 39: 1193–205.

45. Melton LJ, Crowson CS, Khosla S et al. Fracture risk among patients with urolithiasis: a population-based cohort study. Kidney Int 1998; 53: 459–64.

46. Lauderdale DS, Thisted RA, Wen M, Favus MJ. Bone mineral density and fracture among prevalent kidney stone cases in the Third National Health and Nutrition Examination Survey. J Bone Miner Res 2001; 16: 1893–8.

47. Zerwekh JE. Bone disease and idiopathic hypercalciuria. Semin Nephrol 2008; 28: 133–42.

48. Gomes SA, dos Reis LM, Noronha IL et al. RANKL is a mediator of bone resorption in idiopathic hypercalciuria. Clin J Am Soc Nephrol 2008; 3: 1446–52.

49. Goldfarb DS, Coe FL. Beverages, diet, and prevention of kidney stones. Am J Kidney Dis 1999; 33: 398–400.

50. Borghi L, Schianchi T, Meschi T et al. Comparison of two diets for the prevention of recurrent stones in idiopathic hypercalciuria. N Engl J Med 2002; 346: 77–84.

51. Hiatt RA, Ettinger B, Caan B et al. Randomized controlled trial of low animal protein, High fiber diet in the prevention of recurrent calcium oxalate kidney stones. Am J Epidemiol 1996; 144: 25–33.

52. Sacks FM, Svetkey LP, Vollmer WM et al. Effects on blood pressure of reduced dietary sodium and the Dietary Approaches to Stop Hypertension (DASH) diet. DASH-Sodium Collaborative Research Group. New Engl J Med 2001; 344: 3–10.

53. Coe FL, Parks JH, Bushinsky DA et al. Chlorthalidone promotes mineral retention in patients with idiopathic hypercalciuria. Kidney Int 1988; 33: 1140–6.

54. Silverberg SJ, Shane E JT. A 10-year prospective study of primary hyperparathyroidism with or without parathyroid surgery. N Engl J Med 1999; 341: 1249–55.

55. Parks JH, Coe FL, Evan AP, Worcester EM. Clinical and laboratory characteristics of calcium stone formers with and without primary hyperparathyroidism. BJU International epub 2009; 103(5): 670–8.

56. Kaplan EL, Tanaka R, Younes N. Primary Hyperparathyroidism, chap. 35, in Kidney stones: Medical and surgical management, 1 ed., edited by Coe FL, Favus MJ, Pak CYC et al., Philadelphia, Lippincott-Raven Publishers, 1996: 803–20.

57. Rizzato G, Colombo P. Nephrolithiasis as a presenting feature of chronic sarcoidosis: a prospective study. Sarcoidosis Vasc Diffuse Lung Dis 1996; 13: 167–72.

58. Sharma OP. Vitamin D, calcium, and sarcoidosis. Chest 1996; 109: 535–9.

59. Parks JH, Ruml LA, Pak CYC. Hypocitraturia, chap. 40, in Kidney stones: Medical and surgical management, 1 ed., edited by Coe FL, Favus MJ, Pak CYC et al., Philadelphia, Lippincott-Raven, 1996: 905–20.

60. Hamm LL, Hering-Smith KS. Pathophysiology of hypocitraturic nephrolithiasis. Endocrinol Metab Clin N Am 2002; 31: 885–93.

61. Barcelo P, Wuhl O, Servitge E et al. Randomized double-blind study of potassium citrate in idiopathic hypocitraturic calcium nephrolithiasis. J Urol 1993; 150: 1761–4.

62. Ettinger B, Pak CY, Citron JT et al. Potassium-magnesium citrate is an effective prophylaxis against recurrent calcium oxalate nephrolithiasis. J Urol 1997; 158: 2069–73.

63. Hofbauer J, Hobarth K, Szabo N, Marberger M. Alkali citrate prophylaxis in idiopathic recurrent calcium oxalate urolithiasis - a prospective randominzed study. Br J Urol 1994; 73: 362–5.

64. Nicar MJ, Peterson R, Pak CYC. Use of potassium citrate as potassium supplement during thiazide therapy of calcium nephrolithiasis. J Urol 1984; 131: 430–3.

65. Holmes RP, Goodman HO, Assimos DG. Contribution of dietary oxalate to urinary oxalate excretion. Kid Int 2001; 59: 270–6.

66. Jiang Z, Asplin JR, Evan AP et al. Calcium oxalate urolithiasis in mice lacking anion transporter Slc26a6. Nat Genet 2006; 38: 474–8.
67. von Unruh GE, Voss S, Sauerbruch T, Hesse A. Dependence of oxalate absorption on the daily calcium intake. J Am Soc Nephrol 2004; 15: 1567–73.
68. Kaufman DW, Kelly JP, Curhan GC et al. Oxalobacter formigenes may reduce the risk of calcium oxalate kidney stones. J Am Soc Nephrol 2008; 19: 1197–203.
69. Goldfarb DS, Modersitzki F, Asplin JR. A randomized, controlled trial of lactic acid bacteria for idiopathic hyperoxaluria. Clin J Am Soc Nephrol 2007; 2: 745–9.
70. Campieri C, Campieri M, Bertuzzi V et al. Reduction of oxaluria after an oral course of lactic acid bacteria at high concentration. Kidney Int 2008; 60: 1097–105.
71. Taylor EN, Curhan GC. Oxalate intake and the risk for nephrolithiasis. J Am Soc Nephrol 2007; 18: 2198–204.
72. Worcester EM: Stones from bowel disease. Endocrinol Metab Clin North Am 2002; 31: 979–99.
73. Asplin JR, Coe FL. Hyperoxaluria in kidney stone formers treated with modern bariatric surgery. J Urol 2007; 177: 565–9.
74. Lieske JC, Regnier C, Dillon JJ. Use of sevelamer hydrochloride as an oxalate binder. J Urol 2008; 179: 1407–10.
75. Asplin JR. Hyperoxaluric calcium nephrolithiasis. Endocrinol Metab Clin North Am 2002; 31: 927–49.
76. Bobrowski AE, Langman CB. The primary hyperoxalurias. Semin Nephrol 2008; 28: 152–62.
77. Monico CG, Rossetti S, Schwanz HA et al. Comprehensive mutation screening in 55 probands with type 1 primary hyperoxaluria shows feasibility of a gene-based diagnosis. J Am Soc Nephrol 2007; 18: 1905–14.
78. Milliner DS. The primary hyperoxalurias: An algorithm for diagnosis. Am J Nephrol2005; 25: 154–60.
79. Milliner DS, Eickholt JT, Bergstralh EJ et al. Results of long-term treatment with orthophosphate and pyridoxine in patients with primary hyperoxaluria. N Engl J Med 1994; 331(23): 1553–8.
80. Lieske JC, Monico CG, Holmes WS et al. International registry for primary hyperoxaluria. Am J Nephrol 2005; 25, 290–6.
81. Sorensen CMCPS. Hyperuricosuric calcium nephrolithiasis. Endocrinol Metab Clin N Am 2002; 31: 915–25.
82. Ettinger B, Tang A, Citron JT et al. Randomized trial of allopurinol in the prevention of calcium oxalate calculi. N Engl J Med 1986; 315: 1386–9.
83. Parks JH, Coe FL, Evan AP, Worcester EM. Urine pH in renal calcium stone formers who do and do not increase stone phosphate content with time. Nephrol Dial Transplant 2009; 24(1):130–6.
84. Lash JP, Cowell G, Arruda JAL. Calcium nephrolithiasis and renal tubular acidosis. Chap. 32 in Disorders of bone and mineral metabolism, 2nd ed. Coe FL, Favus MJ, eds. Philadelphia, Lippincott Williams & Wilkins, 2002: 717–40.
85. Soriano JR. Renal tubular acidosis: the clinical entity. J Am Soc Nephrol 2002; 13: 2160–70.

8 | Uric acid nephrolithiasis: Pathogenesis, diagnosis, and treatment

Khashayar Sakhaee

INTRODUCTION

Uric acid (UA) was first identified two centuries ago as one of the main compositions of kidney stones.(1) The pathophysiologic mechanisms responsible for UA stone formation are complex and can be divided into congenital, acquired, and idiopathic causes.(2) There has been a recent interest in the pathogenesis of idiopathic UA nephrolithiasis (IUAN), since the majority of cases of UA stone formation are comprised of IUAN subjects. It has recently been shown that IUAN and the metabolic syndrome (MS) share many of the same characteristic features. Specifically unduly low urinary pH, the principle abnormality responsible for the formation of UA stones, has been directly related to the number of features of the MS.(3)

EPIDEMIOLOGY OF UA NEPHROLITHIASIS AND ITS LINK TO THE MS

The global distribution of UA nephrolithiasis is heterogeneous and the prevalence of UA stones varies throughout different areas of the world. This distribution is highest in the Middle East (4) and certain regions in Europe.(5) With the exception of the Midwestern section of the U.S., due to its widespread Hmong immigrant population (6), UA nephrolithiasis is responsible for 10% of the entire kidney stone burden of the United States.(7)

The MS is an aggregate of features that increases the risk of type 2 diabetes mellitus (T2DM) and atherosclerotic cardiovascular disease. A retrospective analysis of the University of Texas Southwestern Medical Center's stone registry in Dallas, Texas, displayed a high prevalence of MS characteristics present in patients with IUAN.(8–11) This registry also reported a higher prevalence of UA stones among patients with T2DM (12) (Figure 8.1). The result of this study was later confirmed by numerous epidemiologic studies that displayed an association between obesity, weight gain, and T2DM (all of which are characteristics of the MS) and an increased risk for nephrolithiasis.(13, 14) One limitation of these large epidemiologic studies was their lack of identification of stone type. However, T2DM and greater body mass index (BMI) have been shown to be independent risk factors for nephrolithiasis, specifically for UA stones.(15)

ETIOLOGIC MECHANISMS OF UA STONE FORMATION

Low urine volume, unduly acidic urine pH, and hyperuricosuria are three main factors necessary in the development of UA stones. Unduly acidic urine is an invariant feature in UA stone formation. UA nephrolithiasis may develop due to an inborn error in metabolism (2, 16, 17) or secondary causes such as chronic diarrhea (18), strenuous physical exercise (19), and a high purine diet.(20) In IUAN, the most prevalent cause of UA nephrolithiasis, none of the above abnormalities are detected (21) (Figure 8.2).

PHYSICOCHEMICAL PROPERTIES OF UA

In higher mammals, UA is an end product of purine metabolism. In these species, serum UA concentrations and urinary UA levels are high due to the absence of the hepatic enzyme, Uricase, which converts UA into the more soluble compound allantoin.(22) Under normal circumstances, urinary UA solubility is limited to approximately 96 mg/L. In humans, with a

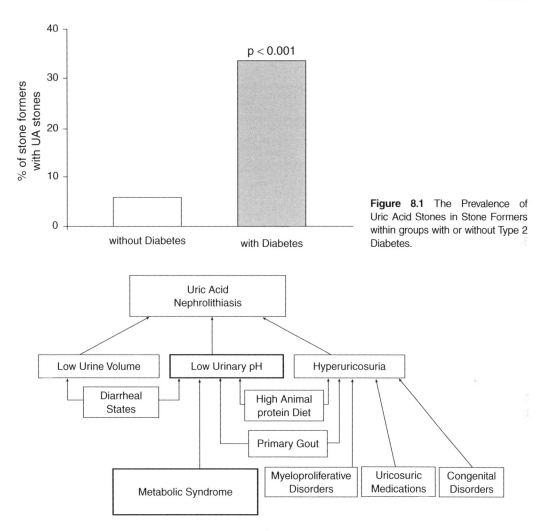

Figure 8.1 The Prevalence of Uric Acid Stones in Stone Formers within groups with or without Type 2 Diabetes.

Figure 8.2 Pathogenesis and Etiologies of Uric Acid Nephrolithiasis.

urinary uric acid excretion of 600 mg/day, this exceeds the limit of solubility and increases the propensity of precipitation.(23) Urine pH also plays a key role in UA solubility. UA is a weak organic acid with an ionization constant (pKa) of 5.5.(24, 25) Therefore, at a urine pH of less than 5.5, the urinary environment becomes supersaturated with poorly soluble, undissociated UA and precipitates to form UA stones (1, 26, 27) (Figure 8.3). In addition, UA crystals may increase the propensity toward the formation of mixed UA and calcium oxalate stones. This occurs through the heterogeneous nucleation and epitaxial crystal growth processes.(28–31) The solubility of urate in the urinary environment is not finite and is influenced by urinary electrolyte composition. The solubility of monopotassium urate has been shown to be higher compared to monosodium urate.(29, 32) The difference in the physicochemical properties of these urate salts has been fundamental in the development of potassium alkali treatment which is far superior to sodium alkali therapy in UA stone formers.(27)

UA Homeostasis

The three major sources of UA production are: 1) de novo synthesis, 2) tissue breakdown, and 3) diet. UA production mainly occurs in the liver and involves the recycling of guanine and hypoxanthine. With an excess in the nucleotide, these bases are converted into xanthine, and consequently into UA mediated by the enzyme xanthine oxidase.(23) Although endogenous purine turnover may affect the production of UA, in a steady state and under normal conditions, endogenous purine turnover does not change significantly. Therefore, UA

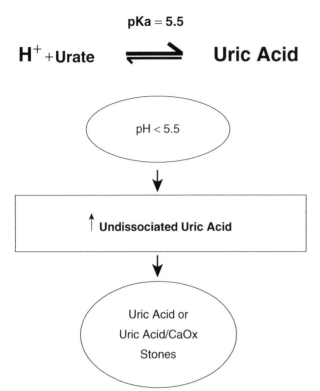

pKa = 5.5

$H^+ + $Urate $\rightleftharpoons$ **Uric Acid**

pH < 5.5

↑ **Undissociated Uric Acid**

Uric Acid or

Uric Acid/CaOx

Stones

Figure 8.3 Physicochemical Scheme for the Development of Uric Acid Stones.

production is minimally influenced by this process.(33) However, with increased tissue breakdown as detected in certain disease states such as myeloproliferative conditions, hematologic disorders, and after chemotherapeutic regimens, purine turnover increases and substantially increases the UA load to the blood and its excretion into the urine.(34) De novo UA synthesis and tissue catabolism makes up half of the daily urate load. The remaining half is acquired from dietary intake. The dietary influence on serum UA and urinary UA is generally very small. However, overindulgence of a high purine diet can significantly increase the serum and urinary UA concentrations.(35, 36) Enteric UA excretion comprises ¼ of daily UA excretion, with the remaining ¾ excreted into the urine.(37)

Renal UA excretion

The processes involved in the renal handling of UA are intricate, involving glomerular filtration, tubular reabsorption, secretion, and post-secretory reabsorption. Normally, 90% of filtered UA is reclaimed and reabsorbed by the proximal renal tubule. Despite the complexity of UA handling, recent advanced have been made in defining various transporters influencing renal tubular reabsorption. UA transporter URAT1 (encoded by SLC22A12) has recently been identified as a major influence in renal tubular UA reabsorption.(38, 39) Certain organic anions including lactate, nicotinate, and pyrazinamide (PZA) have been shown to enhance URAT1-mediated urate absorption by the proximal renal tubular cell.(38) However, the activity of this transporter has also been shown to be inhibited by uricosuric agents such as Probenecid, Benzbromarone, and non-steroid anti-inflammatory drugs. Unfortunately, the mechanism responsible for UA secretion has not been fully elucidated. An increased UA excretion in excess of the glomerular filtration rate has been reported in certain patients with URAT1 mutations. (40) Since UA is not known to be produced in the renal proximal tubular cell, it has been suggested that its apical secretion may initially involve a basolateral uptake of UA. Certain organic anion transporters (OATs) are expressed in the basolateral membrane, and may be the candidate which increase UA uptake into the renal proximal tubular cell, increasing its secretion. (39, 41, 42) Other transporters which may be candidates in the mediation of urate secretion are: OAT1 (which is expressed in the apical membrane of porcine renal proximal tubular cells) (43), and multiresistant-associated protein 4.(44) The contribution of OAT1 in human urate secretion

Table 8.1   Risk Factors for Uric Acid Nephrolithiasis.

Low Urinary Volume		• Chronic Diarrhea • Excessive Perspiration/Exercise • Chronic Dehydration
Hyperuricosuria	Enzymatic Deficiencies	• Hypoxanthine Guanine Phosphoribosyl Transferase Deficiency: Lesch Nyhan Syndrome • Phosphoribosylpyrophosphate Synthetase Overactivity • Glucose-6-Phosphatase Deficiency: Type I Glycogen Storage Disease • Xanthine Oxidase Deficiency
	URAT 1 Mutations	• Hypouricemic Hyperuricosuria
	Urate Overproduction	• Gout • High Dietary Purine Intake • Myeloproliferative Disorders • Hemolytic Anemia • Chemotherapy-Induced Tumor Lysis
	Uricosuric Drugs	• Probenecid • High Dose Salicylates • Radiocontrast Agents • Losartan
Low Urinary pH	Increased Base Loss	• Diarrhea
	Increased Acid Intake	• High animal protein consumption
	Increased Endogenous Acid Production	• Insulin Resistance • Exercise-Induced Lactic Acidosis
	Decreased Urinary Ammonium Excretion	• Insulin Resistance • Gout

Source: Previously Published as a modification of: Cameron et al. *Urol CNn North Am*, 2002.

is unknown at this time. A urate channel has also been proposed in the mediation of UA transport.(45, 46) However, its relevance to the UA handling in humans also remains unknown.

PATHOPHYSIOLOGY OF UA NEPHROLITHIASIS

The three most important factors in the development of UA nephrolithiasis are low urine volume, hyperuricosuria, and abnormally acidic urine pH (Table 8.1).

Low urine volume
Low urine volume is one of the major factors contributing to the development of UA nephrolithiasis. The supersaturation of urine with respect to stone-forming substances occurs more readily with low urine volume.(47) This mechanism is likely responsible for stone formation in patients with chronic diarrhea, excessive sweating in hot environments, or following strenuous exercise.(18, 19) This usually occurs when low urinary volume is associated with excessively acidic urine due to diarrheal alkali loss and following excessive acid production as occurs with strenuous physical exercise.(18, 19)

Hyperuricosuria
Hyperuricosuria is encountered as the result of dietary influences and/or genetic disorders. Certain patients with primary gout are an example in which dietary influences and urate overproduction both contribute to increased serum UA concentrations and urinary UA excretion. However, it has been argued that this abnormality may not be seen in all gouty patients.(26, 48)

Hyperuricosuria is an invariant feature in certain rare hereditary enzymatic UA pathway mutations including: 1) X-linked hypoxanthine guanine phosphoribosyl transferase deficiency, 2) X-linked phosphoribosylpyrophosphate synthetase overactivity, and 3) autosomal recessive glucose-6-phosphatase deficiency.(16) Typically, these patients present significantly elevated serum UA (>10mg/dl) and significantly elevated urinary UA (>1000mg/day) with an increased risk of kidney stones, renal failure, and gout. The affected subjects may present these abnormalities during childhood. However, serum UA concentrations may remain normal until puberty.(49) A recently described genetic mutation of the URAT1 has also reportedly been associated with hyperuricosuria, hypouricemia, a high risk of kidney stones, and exercise-induced acute renal failure.(40, 50)

UA overproduction may occur due to secondary causes as well, and eventually lead to hyperuricosuria. This ensues as a result of high dietary protein intake and/or increased tissue catabolism seen malignancies and chemotherapy. Certain drugs such as Probenecid, high-dose salicylates, and radiocontrast agents may also increase urinary UA excretion. The risk of kidney stones augments early after the institution of these drugs or when in association with hyperuricemia.(23) Therefore, the limitation of these agents is suggested in patients who are in a state of UA overproduction.

Acidic urine pH

Low urinary pH is the principle metabolic abnormality in patients with IUAN (26), the most common cause of UA stone formation.(2) It has been revealed that IUAN shares similar phenotypic characteristics with the MS.(26, 51) Cross-sectional studies conducted independently in kidney stone formers and normal subjects have displayed an inverse relationship between urinary pH, body weight, and features of the MS.(3, 52) Low urinary pH as a factor in UA stone formation was first described in the early 1960s (53) with low ammonium (NH_4^+) excretion attributed as the principle defect. This defect was suggested to be due to the impaired enzymatic conversion of glutamine to α-ketogluatrate, which ultimately results in lower urinary NH_4^+ excretion.(54–57) However, the validity of this metabolic pathway was refuted by further investigation. A major breakthrough elucidating the pathogenic mechanism of abnormal urinary acidity in patients with IUAN has emerged over the past 10 years. Metabolic studies have shown that unduly acidic urine may be due to a combination of lowered NH_4^+ excretion and increased endogenous acid production.(12, 26, 51)

Impaired NH_4^+ excretion

NH_4^+, a major urinary buffer, is known to be tightly regulated by an alteration in acid-base balances.(58) Under normal circumstances, most protons are buffered by ammonia to form NH_4^+. The remaining protons are buffered by titratable acids (TA). Therefore, urinary pH remains within a normal range. In IUAN patients with defective NH_4^+ excretion, most protons are buffered by TA to maintain an acid-base homeostasis. However, this occurs at the expense of low urinary pH, a conducive environment for UA precipitation. A recent metabolic balance study performed in IUAN patients found a significantly lower ratio of urinary NH_4^+ excretion to net acid excretion (NAE) compared to normal subjects (26) (Figure 8.4). This defect was further unmasked with an oral acid load following a single dose of ammonium chloride.(26) These results propose that impaired NH_4^+ excretion may play an important role in influencing the abnormally acidic urine found in IUAN. Furthermore, it also suggests that defective renal ammoniagenesis and low urinary pH may be general features of the MS rather than solely in association with IAUN.(3, 51, 52, 58) In addition, a hyperinsulinemic euglycemic clamp study was found to support a causal relationship between peripheral insulin resistance, urinary NH_4^+ excretion, and low urinary pH.(59) In this study, urinary NH_4^+ excretion was shown to increase in lean normal subjects but did not change in patients with IUAN. These discoveries help substantiate the potential role of insulin resistance in urinary acidification.(59)

Additional experimental evidence has shown that insulin plays an important role both in renal ammonia synthesis and renal NH_4^+ excretion.(60–63) It has been demonstrated that insulin receptors are expressed in various segments of the kidney.(64, 65) Furthermore, it has also been shown that the increased circulating concentration of free fatty acids found in the MS may also act as a substitute substrate for glutamine as an energy source for the kidney, thereby reducing the production of NH_4^+.(66)

Increased endogenous acid production

A metabolic study comparing IUAN subjects and normal control subjects, both on fixed, low acid-ash diets, found a higher NAE in IUAN.(23) A further study comparing subjects with varying degrees of insulin sensitivity also showed a higher NAE in IUAN and nonstone-forming

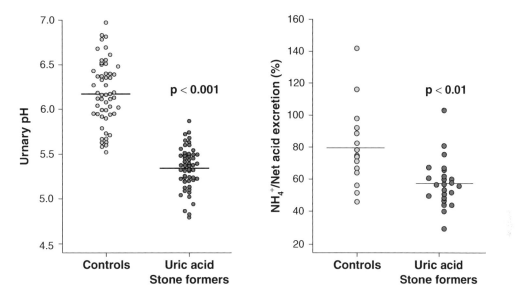

Figure 8.4 Renal Acidification in Uric Acid Stone Formers.

T2DM, compared to normal subjects.(51) This high NAE was shown to persist on both ad-lib and fixed, low acid-ash diets. These studies imply that increased NAE may not only be related to dietary influences, but is potentially attributed to increased endogenous acid production perhaps as a result of obesity and/or insulin resistance.(51) However, the exact source and the nature of this putative endogenous acid has yet to be fully explored.

Renal lipotoxicity

Impaired insulin sensitivity has been shown to occur as a result of fat redistribution in certain organs including the heart (67), liver (68, 69), skeletal muscles, and in the pancreatic β cells.(67, 68, 70–73) This process of fat redistribution into nonadipocyte tissue has been termed lipotoxicity.(70) Cellular injury following the deposition of fat in these target organs may result from the accumulation of certain toxic byproducts, including nonesterified fatty acids and their toxic metabolites including fatty acyl CoA, diacylglycerol, and ceramide.(74–76) Recent studies have shown a potential role of lipotoxicity in the pathogenesis of renal disease.(75, 77, 78) However, it is unknown whether renal lipotoxicity plays a role in defective NH_4^+ excretion and increased endogenous acid production (Figure 8.5) .

DIAGNOSIS

General diagnosis

An initial step in the diagnosis of UA stones is a complete metabolic evaluation to exclude secondary causes that may contribute to UA stone formation.(79) This evaluation must begin with a stone analysis to identify the nature of the kidney stone. Unfortunately, in most occasions, the kidney stone may not be available. Under such circumstances, the physician must rely on an extensive metabolic workup involving full blood and 24-hour urine profiles.(33) The 24-hour urinary chemistries must include total volume, pH, creatinine, sodium, potassium, calcium, magnesium, oxalate, citrate, sulfate, and chloride. This panel is required in order to assess dietary influences and/or the presence of other associated metabolic abnormalities. Urinary sulfate is a surrogate acid-ash diet marker. A high acid-ash diet exaggerates underlying urinary acidification defects and can further influence urinary pH. Moreover, hyperuricosuria can ensue from the overindulgence of a purine-rich diet found in meat, poultry, and fish. This may exacerbate UA stone formation or increase the risk of mixed UA and calcium oxalate stones. A radiologic evaluation is also important since radiolucent UA stones can be readily shown by computerized tomography.

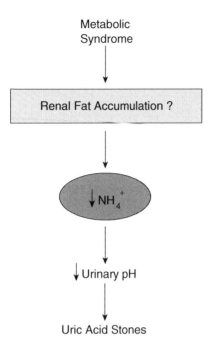

Metabolic Syndrome

Renal Fat Accumulation ?

$\downarrow NH_4^+$

$\downarrow$ Urinary pH

Uric Acid Stones

Figure 8.5 Pathogenesis of Idiopathic Uric Acid Nephrolithiasis.

Table 8.2 Differential Diagnosis of UA Stones.

| Stone Type | Ragiographic Findings | Urinary Findings | | | | Serum UA Findings | Response to Alkali Therapy |
		pH	UA	$FE_{uric\ acid}$	Calcium		
UA Stones	Radiolucent	Decreased	Normal	Decreased	Normal	Increased	Positive
Mixed UA/ Calcium Oxalate Stones	Mixed Radiolucent and Radioopaque	Normal to Decreased	Normal to Increased	Normal to Decreased	Normal to Increased	Normal to Increased	Positive
Hyperuricosuric Calcium Stones	Radioopaque	Normal	Increased	Normal	Normal	Normal	Positive
Xanthine Stones	Radiolucent	Normal	Increased to Normal	Normal	Normal	Decreased	Negative
2, 8-DHA Stones	Radiolucent	Normal	Normal	Normal	Normal	Normal	Negative

UA: Uric Acid.
FE: Fractional Excretion.
Source: Previously published as a modification of: Cameron et al. *Urol Cliri North Am*, 2002.

Differential diagnosis

Xanthine and 2,8-dihydroxyadenine (2,8-DHA) stones are radiolucent and can only be diagnosed with a stone analysis. Xanthine stones are found in patients on allopurinol treatment and in certain inherited disorders such as Lesch-Nyhan Syndrome or hereditary xanthinuria. 2,8-DHA stones are also seen in patients with adenine phosphoribosyl transferase deficiencies. (1, 49) One important diagnostic deficiency usually ignored by practicing physicians is distinguishing between hyperuricosuric calcium oxalate stone formation and UA stone formation. (80, 81) Urinary pH differs between these two presentations. Urinary pH is usually above 5.5 in hyperuricosuric calcium oxalate stone formers, where urinary pH is normally below 5.5 in patients with UA stones. Moreover, hyperuricosuria may not be detected in patients with pure UA stones (Table 8.2).

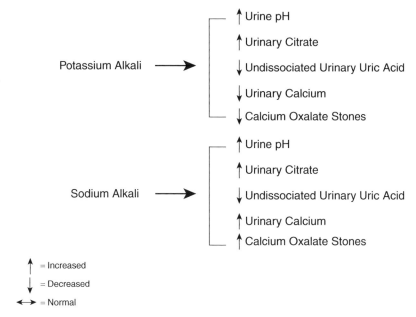

Potassium Alkali ⟶ ⎰ ↑ Urine pH
⎪ ↑ Urinary Citrate
⎨ ↓ Undissociated Urinary Uric Acid
⎪ ↓ Urinary Calcium
⎩ ↓ Calcium Oxalate Stones

Sodium Alkali ⟶ ⎰ ↑ Urine pH
⎪ ↑ Urinary Citrate
⎨ ↓ Undissociated Urinary Uric Acid
⎪ ↑ Urinary Calcium
⎩ ↑ Calcium Oxalate Stones

↑ = Increased
↓ = Decreased
↔ = Normal

Figure 8.6   A Comparison of Various Alkali Treatments.

TREATMENT

Conservative treatment

Conservative treatment for UA stones involves strict dietary and fluid modifications. Sufficient fluid intake of 3 L per day is necessary to attain at least 2 liters of urine per day. Additional fluid intake must be considered in those individuals who work outside in a hot environment and those who perform strenuous physical exercise.(19) Additionally, a rigid restriction of dietary protein consumption should be encouraged. The daily Recommended Dietary Allowances are 0.8g/kg per day. It is unknown whether proteins from varying sources have differential effects on urinary pH and/or urinary UA excretion.

Pharmacological treatment

The most important factor in the treatment of UA stone formers is low urine pH. Both potassium and sodium alkali treatment can effectively raise urinary pH and prevent stone recurrence.(27, 82, 83) However, it has been shown that potassium alkali is advantageous since it reduces urinary calcium excretion and therefore may decrease the risk of calcium oxalate stone formation as well.(27, 82) Sodium alkali may be an appropriate choice for those patients with impaired renal function and in those with a GI intolerance for potassium salt. The recommended daily dose for both of these treatments depends on the size of the patient and the rise in their urinary pH. However, the recommended initial dose is between 30 and 40mEq/day. Urinary pH should be monitored after three months of treatment in order to avoid the propensity of calcium phosphate stones by maintaining a urinary pH above 6.1 and below 6.7 (84) (Figure 8.6). In rare instances, carbonic anhydrase inhibitors (Diamox®) can be used as an alternative alkalinizing agent. However, the physician should be aware of its complications including systemic metabolic acidosis, hypocitraturia, and a highly alkaline urine that may increase the risk of calcium phosphate stones.(85–87) Allopurinol treatment should be considered in women with a urinary UA excretion higher than 600mg/day and in men with urinary UA higher than 700mg/day. Allopurinol treatment is a main-stay treatment in patients with primary gout, inherited UA metabolism disorders, and in a state of increased tissue turnover. Side effects of this treatment are infrequent; however, careful consideration should be made in its use in patients with renal insufficiency.(88) There is no alternative treatment to allopurinol to date. Febuxostate®, a treatment which has not been approved by the FDA, is a related purine analog inhibitor of xanthine oxidase. Febuxostate® may be used in those patients who do not tolerate Allopurinol treatment. However, its potential beneficial effect against UA stone formation has yet to be studied.

CONCLUSION

In the Unites States, the increased prevalence of obesity parallels the rise in nephrolithiasis.(89) Several cross-sectional studies have suggested that the increased prevalence of UA stones is associated with the MS, obesity, and T2DM.(12, 15, 90, 91) Two abnormalities have been shown to be the primary features in the underlying abnormal urinary pH in patients with IUAN. These abnormalities include defective urinary NH_4^+ excretion and increased endogenous acid production. There is emerging data suggesting that renal lipotoxicity may have a role in certain renal diseases. It is also possible that such a defect may play a role in the pathogenesis of IUAN as well. Further understanding of these pathophysiological mechanisms may lead to the development of future treatments.

ACKNOWLEDGMENTS

The author was supported by the National Institutes of Health Grants P01-DK20543 and M01-RR00633.
The author acknowledges the editorial assistance of Ms. Hadley Armstrong.

DISCLOSURES

The author has nothing to disclose.

REFERENCES

1. Riese RJ, Sakhaee K. Uric acid nephrolithiasis: pathogenesis and treatment. J Urol 1992; 148(3): 765–71.
2. Maalouf NM, Cameron MA, Moe OW, Sakhaee K. Novel insights into the pathogenesis of uric acid nephrolithiasis. Curr Opin Nephrol Hypertens 2004; 13(2): 181–9.
3. Maalouf NM, Cameron MA, Moe OW, Adams-Huet B, Sakhaee K. Low urine pH: A novel feature of the metabolic syndrome. Clin J Am Soc Nephrol 2007; 2(5): 883–8.
4. Atsmon A, DeVries A, Frank M. Uric acid lithiasis. Elsevier: Amsterdam; 1963.
5. Hesse A, Schneider HJ, Berg W, Hienzsch E. Uric acid dihydrate as urinary calculus component. Invest Urol 1975; 12(5): 405–9.
6. Portis AJ, Hermans K, Culhane-Pera KA, Curhan GC. Stone disease in the Hmong of Minnesota: initial description of a high-risk population. J Endourol 2004; 18(9): 853–7.
7. Mandel NS, Mandel GS. Urinary tract stone disease in the United States veteran population. II. Geographical analysis of variations in composition. J Urol 1989; 142: 1516–21.
8. Executive Summary of the third report of The National Cholesterol Education Program (NCEP) expert panel on detection, evaluation, and treatment of high blood cholesterol in adults (Adult Treatment Panel III). JAMA 2001; 285(19): 2486–97.
9. Alberti KG, Zimmet PZ. Definition, diagnosis and classification of diabetes mellitus and its complications. Part 1: diagnosis and classification of diabetes mellitus provisional report of a WHO consultation. Diabet Med 1998; 15(7): 539–53.
10. Eckel RH, Grundy SM, Zimmet PZ. The metabolic syndrome. Lancet 2005; 365(9468): 1415–28.
11. Reaven GM. The kidney: an unwilling accomplice in syndrome X. Am J Kidney Dis 1997; 30(6): 928–31.
12. Pak CY, Sakhaee K, Moe O et al. Biochemical profile of stone-forming patients with diabetes mellitus. Urology 2003; 61(3): 523–7.
13. Taylor EN, Stampfer MJ, Curhan GC. Obesity, weight gain, and the risk of kidney stones. JAMA 2005; 293(4): 455–62.
14. Taylor EN, Stampfer MJ, Curhan GC. Diabetes mellitus and the risk of nephrolithiasis. Kidney Int 2005; 68(3): 1230–5.
15. Daudon M, Traxer O, Conort P, Lacour B, Jungers P. Type 2 diabetes increases the risk for uric acid stones. J Am Soc Nephrol 2006; 17(7): 2026–33.
16. Moe OW, Abate N, Sakhaee K. Pathophysiology of uric acid nephrolithiasis. Endocrinol Metab Clin North Am 2002; 31(4): 895–914.

17. Mineo I, Kono N, Hara N et al. Myogenic hyperuricemia. A common pathophysiologic feature of glycogenosis types III, V, and VII. N Engl J Med 1987; 317(2): 75–80.

18. Grossman MS, Nugent FW. Urolithiasis as a complication of chronic diarrheal disease. Am J Dig Dis 1967; 12(5): 491–8.

19. Sakhaee K, Nigam S, Snell P, Hsu MC, Pak CY. Assessment of the pathogenetic role of physical exercise in renal stone formation. J Clin Endocrinol Metab 1987; 65(5): 974–9.

20. Reddy ST, Wang CY, Sakhaee K, Brinkley L, Pak CY. Effect of low-carbohydrate high-protein diets on acid-base balance, stone-forming propensity, and calcium metabolism. Am J Kidney Dis 2002; 40(2): 265–74.

21. Pak CY. Medical management of nephrolithiasis in Dallas: update 1987. J Urol 1988; 140(3): 461–7.

22. Rafey MA, Lipkowitz MS, Leal-Pinto E, Abramson RG. Uric acid transport. Curr Opin Nephrol Hypertens 2003; 12(5): 511–6.

23. Asplin JR. Uric acid stones. Semin Nephrol 1996; 16(5): 412–24.

24. Coe FL, Strauss AL, Tembe V, Le Dun S. Uric acid saturation in calcium nephrolithiasis. Kidney Int 1980; 17(5): 662–8.

25. Finlayson B, Smith L. Stability of first dissociable proton of uric acid. J Chem Engl Data 1974; 19: 94–7.

26. Sakhaee K, Adams-Huet B, Moe OW, Pak CY. Pathophysiologic basis for normouricosuric uric acid nephrolithiasis. Kidney Int 2002; 62(3): 971–9.

27. Sakhaee K, Nicar M, Hill K, Pak CY. Contrasting effects of potassium citrate and sodium citrate therapies on urinary chemistries and crystallization of stone-forming salts. Kidney Int 1983; 24(3): 348–52.

28. Coe FL, Kavalach AG. Hypercalciuria and hyperuricosuria in patients with calcium nephrolithiasis. N Engl J Med 1974; 291(25): 1344–50.

29. Pak CY, Waters O, Arnold L et al. Mechanism for calcium urolithiasis among patients with hyperuricosuria: supersaturation of urine with respect to monosodium urate. J Clin Invest 1977; 59(3): 426–31.

30. Pak CY, Hayashi Y, Arnold LH. Heterogeneous nucleation with urate, calcium phosphate and calcium oxalate. Proc Soc Exp Biol Med 1976; 153(1): 83–7.

31. Pak CY, Arnold LH. Heterogeneous nucleation of calcium oxalate by seeds of monosodium urate. Proc Soc Exp Biol Med 1975; 149(4): 930–2.

32. Wilcox WR, Khalaf A, Weinberger A, Kippen I, Klinenberg JR. Solubility of uric acid and monosodium urate. Med Biol Eng 1972; 10(4): 522–31.

33. Cameron MA, Sakhaee K. Uric acid nephrolithiasis. Urol Clin North Am 2007; 34(3): 335–46.

34. Sorensen L. Extrarenal disposal of uric acid. In: Kelley W, Weiner I, editors. Uric acid Springer-Verlag: New York, 1978: 325–36.

35. Pak CY, Barilla DE, Holt K et al. Effect of oral purine load and allopurinol on the crystallization of calcium salts in urine of patients with hyperuricosuric calcium urolithiasis. Am J Med 1978; 65(4): 593–9.

36. Fellstrom B, Danielson BG, Karlstrom B et al. The influence of a high dietary intake of purine-rich animal protein on urinary urate excretion and supersaturation in renal stone disease. Clin Sci (Lond) 1983; 64(4): 399–405.

37. Sorensen LB. Role of the intestinal tract in the elimination of uric acid. Arthritis Rheum 1965; 8(5): 694–706.

38. Enomoto A, Kimura H, Chairoungdua A et al. Molecular identification of a renal urate anion exchanger that regulates blood urate levels. Nature 2002; 417(6887): 447–52.

39. Hediger MA, Johnson RJ, Miyazaki H, Endou H. Molecular physiology of urate transport. Physiology (Bethesda) 2005; 20: 125–33.

40. Ichida K, Hosoyamada M, Hisatome I et al. Clinical and molecular analysis of patients with renal hypouricemia in Japan-influence of URAT1 gene on urinary urate excretion. J Am Soc Nephrol 2004; 15(1): 164–73.

41. Sekine T, Watanabe N, Hosoyamada M, Kanai Y, Endou H. Expression cloning and characterization of a novel multispecific organic anion transporter. J Biol Chem 1997; 272(30): 18526–9.

42. Cha SH, Sekine T, Fukushima JI et al. Identification and characterization of human organic anion transporter 3 expressing predominantly in the kidney. Mol Pharmacol 2001; 59(5): 1277–86.

43. Jutabha P, Kanai Y, Hosoyamada M et al. Identification of a novel voltage-driven organic anion transporter present at apical membrane of renal proximal tubule. J Biol Chem 2003; 278(30): 27930–8.

44. van Aubel RA, Smeets PH, van den Heuvel JJ, Russel FG. Human organic anion transporter MRP4 (ABCC4) is an efflux pump for the purine end metabolite urate with multiple allosteric substrate binding sites. Am J Physiol Renal Physiol 2005; 288(2): F327–F333.

45. Lipkowitz MS, Leal-Pinto E, Rappoport JZ, Najfeld V, Abramson RG. Functional reconstitution, membrane targeting, genomic structure, and chromosomal localization of a human urate transporter. J Clin Invest 2001; 107(9): 1103–15.

46. Uchino H, Tamai I, Yamashita K et al. p-aminohippuric acid transport at renal apical membrane mediated by human inorganic phosphate transporter NPT1. Biochem Biophys Res Commun 2000; 270(1): 254–9.

47. Pak CY, Skurla C, Harvey J. Graphic display of urinary risk factors for renal stone formation. J Urol 1985; 134(5): 867–70.

48. Alvarez-Nemegyei J, Medina-Escobedo M, Villanueva-Jorge S, Vazquez-Mellado J. Prevalence and risk factors for urolithiasis in primary gout: is a reappraisal needed? J Rheumatol 2005; 32(11): 2189–91.

49. Cameron JS, Moro F, Simmonds HA. Gout, uric acid and purine metabolism in paediatric nephrology. Pediatr Nephrol 1993; 7(1): 105–18.

50. Tanaka M, Itoh K, Matsushita K et al. Two male siblings with hereditary renal hypouricemia and exercise-induced ARF. Am J Kidney Dis 2003; 42(6): 1287–92.

51. Cameron MA, Maalouf NM, Adams-Huet B, Moe OW, Sakhaee K. Urine composition in type 2 diabetes: predisposition to uric acid nephrolithiasis. J Am Soc Nephrol 2006; 17(5): 1422–8.

52. Maalouf NM, Sakhaee K, Parks JH et al. Association of urinary pH with body weight in nephrolithiasis. Kidney Int 2004; 65(4): 1422–5.

53. Henneman PH, Wallach S, Dempsey EF. The metabolism defect responsible for uric acid stone formation. J Clin Invest 1962; 41: 537–42.

54. Gutman AB, Yue TF. An Abnormality of Glutamine Metabolism in Primary Gout. Am J Med 1963; 35: 820–31.

55. Pagliara AS, Goodman AD. Elevation of plasma glutamate in gout. Its possible role in the pathogenesis of hyperuricemia. N Engl J Med 1969; 281(14): 767–70.

56. Pollak VE, Mattenheimer H. Glutaminase activity in the kidney in gout. J Lab Clin Med 1965; 66(4): 564–70.

57. Sperling O, Wyngaarden JB, Starmer CF. The kinetics of intramolecular distribution of 15N in uric acid after administration of (15N) glycine. A reappraisal of the significance of preferential labeling of N-(3+9) of uric acid in primary gout. J Clin Invest 1973; 52(10): 2468–85.

58. DuBose TD Jr, Good DW, Hamm LL, Wall SM. Ammonium transport in the kidney: new physiological concepts and their clinical implications. J Am Soc Nephrol 1991; 1(11): 1193–203.

59. Abate N, Chandalia M, Cabo-Chan AV Jr, Moe OW, Sakhaee K. The metabolic syndrome and uric acid nephrolithiasis: novel features of renal manifestation of insulin resistance. Kidney Int 2004; 65(2): 386–92.

60. Krivosikova Z, Spustova V, Dzurik R. Participation of P-dependent and P-independent glutaminases in rat kidney ammoniagenesis and their modulation by metabolic acidosis, hippurate and insulin. Physiol Res 1998; 47(3): 177–83.

61. Chobanian MC, Hammerman MR. Insulin stimulates ammoniagenesis in canine renal proximal tubular segments. Am J Physiol 1987; 253: F1171–F1177.

62. Klisic J, Hu MC, Nief V et al. Insulin activates Na(+)/H(+) exchanger 3: Biphasic response and glucocorticoid dependence. Am J Physiol Renal Physiol 2002; 283(3): F532–F539.

63. Nagami GT. Luminal secretion of ammonia in the mouse proximal tubule perfused in vitro. J Clin Invest 1988; 81(1): 159–64.

64. Meezan E, Freychet P. Specific insulin receptors in rat renal glomeruli. Ren Physiol 1980; 3(1-6): 72–8.

65. Nakamura R, Emmanouel DS, Katz AI. Insulin binding sites in various segments of the rabbit nephron. J Clin Invest 1983; 72(1): 388–92.

66. Vinay P, Lemieux G, Cartier P, Ahmad M. Effect of fatty acids on renal ammoniagenesis in in vivo and in vitro studies. Am J Physiol 1976; 231(3): 880–7.

67. Szczepaniak LS, Dobbins RL, Metzger GJ et al. Myocardial triglycerides and systolic function in humans: in vivo evaluation by localized proton spectroscopy and cardiac imaging. Magn Reson Med 2003; 49(3): 417–23.

68. Szczepaniak LS, Nurenberg P, Leonard D et al. Magnetic resonance spectroscopy to measure hepatic triglyceride content: prevalence of hepatic steatosis in the general population. Am J Physiol Endocrinol Metab 2005; 288(2): E462–E468.

69. Browning JD, Szczepaniak LS, Dobbins R et al. Prevalence of hepatic steatosis in an urban population in the United States: Impact of ethnicity. Hepatology 2004; 40(6): 1387–95.

70. Lee Y, Hirose H, Ohneda M et al. Beta-cell lipotoxicity in the pathogenesis of non-insulin-dependent diabetes mellitus of obese rats: impairment in adipocyte-beta-cell relationships. Proc Natl Acad Sci U S A 1994; 91(23): 10878–82.

71. Bachmann OP, Dahl DB, Brechtel K et al. Effects of intravenous and dietary lipid challenge on intramyocellular lipid content and the relation with insulin sensitivity in humans. Diabetes 2001; 50(11): 2579–84.

72. McGavock JM, Victor RG, Unger RH, Szczepaniak LS. Adiposity of the heart, revisited. Ann Intern Med 2006; 144(7): 517–24.

73. McGarry JD. Banting lecture 2001: Dysregulation of fatty acid metabolism in the etiology of type 2 diabetes. Diabetes 2002; 51(1): 7–18.

74. Unger RH. Lipotoxic diseases. Annu Rev Med 2002; 53: 319–36.

75. Weinberg JM. Lipotoxicity. Kidney Int 2006; 70(9): 1560–6.

76. Schaffer JE. Lipotoxicity: When tissues overeat. Curr Opin Lipidol 2003; 14(3): 281–7.

77. Bagby SP. Obesity-initiated metabolic syndrome and the kidney: a recipe for chronic kidney disease? J Am Soc Nephrol 2004; 15(11): 2775–91.

78. Wahba IM, Mak RH. Obesity and obesity-initiated metabolic syndrome: mechanistic links to chronic kidney disease. Clin J Am Soc Nephrol 2007; 2(3): 550–62.

79. Cameron MA, Pak CY. Approach to the patient with the first episode of nephrolithiasis. Clin Rev Bone Miner Metab 2004; 2: 265–78.

80. Sorensen CM, Chandhoke PS. Hyperuricosuric calcium nephrolithiasis. Endocrinol Metab Clin North Am 2002; 31(4): 915–25.

81. Pak CY, Poindexter JR, Peterson RD, Koska J, Sakhaee K. Biochemical distinction between hyperuricosuric calcium urolithiasis and gouty diathesis. Urology 2002; 60(5): 789–94.

82. Pak CY, Sakhaee K, Fuller C. Successful management of uric acid nephrolithiasis with potassium citrate. Kidney Int 1986; 30(3): 422–8.

83. Freed SZ. The alternating use of an alkalizing salt and acetazolamide in the management of cystine and uric acid stones. J Urol 1975; 113(1): 96–9.

84. Coe FL, Evan A, Worcester E. Kidney stone disease. J Clin Invest 2005; 115(10): 2598–08.

85. Gordon EE, Sheps SG. Effect of acetazolamide on citrate excretion and formation of renal calculi. N Engl J Med 1957; 256(26): 1215–9.

86. Lamb EJ, Stevens PE, Nashef L. Topiramate increases biochemical risk of nephrolithiasis. Ann Clin Biochem 2004; 41: 166–9.

87. Kuo RL, Moran ME, Kim DH et al. Topiramate-induced nephrolithiasis. J Endourol 2002; 16(4): 229–31.

88. Becker MA, Schumacher HR Jr, Wortmann RL et al. Febuxostat compared with allopurinol in patients with hyperuricemia and gout. N Engl J Med 2005; 353(23): 2450–61.

89. Stamatelou KK, Francis ME, Jones CA, Nyberg LM, Curhan GC. Time trends in reported prevalence of kidney stones in the United States: 1976-1994. Kidney Int 2003; 63(5): 1817–23.

90. Daudon M, Lacour B, Jungers P. Influence of body size on urinary stone composition in men and women. Urol Res 2006; 34(3): 193–9.

91. Daudon M, Lacour B, Jungers P. High prevalence of uric acid calculi in diabetic stone formers. Nephrol Dial Transplant 2005; 20(2): 468–9.

9 | Pathophysiology and management of cystine stones

John R Asplin

Cystinuria is an inherited disorder of amino acid metabolism (OMIM 220100) in which there is reduced renal and intestinal transport of cystine and the dibasic amino acids lysine, arginine, and ornithine. Cystine is an amino acid formed by the linkage of two cysteine molecules via a disulfide bond. Cystine has a much lower solubility than cysteine, which leads to the clinically relevant feature of cystinuria, cystine urolithiasis. Cystine stones were first described by Wollaston in 1810 when he reported two bladder stones composed of a previously unrecognized substance.(1) He believed the substance was an oxide and named it cystic oxide in honor of its origin in the bladder. Berzelius later demonstrated the substance was not an oxide and renamed the new compound cystine.(2)

Cystinuria is one of the most common inherited diseases, with an estimated prevalence of 1:7,000.(3) The prevalence of cystine stones varies depending on the population being studied, ranging from 1:2,500 in Libyan Jews to 1:100,000 in Sweden.(4) In the United States the prevalence is estimated as 1:15,000.(5) Prevalence studies may underestimate the level of disease as not all people homozygous for the gene defect will develop kidney stones. Neonatal screening programs provide higher prevalence estimates. In Quebec, 1:1,800 newborns tested positive for cystinuria, a much higher rate than found in the Quebec adult population.(6) Whether this discrepancy is due to identifying large numbers of heterozygotes who will never develop the cystinuric phenotype or if it is due to the fall in urine cystine excretion as children age is not clear.(7) Cystinuria accounts for less than 1% of kidney stone disease in adults (8), though the relatively early onset of the disease makes it more common in the pediatric population, 6–8% of children with stones have cystinuria.(9, 10)

PHENOTYPE

The original phenotypic classification system for cystinuria was developed before knowledge of the genetics of the disease. Three phenotypes were described based on the level of urine excretion of cystine in obligate heterozygotes (i.e. parents) of the proband.(11) Type I patients had parents with normal cystine excretion. Thus type I is an autosomal recessive disorder in which the parents phenotype is normal and they each carry one normal and one mutant gene. Probands with type II and type III phenotypes have parents with elevated cystine excretion. Type II heterozygotes have markedly abnormal cystine excretion (>990 µmol/g creatinine), approaching that of some homozygotes and on occasion they can form cystine stones. Type III heterozygotes have only modest elevations of urine cystine excretion, 100–660 µmol/g creatinine, not high enough for stone formation. However, it was recognized that the classification of subjects into type II and type III phenotypes was somewhat arbitrary and that the distinction was not always clear, especially for subjects whose excretion rates fell between those defined for type II and type III.

After identification of the genetic defects that cause cystinuria, it became clear that the phenotype classification needed to be changed as only two gene defects accounted for the three known phenotypes. The majority of patients with type I phenotype had defects in the SLC3A1 gene while both types II and III resulted from defects in the SLC7A9 gene. This has led to reclassification of the phenotypes into type I, probands whose parents have normal cystine excretion and nontype I, probands whose parents have elevated cystine excretion.(12) Nontype I is an autosomal dominant disorder with incomplete penetrance.

GENETICS

In 1993, a human cDNA was isolated that stimulated uptake of cystine and dibasic amino acids when expressed in Xenopus oocytes.(13) The corresponding gene was identified as SCL3A1 and localized to the short arm of chromosome 2 (2p21).(14) Calonge et al reported the first cystinuria-inducing mutations in the SCL3A1 gene.(15) The gene encodes a 685 amino acid glycoprotein that forms the heavy subunit of the cystine transporter. The protein is referred to as rBAT, an abbreviation for "related to $b^{0,+}$ amino acid transporter". Since the original report numerous other gene defects have been found, with a total of 103 mutations being reported as of 2005.(16) Chromosome deletions, insertions, rearrangements, as well as missense, nonsense, and frameshift mutations have been reported. The most common mutation is M467T, which replaces a methionine with a threonine in the peptide chain. It accounts for 26% of cystinuria cases around the world but prevalence of this mutation varies within population groups.

Since mutations in SLC3A1were not found in all patients with cystinuria, the search for other genes continued.(17–19) In 1999, the second cystinuria gene, SLC7A9, was localized to the long arm of chromosome 19 (19q12–13). (20, 21) The gene encodes a 487 amino acid protein called $b^{0,+}$ AT, which forms the light subunit of the cystine transporter. A total of 60 mutations in SLC7A9 had been reported as of 2005.(16)

An alternative classification system has been proposed based on the genes affected in an individual. Patients with type A cystinuria are homozygous for mutations in the SLC3A1 and patients homozygous with mutations in SCL7A9 are type B. If a patient has a defect in both genes, they are classified as type AB. In 2005 the International Cystinuria Consortium (ICC) reported genotypes on 164 probands, of which 97 had also been phenotyped as type I or nontype I.(16) Of the 97 probands who were phenotyped, 38% were type I, 47% were nontype I and 14% were of mixed phenotype, one parent type I and the other parent nontype I. In the probands, 90% of the expected mutations were identified, 44% of mutations were type A and 56% were type B. Type A mutations were always phenotype I except one notable exception. A duplication of exons 5 to 9 of gene SLC3A1 was shown to produce a nontype I phenotype in 4 of 6 heterozygotes who had the abnormality. Type B mutations account for all other nontype I phenotypes. Type B mutations usually present as nontype 1 phenotype, though 14% of type B heterozygotes will have normal cystine excretion, a type I phenotype.(16, 22) Of the 14% of probands who were found to have obligate heterozygotes with mixed phenotypes, most were eventually found to have two type B mutations, not the AB genotype that would be expected. In fact, type AB genotypes are rarely associated with a stone-forming phenotype. This is surprising since type A and type B mutations have a similar prevalence which would make one predict type AB to be the most common of the genotypes; yet in the ICC database AB genotypes were quite rare and none had formed cystine stones. Perhaps the rarity of AB genotypes in the disease reflects a lower cystine excretion in these subjects with much less risk of stone formation.

Despite the recent success of genetic research in understanding cystinuria, 3% of cystinuric probands have no mutation identified in either gene and in 20% only one mutant allele was found. (16) Whether these cases represent mutations outside the open reading frames of the genes or are due to mutations in as yet unidentified other genes involved in cystinuria remains to be seen.

Isolated cystinuria, where cystine excretion and stone disease is found without the expected abnormal excretion of the dibasic amino acids, has been reported.(23) It led to speculation that there may be an additional cystine transport system separate from that of the combined cystine and dibasic amino acid transporter. However, a recent study showed that two siblings with isolated cystinuria were both heterozyogotes for a mutation in SLC7A9, T123M.(24) This mutation has been reported to cause both type 1and nontype 1 phenotypes in other families.

PATHOPHYSIOLOGY

In normal physiology, greater than 99% of cystine and the dibasic amino acids that are filtered by the glomerulus are reabsorbed in the proximal tubule. In cystinuria, the fractional excretion of cystine can reach 100%.(25) Cystine and the dibasic amino acids are transported across the apical membrane of the proximal tubule by the sodium-independent heteromeric amino acid transporter rBAT/ $b^{0,+}$AT in exchange for neutral amino acids in a 1:1 stoichiometry (Figure 9.1).(26)

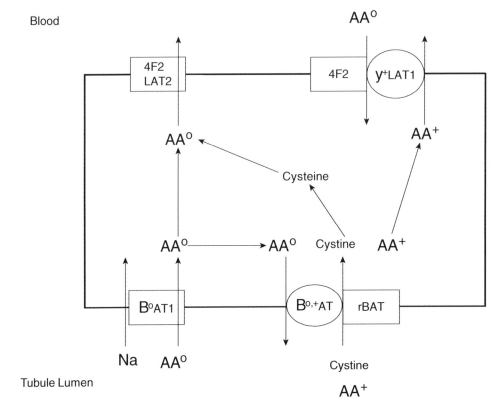

Figure 9.1 Reabsorption of amino acids across the proximal tubule. Neutral amino acids (AA°) are absorbed by a sodium-dependent process by the apical transporter B°AT1. Dibasic amino acids (AA⁺) and cystine are reabsorbed in a sodium independent process by rBAT/ b⁰,⁺AT in exchange for intracellular neutral amino acids. Once in the cell, cystine is reduced to cysteine and transported across the basolateral membrane by the neutral amino acid transporter 4F2/LAT2. The dibasic amino acids are transported across the basolateral membrane by the heterodimeric amino acid transporter, 4F2/y⁺LAT1.

There is also a sodium-dependent neutral amino acid transporter, B°AT1 in the apical membrane which maintains a high intracellular concentration of neutral amino acids.(27) Once transported into the cell, cystine is reduced to its component cysteine molecules, keeping intracellular cystine levels low, providing a favorable chemical gradient for cystine reabsorption. Cysteine is transported across the basolateral membrane via a neutral amino acid transporter. The dibasic amino acids exit across the basolateral membrane via another heteromeric amino acid transporter, which consists of the 4F2 heavy chain and the y+LAT1 light chain.(28, 29)

The cystine transporter is a heterodimer composed of the heavy subunit, rBAT, and the light subunit, b⁰,⁺AT. The two proteins are linked by a disulfide bond. The light chain is the catalytic unit that directs the exchange of neutral amino acids for dibasic amino acids and cystine.(30) The heavy chain transports the light chain to the apical membrane.(31) If the light chain is defective, then no amino acid transport occurs. If the heavy chain is defective, the light chain never reaches the apical membrane, leading to loss of apical cystine transport. In *in vitro* systems, the light chain does not require the heavy chain to transport amino acids.(30) The light chain is expressed predominantly in the S1 and S2 segments of the proximal tubule apical membrane, it is always associated with rBAT.(26) rBAT has the opposite expression characteristic, being expressed at the highest levels in S3 and lowest levels in S1. It is likely that rBAT in the proximal straight tubule is complexed to a different light chain than b⁰,⁺AT, but at this time none have been identified.(27) It has been speculated that there is an additional cystine transporter in addition to the rBAT/ b⁰,⁺AT system, perhaps the other rBAT light chain complex. However, since most transport appears to be via the rBAT/ b⁰,⁺AT system, if there is a second system it appears to be of minor importance.

Since cystine transport mechanisms are similar in the gut and the kidney, cystine is not absorbed normally from the intestinal lumen. However, patients do not become cystine deficient despite increased urine losses. Cystine is not an essential amino acid, so cystine can be synthesized from methionine. In addition, cystine is absorbed from the intestinal tract in the form of small peptide fragments, where transport is not dependent on specific amino acid configurations. The net result is that cystinuric patients have basically normal serum levels of cystine and dibasic amino acids and show no overt signs of amino acid deficiencies.(32)

CLINICAL PRESENTATION

Cystinuria usually presents during childhood or adolescence, though the disease may be diagnosed soon after birth or escape diagnosis well into adulthood. A report from the Mayo Clinic revealed a median age of onset of 19 years while the ICC reports the median age of onset was 13 for type 1 patients and 12 years for nontype 1.(12, 33) There was not a difference between genders in the age of onset in either study. Since the formation of cystine stones is not dependent solely on elevated cystine excretion but is modified by diet, fluid intake, and lifestyle, some subjects may never form stones even though they have cystinuria and others may not form stones until their sixth or seventh decade of life.(33) Renal colic or hematuria, either gross or microscopic, are the usual presenting features of the disease. Stones may be present in the renal pelvis, ureter, or bladder, though bladder stones are more common in children than adults. Unfortunately, some patients can develop a large stone burden without significant symptoms, such that by the time their stone disease comes to medical attention, a staghorn stone may have formed and damaged the kidney. Some cases of cystinuria are identified before forming kidney stones, either through neonatal screening programs or through screening of siblings of a patient who has developed symptoms.

Stone disease is often more severe and unrelenting than in typical calcium stones. Data from 224 patients in the ICC registry shows males have 0.42 and females 0.21 stone events per year.(12) Cystinuric patients require urologic procedures to remove stones at more than twice the rate of patients with routine kidney stone disease.(34) The level of cystine excretion and rate of stone formation is the same regardless of genotype classification so at the present time there is no role for genotyping patients in the routine management of cystinuria.(12, 16)

Patients with cystinuria may also develop stones composed of other more common stone-forming salts such as calcium or uric acid or they may have stones of mixed composition. In a study from Dallas, 29% of cystinuric patients had at least one stone containing calcium salts.(35) Upon further study, they found a surprisingly high rate of metabolic abnormalities in these patients, with 18% having hypercalciuria, 44% hypocitraturia, and 22% hyperuricosuria. For this reason, all stone formers should be screened for cystinuria rather than assume they do not have the disease after an initial stone analysis reveals a more routine type of stone.

A more unusual presentation of cystinuria has recently been described in which patients have neurologic symptoms as well as classic cystinuria. Parvari et al. described seven patients from a Bedouin clan who presented with type A cystinuria, hypotonia, neonatal seizures, and mental retardation.(36) These patients were found to have a deletion in chromosome 2p21 which included the SLC3A1 gene among others. Jaeken et al. reported 11 patients of Flemish or French descent who presented with a milder form of the disease described by Pavari et al. where the only significant neurologic feature was hypotonia.(37) Discrete deletions of SLC3A1 and PREPL, a gene that encodes an oligopeptidase, account for the cystinuria and hypotonia, respectively.

KIDNEY DAMAGE

Urinary tract obstruction and infection are common consequences of cystinuria. In addition, frequent stone formation leads to repeated surgical intervention to relieve obstruction or reduce stone burden. Cystine stones are more difficult to fragment with shock-wave lithotripsy (SWL) than calcium stones.(38, 39) When SWL is not successful, it may lead to repeated SWL for a single stone. SWL has been shown to cause renal scarring and though the extent of injury with a single SWL in a human is not well quantified, the cumulative effect of multiple SWL would be expected to result in some level of kidney damage.(40) The persistent nature of stone disease in cystinuria increases the risk of kidney damage from recurrent procedures.

Recent anatomic studies also suggest that renal damage may occur in the absence of ureteral obstruction or surgical procedures. Evan et al have combined visualization of the renal pelvis with renal biopsy of the medulla and the cortex in order to better define the mechanism of stone formation.(41) During endoscopy they found obstruction of the terminal collecting duct with small cystine stones. On biopsy, dilation of the collecting duct proximal to the obstruction and upstream nephron drop out and fibrosis show how local obstruction at the nephron level can lead to silent loss of renal function. Since each terminal collecting duct may provide drainage for over 1,000 nephrons, even this seemingly mild lesion can have significant clinical consequences.

There have been numerous studies that show cystine stone disease is associated with a more rapid loss of renal function then other forms of stone disease. Bostrom and Hambraus reported the clinical outcome of 98 cystinuric patients from Sweden.(42) Elevated serum creatinine or urea nitrogen was present in 40% of the patients, and 21% had been subjected to nephrectomy or partial kidney resection. In 1977 Dahlberg et al reported the Mayo Clinic experience with 89 cystinuric patients and noted that 50% had abnormal serum creatinine and two of the 89 patients developed advanced kidney disease.(33) However, much of the data from these two studies was collected before current medical therapy and may not reflect the risk patients face today.

Lindell et al reported glomerular filtration rates measured by renography on 34 cystinuric patients, none of whom had nephrectomy.(43) They found 24% had GFR below the age adjusted normal range. They also found that presence of a staghorn stone correlated with greater loss of GFR in the involved kidney. Worcester et al reported creatinine clearance measurements of 52 patients with cystinuria and 3,215 routine kidney stone patients.(44) The creatinine clearance at presentation was 160 L/d in the routine stone patients compared to 91 L/d in the cystinuric patients. They also noted that cystine stone patients were twice as likely to have a nephrectomy as routine stone formers. Assimos et al reported that 5.8% of 85 cystine patients had an abnormal elevation of serum creatinine compared to 2.2% of calcium stone-forming patients.(45) Nephrectomy had been performed in 14.1% of cystinuric patients, but only 2.9% of the calcium stone formers.

Though chronic kidney disease does occur, it is unusual for a patient to progress to end-stage kidney disease. If kidney failure occurs, kidney transplant is the desired treatment option. The transplanted kidney will have normal amino acid transport, so the patient will not have clinical cystinuria and no risk of losing the graft due to recurrent cystine stone disease.(46, 47)

LABORATORY AND RADIOLOGIC EVALUATION

Most commonly cystinuria is diagnosed by crystallographic analysis of stones that have been passed spontaneously or removed surgically. Alternatively, cystinuria can be diagnosed by the finding of the classic hexagonal shape crystals on urinalysis (Figure 9.2). A first morning void is the most likely to contain cystine crystals as it is usually the most concentrated and acidic urine sample of the day. Identification of cystine crystals in urine is always abnormal, it never occurs in a normal subject no matter how concentrated the urine sample.(48) However, a subject with cystine crystals in the urine may have only modest elevations in urine cystine excretion, such as a nontype I heterozygote. An alternative method to screen for cystinuria in kidney stone patients is a qualitative nitroprusside test. The test can detect cystine down to concentrations of 75 mg/l with a sensitivity of 72% and specificity of 95%.(49)

Once cystinuria is suspected, daily cystine excretion should be quantified in a 24-hour urine specimen. Cystine can be measured by a variety of methods, though usually it is measured by colormetric methods such as nitroprusside reaction or by column chromatography.(50–52) Cystine excretion of less than 30 mg/d is generally recognized as normal, though normal range varies with the type of assay used. A critical issue often ignored in the measurement of cystine is the risk of crystallization during collection and processing of the sample.(53) Whatever cystine precipitates out of solution will not be measured by the assay, leading to an underestimate of cystine concentration and excretion. At one time it was commonplace to either acidify or alkalinize urine collections performed for cystine, as cystine solubility increases at extremes of pH. However, the desire to obtain the maximum number of chemistries from a single 24-hour urine collection has led many laboratories to abandon this practice. Figure 9.3 shows the results

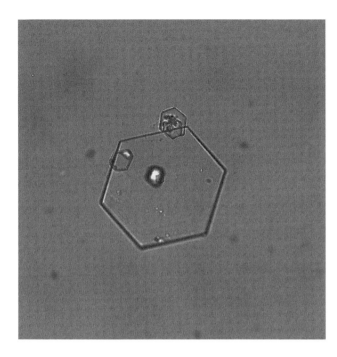

Figure 9.2 Cystine crystals. Hexagonal cystine crystals of varying size in human urine (400x).

of an experiment in which urine was collected for 24 hours at room temperature without taking precautions to prevent precipitation. At the end of the collection, cystine concentration was measured and then the entire sample alkalinized and cystine concentration re-measured. As can be seen, a number of the samples have cystine concentration well above the line of identity, showing that cystine had crystallized and had been brought back into solution by alkalinization. If 24-hour urine samples are refrigerated during collection, as many laboratories recommend, then risk of crystallization is even higher. It is not uncommon for cystine excretion to apparently increase during therapy, frustrating the clinician as the patient appears to be getting worse. As effective therapy improves solubility of cystine, spontaneous crystallization is halted and cystine excretion appears to increase.

Since the level of saturation of cystine in the urine is the driving force for stone formation, the goal of therapy is to keep cystine saturation as low as possible. In general, cystine solubility is around 250 to 300 mg/l at urine pH above 7.0, so the goal of therapy is to keep urine cystine concentration below this level. There are refinements of this approach in which a nomogram provides a relationship of solubility to pH, so the clinician can adjust pH and cystine concentration to keep urine undersaturated.(54) The other alternative is to do a direct measurement of cystine saturation.(55) As can be seen in Figure 9.4 there is considerable variability in cystine solubility at any given level of urine pH.(53, 56) A direct measure of supersaturation will provide a cystine solubility for that particular patient's urine, presumably making therapeutic goals patient specific. Although theoretically a sound approach, direct measurements of saturation have not yet been shown to enhance patient management in prospective trials, nor have saturation measurements been shown to correlate with stone growth or formation.

Other critical variables of interest in 24-hour urine collections include urine pH which is a major determinant of cystine solubility (Figure 9.4). Since alkalinization is a goal of therapy, urine pH must be monitored to make sure the dose of alkali is adequate. A single-spot urine pH is not adequate to determine success of alkali therapy as urine pH varies considerably during the course of the day. Either repetitive measures of urine pH can be made at home by the patient using litmus paper or a urine pH can be measured on a 24-hour urine sample, which provides a time average of the patients urine pH. Other important values from the 24-hour urine include the urine volume, which is critical in diluting cystine below its saturation concentration, urine sodium which provides an estimate of diet sodium and urea nitrogen which provides an estimate of dietary protein intake.(57) Using these urine dietary markers greatly improves a clinician's ability to judge the adherence to and effectiveness of any dietary intervention.

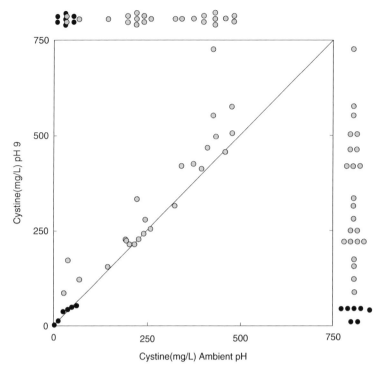

Figure 9.3 Effect of alkalinization on urine cystine concentration. The urine cystine concentration at the ambient pH of the urine increases when the urine pH is raised to 9 by the addition of alkali *in vitro*. Open circles are samples from cystinuric patients, closed circles are normal subjects. All points above the line of identity (diagonal line) had crystallization of cystine during the urine collection. Reproduced with permission.(53)

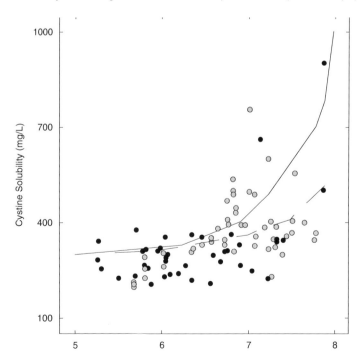

Figure 9.4 Urine pH and cystine solubility. As urine pH increases, cystine solubility increases. Note the variability in solubility at any given urine pH. Open circles are cystinuric patients, closed circles are normal subjects. Reproduced with permission.(53)

All siblings of an affected individual should be screened for abnormal excretion of cystine. If screening tests are positive, quantification of cystine excretion should be performed. If a subject has cystine excretion that is abnormal, but in the range expected of a nontype I heterozygote, they can usually be treated with consistent high fluid intake and they should have radiologic studies to make sure they do not have clinically silent urolithiasis. If cystine excretion is in the range expected for a homozygote, then more aggressive treatment and monitoring may be warranted.

As part of the basic management of a cystinuric patient, radiologic evaluation is required to determine the extent of stone burden and the location of stones in the urinary system. Cystine stones are radio-opaque due to the sulfur atom in the molecular structure. Therefore cystine stones can be seen on a plain film of the abdomen, though the radiodensity is not as great as that of calcium stones, so small stones may be missed. CT scan is now the preferred radiologic technique for assessing stone disease, including stones in the ureter. Cystine stones are easily visible on CT scans, and the identification of stones as cystine may be suggested by the attenuation values obtained on the stones. However, attenuation values can be misleading in small stones. Ultrasound can also be used to evaluate cystine stone formers, though it is not as reliable as CT scan in identifying stones in the ureters and may also miss small stones in the renal pelvis. However, due to the recurrent nature of cystine stone disease ultrasound may be a useful technique for repeated evaluation over time, due to the lack of radiation exposure. Repeated CT scans may lead to an unacceptable level of radiation over the years of follow up.(58)

MEDICAL MANAGEMENT

When initiating medical therapy, consideration must be given as to the goals of the treatment. The aim of treatment is to prevent new stone formation and reduce the rate of growth of any existing stones. In some patients, aggressive therapy can also lead to dissolution of cystine stones. Radiologic evaluation is a critical component of any treatment regimen. Knowledge of the number and location of all stones at the time treatment is initiated is required to monitor the success of therapy. If a patient develops renal colic and the stone passing is clearly new, then medical therapy has not been successful. Adherence of the patient to the treatment protocol should be confirmed and the treatment regimen re-evaluated. Changes in diet and lifestyle should also be considered in assessing failure of medical management. If a symptomatic stone is clearly a stone that had been present before initiating therapy but now has moved and caused obstruction, then a change in medical therapy may not be required, especially if new stones or stone growth are not observed on X-ray. Not only is the knowledge of old vs. new stone important for the physician, but also for the patient. Patients who pass a stone despite adhering to their therapeutic plan will become discouraged and stop therapy unless they understand that the stone they passed was present before the initiation of therapy. Serial radiologic evaluation is needed to ensure that new asymptomatic stones are not forming during treatment, as growth or formation of clinically silent stones is an indication to intensify medical therapy.

Cystine stone formation is directly related to the level of cystine saturation of the urine. Cystine saturation is a function of cystine solubility, cystine excretion, and urine flow rate; the last two factors determine the urine cystine concentration. Therapy to reduce stone formation is focused on lowering cystine concentration in the urine or increasing urine cystine solubility. There are no controlled prospective trials, using stone formation as an endpoint, for any therapy for cystine stones. However, studies using endpoints of cystine excretion and studies of stone passage using patients as their own historical controls provide reasonable data on which to base therapeutic choices.

Dietary Therapy

Fluids

Cystinuric patients are routinely instructed to increase fluid intake and maintain a high urine flow rate in order to lower urine cystine concentration and therefore urine cystine saturation. The level of urine flow required is dependent on the patient's cystine excretion, a rough guide should be a urine flow high enough to keep cystine concentration below 240 mg/l (1 mmol/l). However, as noted above cystine solubility is variable but this guideline should suffice when

Table 9.1 Effect of low sodium diet on urine cystine excretion.

	n	Diet Sodium	Urine Cystine	Comment
Norman et al (60)	5	122 ± 8 mmol/g creat	1.6 ± 0.7 mmol/g creat	
		76 ± 9 mmol/g creat	1.0 ± 0.3 mmol/g creat	
Peces et al (61)	3	227 ± 36 mmol/d	1.7 ± 0.3 mmol/g creat	
		51 ± 11 mmol/d	0.7 ± 0.3 mmol/g creat	
Lindell et al (63)	13	129 + 48 mmol/g creat	2.3 ± 0.7 mmol/g creat	Seven of the thirteen subjects were
		37 ± 16 mmol/g creat	1.7 ± 0.7 mmol/g creat	on a stable dose of tiopronin.
Rodriguez et al (62)	5	6.0 ± 2.1 mmol/kg/d	19 ± 7 mg/kg/d	Subjects were children, ages six
		1.5 ± 0.5 mmol/kg/d	1.0 ± 0.2 mg/kg/d	to ten.

Diet sodium was estimated from diet records by Peces et al and from urine sodium excretion in all other studies.

saturation measurements are not available. Certainly the higher the urine volume the better, and some patients maintain urine flows of 5–6 L/day. Patients should awaken at least once per night to void and drink additional water in order to avoid the usual nocturnal concentration of urine. There have been no studies as to whether all beverages are equally effective in preventing cystine stone formation. Theoretically, citrus juices and other beverages containing citrate will raise urine pH and could reduce stone risk (59), but it is probably more important to focus on the amount of fluid the patient drinks rather than the specific beverage.

Sodium
Amino acids are freely filtered by the glomerulus and reabsorbed in the proximal tubule. Proximal tubule reabsorption of sodium and water provide the electrochemical gradient for the reabsorption of cystine. In a cross-sectional study of 69 cystine patients, dietary intake of sodium, as assessed by urine sodium excretion, was positively correlated with urine cystine excretion.(55) Low sodium diets, which lead to slight volume depletion and subsequent increased proximal tubule reabsorption of sodium, have been used to lower urine cystine excretion.(60–63) These studies have been summarized in Table 9.1. The number of subjects in each study is fairly small, but all show a significant fall in urine cystine when diet sodium is lowered.

Protein
Cystine is a nonessential amino acid that can be obtained from a normal diet, or can be produced endogenously using the sulfur from the essential amino acid methionine. There is a correlation of urine cystine excretion with dietary protein intake, as judged by urine urea nitrogen excretion.(55) Thus, restricting dietary protein intake is a potentially attractive therapy for cystinuric patients. There has been only a single study of low-protein diet in cystinuria. Rodman et al studied seven patients on low-protein (mean of 54 g/d) and high-protein diet (mean of 140 g/ d), five days on each diet.(64) They found a 20% reduction in cystine excretion on the low-protein diet.

The effectiveness and safety of long term low-protein diets in cystinuria has not been established. The reduction in urine cystine in the Rodman study is modest despite a large change in dietary protein. Lowering the intake of the essential amino acid methionine in patients who already have a defect in sulfur amino acid metabolism could theoretically lead to a nutritional deficiency, though there has not been definitive evidence of such.(65) Rather than placing patients on low-protein diets, it seems prudent to have patients maintain normal protein intake and avoid protein gluttony. An additional benefit of avoiding high-protein diets is lowering diet acid load, thus increasing urine pH and cystine solubility.

Pharmacologic Therapy

Urine Alkalinization
One of the main factors controlling cystine solubility is urine pH. Unfortunately, solubility does not begin to increase significantly until pH is above 7 to 7.5, a level that requires significant and frequent dosing of alkali. Unfortunately, the effect of urine pH on solubility varies considerably amongst individuals (Figure 9.4), making it difficult to determine the optimal dose of alkali in any given patient.(53, 56) Whether the variation in solubility at a given pH is due to the ionic

Table 9.2   Common side effects of d-penicillamine and tiopronin.

Nausea/Vomiting
Diarrhea
Skin Rash
Fever
Proteinuria
Fatigue
Anorexia

composition of the urine or the macromolecular fraction of the urine such as proteins and gly-cosoaminoglycans is not known.(56) To avoid the uncertainty of urine cystine solubility when managing patients, urine cystine saturation can be directly measured.(55)

Alkali salts are routinely used to increase urine pH. Since diet sodium restriction is part of the basic therapy for cystinuria, potassium alkali salts are generally favored over sodium salts. Potassium citrate is the most commonly used potassium alkali, though potassium bicarbonate should be equally as effective in raising urine pH. If the patient develops hyperkalemia due to renal insufficiency or Type IV RTA, then sodium alkali would be preferred. When bicarbonate is used as the alkali, it may be necessary to dose four times per day; when citrate is used as the alkali, it may be provided in two or three doses per day, as the citrate requires metabolism by the liver to be converted into bicarbonate. Fjellstedt et al have shown potassium citrate and sodium bicarbonate to be equally effective in alkalinizing urine in cystinuric patients.(66) In patients who have developed significant renal insufficiency, bicarbonate should be used in preference to citrate, as citrate can increase intestinal absorption of aluminum and lead to sys-temic aluminum toxicity.(67) Many patients with cystinuria have urine pH that is higher than a healthy population, even when not treated with alkali, so the dose of alkali required may not be excessive even though the urine pH goal is at the upper end of the range of urine pH.(34, 35) The mechanism of the elevated urine pH in cystinuria is not known.(35)

Thiol-binding Drugs

Cystine is comprised of two cysteine molecules, combined via a covalent disulfide bond. Cysteine is quite soluble and if all urinary cystine could be reduced to individual cysteine molecules, no kidney stones would form. Unfortunately, this cannot be done, but an alternative approach is to provide other compounds with a free thiol group which can solublize cystine. Tiopronin and d-penicillamine are the two most commonly used thiol drugs. When present in solution with cystine, a disulfide exchange reaction can occur and a drug-cysteine complex will form. The drug-cysteine complexes for both of these thiol-binding drugs are much more soluble than cys-tine, effectively increasing cystine solubility. Thiol drugs have been shown to lower urine cystine saturation in cystinuric patients.(68–71) The drugs do appear to lower cystine stone formation in uncontrolled clinical studies, as judged by pre and post-treatment stone formation rates.(72–75) However, the significant level of side effects of the drugs generally restricts their use to patients who are unable to control stones by high fluid intake, dietary modification and urine alkalini-zation.(Table 9.2) Some investigators have suggested starting at a low dose and increasing the dose over a few weeks to the final desired level, to help minimize adverse reactions. Overall, tiopronin has been reported to have lower rates of side effects than d-penicillamine, though this has not been rigorously studied.(72) The side effects of the thiol drugs appear to be dose related so prescribing these drugs is a balancing act, finding the dose that is both efficacious and yet not excessive so as to limit side effects. Patients treated with thiol-containing drugs should have liver enzymes and hematologic studies performed on a periodic basis.

One common clinical misconception is that the thiol drugs will lower urine cystine excre-tion as cystine is converted to the drug-cysteine complex. Though this is true *in vivo*, the proc-ess of measuring cystine and other urine amino acids may cause the cysteine drug complex to dissociate; or an assay may measure total free sulfhydryl groups in the urine which may not distinguish between drug and cystine. In either of these situations, cystine excretion will not fall during thiol drug therapy. This may lead a physician to increase the dose of thiol drug unnecessarily in the quest of lowering cystine excretion. Alternatively, the optimal dose may be determined by an endpoint of stone formation, a late endpoint which often leads the physician to prescribe the thiol at a maximal dose to avoid under-treating the patient. If urine cystine saturation can be measured, it may provide a better guide as to the optimal dose of thiol drugs; though there has not been a prospective trial of the utility of saturation measurements in patient management.

Captopril has received considerable attention as a potential therapy. There are a few uncontrolled studies which show reduction in stone rates with captopril.(76–78) However, there are conflicting results as to the effect of captopril on urine cystine excretion in these patients. (76, 77, 79, 80) Captopril is generally better tolerated than tiopronin and d-penicillamine, but that is likely due to the much lower dose used, 150 mg/d (0.7 mmol/d) vs 1,000–2,000 mg/d (6–12 mmol/d) for tiopronin and d-penicillamine. In fact, the dose of captopril brings the effectiveness of the drug into question. At a dose of 150 mg/d (0.7 mmol/d) and an estimated absorption of 70%, only 0.5 mmol/d would be excreted in the urine, an amount insufficient to bind the cystine present in the urine of most patients, which is in the range of 1 to 5 mmol/d, equivalent to 2 to 10 mmol/d of cysteine, the molecule that is actually bound by the drug. In contrast, 3 to 6 mmol/d of tiopronin and d-penicillamine would be excreted in the urine during standard therapy. If captopril is effective in reducing cystine stone formation presumably there is an alternate mechanism, such as altering cystine metabolism or increasing proximal tubule reabsorption, in addition to forming a drug-cysteine complex. Until better studies are available, captopril should not be considered the preferred thiol-binding drug, unless the patient also has hypertension.

Alternatives to the current thiol drugs are limited. Cysteamine and 2,3 dimercaptosuccinic acid (DMSA) both contain thiol groups and may be effective therapy for cystinuria. DMSA is particularly attractive as a therapeutic agent as it contains two free thiol groups and could potentially bind twice the amount of cysteine per mole of drug. However, at this time they have not been studied adequately in cystinuria patients to recommend them as therapy outside of formal trials.(81, 82)

One of the problems with designing new drugs for cystinuria is that therapy is being aimed at a molecule intrinsic to human metabolism. Thiol drug therapy is based on the unique characteristic of the cystine molecule, the disulfide bond. Other possible therapies which could be aimed at cystine in the urine include a general change in redox potential of the urine to induce reduction of cystine to two soluble cysteine molecules. However, any compound that could accomplish such a change in urine would likely be too toxic for human use. The only other chemically active sites on the cystine molecule are the amino and carboxy terminus of the amino acid. In theory, a complexation or chemical reaction could be attempted at these sites, but the high levels of ornithine, lysine, and arginine in cystinuric urine would compete with cystine for the drug, requiring very high doses of such a therapy. It seems unlikely that chemical solubilization of cystine in the urine will progress much beyond the use of thiol drugs and any radical improvement in therapy will require new methods to increase cystine reabsorption in the proximal tubule.

REFERENCES

1. Wollaston WH. On cystic oxide: a new species of urinary calculus. Philos Trans R Soc Lond 1810; 100: 223–30.
2. Berzelius J. Calculus urinaire. Traite Chem 1833; 7: 424.
3. Palacin M, Goodyear P, Nunes V, Gasparini P. The Metabolic and Molecular Bases of Inherited Diseases, 8th edition, edited by Scriver CR, Beaudet AL, Sly WS, Valle D, NY, 2001: 4909–32.
4. Weinberger A, Sperling O, Rabinovitz M et al. High frequency of cystinuria among Jews of Libyan origin. Hum Hered 1974; 24: 568–72.
5. Levy HL, Shih VE, Madiga PM. Massachusetts metabolic disorders screening program. I. Techniques and results of urine screening. Pediatrics 1971; 49: 825–36.
6. Scriver CR, Clow CL, Reade TM et al. Ontogeny modifies manifestations of cystinuria genes: implications for counseling. J Pediatr 1985; 106(3): 411–6.
7. Boutros M, Vicanek C, Rozen R, Goodyer P. Transient neonatal cystinuria. Kidney Int 2005; 67(2): 443–8.
8. Mandel NS, Mandel GS. Urinary tract stone disease in the United States veteran population. Geographical analysis of variations in composition. J Urol 1989; 142: 1516–21.
9. Milliner DS, Murphy ME. Urolithiasis in pediatric patients. Mayo Clin Proc 1993; 68(3): 241–8.

10. Polinsky MS, Kaiser BA, Baluarte HJ. Urolithiasis in childhood. Pediatr Clin North Am 1987; 34(3): 683–710.
11. Rosenberg LE, Downing S, Durant JL, Segal S. Cystinuria: biochemical evidence for three genetically distinct diseases. J Clin Invest 1966; 45(3): 365–71.
12. Dello SL, Pras E, Pontesilli C et al. Comparison between SLC3A1 and SLC7A9 cystinuria patients and carriers: a need for a new classification. J Am Soc Nephrol 2002; 13(10): 2547–53.
13. Lee WS, Wells RG, Sabbag RV, Mohandas TK, Hediger MA. Cloning and chromosomal localization of a human kidney cDNA involved in cystine, dibasic, and neutral amino acid transport. J Clin Invest 1993; 91(5): 1959–63.
14. Pras E, Arber N, Aksentijevich I et al. Localization of a gene causing cystinuria to chromosome 2p. Nat Genet 1994; 6(4): 415–9.
15. Calonge MJ, Gasparini P, Chillaron J et al. Cystinuria caused by mutations in rBAT, a gene involved in the transport of cystine. Nat Genet 1994; 6(4): 420–5.
16. Font-Llitjos M, Jimenez-Vidal M, Bisceglia L et al. New insights into cystinuria: 40 new mutations, genotype-phenotype correlation, and digenic inheritance causing partial phenotype. J Med Genet 2005; 42(1): 58–68.
17. Saadi I, Chen XZ, Hediger M et al. Molecular genetics of cystinuria: mutation analysis of SLC3A1 and evidence for another gene in type I (silent) phenotype. Kidney Int 1998; 54(1): 48–55.
18. Wartenfeld R, Golomb E, Katz G et al. Molecular analysis of cystinuria in Libyan Jews: exclusion of the SLC3A1 gene and mapping of a new locus on 19q. Am J Hum Genet 1997; 60(3): 617–24.
19. Calonge MJ, Volpini V, Bisceglia L et al. Genetic heterogeneity in cystinuria: the SLC3A1 gene is linked to type I but not to type III cystinuria. Proc Natl Acad Sci U S A 1995; 92(21): 9667–71.
20. Feliubadalo L, Font M, Purroy et al. Non-type I cystinuria caused by mutations in SLC7A9, encoding a subunit (bo,+AT) of rBAT. Nat Genet 1999; 23(1): 52–7.
21. Stoller ML, Bruce JE, Bruce CA et al. Linkage of type II and type III cystinuria to 19q13.1: codominant inheritance of two cystinuric alleles at 19q13.1 produces an extreme stone-forming phenotype. Am J Med Genet 1999; 86(2): 134–9.
22. Leclerc D, Boutros M, Suh D et al. SLC7A9 mutations in all three cystinuria subtypes. Kidney Int 2002; 62(5): 1550–9.
23. Brodehl J, Gellissen K, Kowalewski S. [Isolated cystinuria (without lysin-, ornithin and argininuria) in a family with hypocalcemic tetany]. Monatsschr Kinderheilkd 1967; 115(4): 317–20.
24. Eggermann T, Elbracht M, Haverkamp F, Schmidt C, Zerres K. Isolated cystinuria (OMIM 238200) is not a separate entity but is caused by a mutation in the cystinuria gene SLC7A9. Clin Genet 2007; 71(6): 597–8.
25. Crawhall JC, Scowen EF, Thompson CJ, Watts RW. The renal clearance of amino acids in cystinuria. J Clin Invest 1967; 46(7): 1162–71.
26. Fernandez E, Carrascal M, Rousaud F et al. rBAT-b(0,+)AT heterodimer is the main apical reabsorption system for cystine in the kidney. Am J Physiol Renal Physiol 2002; 283(3): F540–F548.
27. Broer S. Amino acid transport across mammalian intestinal and renal epithelia. Physiol Rev 2008; 88(1): 249–86.
28. Franca R, Veljkovic E, Walter S, Wagner CA, Verrey F. Heterodimeric amino acid transporter glycoprotein domains determining functional subunit association. Biochem J 2005; 388: 435–43.
29. Chillaron J, Estevez R, Mora C et al. Obligatory amino acid exchange via systems bo,+-like and y+L-like. A tertiary active transport mechanism for renal reabsorption of cystine and dibasic amino acids. J Biol Chem 1996; 271(30): 17761–70.
30. Reig N, Chillaron J, Bartoccioni P et al. The light subunit of system b(o,+) is fully functional in the absence of the heavy subunit. EMBO J 2002; 21(18): 4906–14.
31. Bauch C, Verrey F. Apical heterodimeric cystine and cationic amino acid transporter expressed in MDCK cells. Am J Physiol Renal Physiol 2002; 283(1): F181–F189.
32. London DR, Foley TH. Cystine metabolism in cystinuria. Clin Sci 1965; 19: 129–41.
33. Dahlberg PJ, van den B, Kurtz SB, Wilson DM, Smith LH. Clinical features and management of cystinuria. Mayo Clin Proc 1977; 52(9): 533–42.
34. Worcester EM, Coe FL, Evan AP, Parks JH. Reduced renal function and benefits of treatment in cystinuria vs other forms of nephrolithiasis. BJU Int 2006; 97(6): 1285–90.
35. Sakhaee K, Poindexter JR, Pak CY. The spectrum of metabolic abnormalities in patients with cystine nephrolithiasis. J Urol 1989; 141(4): 819–21.
36. Parvari R, Brodyansky I, Elpeleg O et al. A recessive contiguous gene deletion of chromosome 2p16 associated with cystinuria and a mitochondrial disease. Am J Hum Genet 2001; 69(4): 869–75.
37. Jaeken J, Martens K, Francois I et al. Deletion of PREPL, a gene encoding a putative serine oligopeptidase, in patients with hypotonia-cystinuria syndrome. Am J Hum Genet 2006; 78(1): 38–51.
38. Lingeman JE, Newman D, Mertz JH et al. Extracorporeal shock wave lithotripsy: the Methodist Hospital of Indiana experience. J Urol 1986; 135(6): 1134–7.
39. Kim SC, Burns EK, Lingeman JE et al. Cystine calculi: correlation of CT-visible structure, CT number, and stone morphology with fragmentation by shock wave lithotripsy. Urol Res 2007; 35(6): 319–24.

40. McAteer JA, Evan AP. The acute and long-term adverse effects of shock wave lithotripsy. Semin Nephrol 2008; 28(2): 200–13.
41. Evan AP, Coe FL, Lingeman JE et al. Renal crystal deposits and histopathology in patients with cystine stones. Kidney Int 2006; 69(12): 2227–35.
42. Bostrom H, Hambraeus L. Cystinuria in Sweden: clinical, histopathological and medico-social aspects of the disease. Aca Med Scand 1964; 175: 411.
43. Lindell A, Denneberg T, Granerus G. Studies on renal function in patients with cystinuria. Nephron 1997; 77(1): 76–85.
44. Worcester EM, Parks JH, Evan AP, Coe FL. Renal function in patients with nephrolithiasis. J Urol 2006; 176(2): 600–3.
45. Assimos DG, Leslie SW, Ng C, Streem SB, Hart LJ. The impact of cystinuria on renal function. J Urol 2002; 168(1): 27–30.
46. Tuso P, Barnett M, Yasunaga C, Nortman D. Cystinuria and renal transplantation. Nephron 1993; 63(4): 478.
47. Kelly S, Nolan EP. Excretory rates in posttransplant cystinuric patient. JAMA 1978; 239(12): 1132.
48. Labeeuw M, Gerbaulet C, Pozet N, Zech P, Traeger J. Cystine crystalluria and urinary saturation in cystine and non-cystine stone formers. Urol Res 1981; 9(4): 163–8.
49. Finocchiaro R, D'Eufemia P, Celli M et al. Usefulness of cyanide-nitroprusside test in detecting incomplete recessive heterozygotes for cystinuria: a standardized dilution procedure. Urol Res 1998; 26(6): 401–5.
50. Nakagawa Y, Coe FL. A modified cyanide-nitroprusside method for quantifying urinary cystine concentration that corrects for creatinine interference. Clin Chim Acta 1999; 289(1–2): 57–68.
51. Giugliani R, Ferrari I, Greene LJ. An evaluation of four methods for the detection of heterozygous cystinuria. Clin Chim Acta 1987; 164(2): 227–33.
52. Birwe H, Hesse A. High-performance liquid chromatographic determination of urinary cysteine and cystine. Clin Chim Acta 1991; 199(1): 33–42.
53. Nakagawa Y, Asplin JR, Goldfarb D, Parks JH, Coe F.L. Clinical use of cystine supersaturation measurements. J Urol 2000; 164: 1481–5.
54. Marshall RW, Robertson WG. Nomograms for the estimation of the saturation of urine with calcium oxalate, calcium phosphate, magnesium ammonium phosphate, uric acid, sodium acid urate, ammonium acid urate and cystine. Clin Chim Acta 1976; 72(2): 253–60.
55. Goldfarb DS, Coe FL, Asplin JR. Urinary cystine excretion and capacity in patients with cystinuria. Kidney Int 2006; 69(6): 1041–7.
56. Pak CYC, Fuller C. Assessment of cystine solubility and heterogenous nucleation. J Urol 1983; 129: 1066–70.
57. Maroni BJ, Steinman TI, Mitch WE. A method for estimating nitrogen intake of patients with chronic renal failure. Kidney Int 1985; 27(1): 58–65.
58. Brenner DJ, Hall EJ. Computed tomography--an increasing source of radiation exposure. N Engl J Med 2007; 357(22): 2277–84.
59. Odvina CV. Comparative value of orange juice vs. lemonade in reducing stone-forming risk. Clin J Am Soc Nephrol 2006; 1(6): 1269–74.
60. Norman RW, Manette WA. Dietary restriction of sodium as a means of reducing urinary cystine. J Urol 1990; 143(6): 1193–5.
61. Peces R, Sanchez L, Gorostidi M, Alvarez J. Effects of variation in sodium intake on cystinuria. Nephron 1991; 57(4): 421–3.
62. Rodriguez LM, Santos F, Malaga S, Martinez V. Effect of a low sodium diet on urinary elimination of cystine in cystinuric children. Nephron 1995; 71(4): 416–8.
63. Lindell A, Denneberg T, Edholm E, Jeppsson JO. The effect of sodium intake on cystinuria with and without tiopronin treatment. Nephron 1995; 71(4): 407–15.
64. Rodman JS, Blackburn P, Williams JJ et al. The effect of dietary protein on cystine excretion in patients with cystinuria. Clin Nephrol 1984; 22(6): 273–8.
65. Martensson J, Denneberg T, Lindell A, Textorius O. Sulfur amino acid metabolism in cystinuria: a biochemical and clinical study of patients. Kidney Int 1990; 37(1): 143–9.
66. Fjellstedt E, Denneberg T, Jeppsson JO, Tiselius HG. A comparison of the effects of potassium citrate and sodium bicarbonate in the alkalinization of urine in homozygous cystinuria. Urol Res 2001; 29(5): 295–302.
67. Lindberg JS, Copley JB, Koenig KG, Cushner HM. Effect of citrate on serum aluminum concentrations in hemodialysis patients: a prospective study. South Med J 1993; 86(12): 1385–8.
68. Dolin DJ, Asplin JR, Flagel L, Grasso M, Goldfarb DS. Effect of cystine-binding thiol drugs on urinary cystine capacity in patients with cystinuria. J Endourol 2005; 19(3): 429–32.
69. Harbar JA, Cusworth DC, Lawes LC, Wrong OM. Comparison of 2-mercaptopropionylglycine and D-penicillamine in the treatment of cystinuria. J Urol 1986; 136(1): 146–9.
70. Denneberg T, Jeppsson JO, Stenberg P. Alternative treatment of cystinuria with alpha-merkaptopropionyl-glycine, Thiola. Proc Eur Dial Transplant Assoc 1983; 20: 427–33.

71. Coe F.L., Clark C, Parks JH, Asplin JR. Solid phase assay of urine cystine supersaturation in the presence of cystine binding drugs. J Urol 2001; 166(2): 688–93.
72. Pak CY, Fuller C, Sakhaee K, Zerwekh JE, Adams BV. Management of cystine nephrolithiasis with alpha-mercaptopropionylglycine. J Urol 1986; 136(5): 1003–8.
73. Chow GK, Streem SB. Medical treatment of cystinuria: results of contemporary clinical practice. J Urol 1996; 156(5): 1576–8.
74. Tekin A, Tekgul S, Atsu N, Sahin A, Bakkaloglu M. Cystine calculi in children: the results of a metabolic evaluation and response to medical therapy. J Urol 2001; 165: 2328–30.
75. Barbey F, Joly D, Rieu P et al. Medical treatment of cystinuria: critical reappraisal of long-term results. J Urol 2000; 163(5): 1419–23.
76. Perazella MA, Buller GK. Successful treatment of cystinuria with captopril. Am J Kidney Dis 1993; 21(5): 504–7.
77. Cohen TD, Streem SB, Hall P. Clinical effect of captopril on the formation and growth of cystine calculi. J Urol 1995; 154(1): 164–6.
78. Sloand JA, Izzo JL Jr. Captopril reduces urinary cystine excretion in cystinuria. Arch Intern Med 1987; 147(8): 1409–12.
79. Michelakakis H, Delis D, Anastasiadou V, Bartsocas C. Ineffectiveness of captopril in reducing cystine excretion in cystinuric children. J Inherit Metab Dis 1993; 16(6): 1042–3.
80. Dahlberg PJ, Jones JD. Cystinuria: failure of captopril to reduce cystine excretion. Arch Intern Med 1989; 149(3): 713–7.
81. Parvex P, Rozen R, Dziarmaga A, Goodyer P. Studies of urinary cystine precipitation in vitro: ontogeny of cystine nephrolithiasis and identification of meso-2,3-dimercaptosuccinic acid as a potential therapy for cystinuria. Mol Genet Metab 2003; 80(4): 419–25.
82. Belldina EB, Huang MY, Schneider JA, Brundage RC, Tracy TS. Steady-state pharmacokinetics and pharmacodynamics of cysteamine bitartrate in paediatric nephropathic cystinosis patients. Br J Clin Pharmacol 2003; 56(5): 520–5.

10 | Pathophysiology and management of infection stones

Sangtae Park

BACKGROUND

Archaeological records from ancient Egypt, Babylonia, and China show that infection stones have afflicted humans for millennia. In the early 19th century, the chemical composition of infection stones was elucidated as Magnesium Ammonium Phosphate ($MgNH_4PO_4 \cdot 6H_2O$). They are also called struvite (named after the Russian naturalist, Baron von Struve), infection-induced, phosphatic and triple phosphate stones in the medical literature. Struvite calculi often coexist with calcium carbonate apatite crystals ($Ca_{10}(PO_4)_6 \cdot CO_3$) due to their shared propensity for forming in alkaline urine. Struvite/Calcium carbonate apatite crystals in the urinary tract commonly aggregate and grow to form large, branched stones called staghorns. Indeed, they account for approximately 75% of staghorns, whereas uric acid, cystine, and calcium oxalate or phosphate calculi account for the remaining 25%.[1] Although struvite calculi represent less than 10% of urolithiasis cases in North America, their potential for morbidity and mortality make them important for physicians to recognize and treat expeditiously.[2]

Firstly, untreated infection stones are capable of rapidly growing to fill all the calyces in the kidney (staghorn) and causing progressive renal demise. This was illustrated by a study that analyzed 1,391 consecutive patients started on hemodialysis between 1989 and 2000 at the Necker Hospital in Paris.[3] 3.2% of the patients required hemodialysis as a result of chronic nephrolithiasis, with a disproportionate number (42%) occurring in patients with a history of recurrent struvite calculi.

Secondly, inadequately treated struvite stone fragments can serve as niduses for recurrent urinary tract infections and recurrent struvite stone formation. Beck et al. reviewed 53 patients with infection stones treated by extracorporeal shock-wave lithotripsy (SWL) monotherapy and followed for a mean duration of mean 26.6 months.[4] 62% had residual fragments more than 5 millimeters at 3 months by abdominal radiography (KUB) and 78% of these individuals experienced progression of their stone disease. The authors concluded that only a minority of patients can be fully treated with SWL monotherapy alone, and these patients require close follow-up to assure that residual fragments have passed and urine remains sterile. In a similar study by Streem, 43 patients were followed for 12–111 months (mean 41.7) after percutaneous nephrostolithotomy (PCNL) for infection-related staghorn stones.[5] The risk of new stone formation at 5 years after treatment was 36.8%, and the most predictive factor for recurrence was presence of an untreated intrarenal anatomical abnormality ($p = 0.005$).

Thirdly, bacteria reside within these stones, and the combination of obstruction from the calculus, bacteremia, and endotoxemia can lead to life-threatening sepsis. While urosepsis is a well-known complication of PCNL for struvite stones, McAleer et al. also reported on a death after PCNL from overwhelming endotoxemia despite use of appropriate perioperative antibiotics.[6] They performed an endotoxin assay of the stone fragments retrieved during PCNL, and demonstrated an extremely high endotoxin content despite low colony bacterial culture growth.

In this chapter, the pathophysiology, medical and surgical management of upper tract struvite/calcium carbonate apatite calculi are discussed. Pediatric infection stones, struvite bladder calculi, and struvite calculi in continent or incontinent urinary reservoirs will not be discussed in this chapter.

PATHOPHYSIOLOGY

Physicochemistry of struvite stone formation

Infection stones form when the urine pH is > 7.2 and is supersaturated with magnesium, ammonium, and phosphate ions.(7) The relative saturation ratio (RSR) or concentration product ratio (CPR) is defined as the ratio of the concentration product for a given urine to that of the solubility product. For struvite stones, this can be represented as:

$$\text{RSR} = \frac{[Mg^{2+}][NH_4^+][PO_4^{3-}]}{Ksp}$$

Human urine is normally abundant in calcium, magnesium, and phosphate, whereas the ammonium ion NH_4^+ is not present in adequate concentrations for struvite precipitation. The necessary conditions for struvite precipitation are the presence of ammonium and alkaline pH, both of which occur by the action of urease produced by the infecting microorganism. In actively infected urine, NH_4^+ is generated as ammonia (NH_3) by the hydrolytic action of the enzyme urease on urea,

$$(NH_2)_2\text{--}C = O + H_2O \xrightarrow{\text{urease}} 2NH_3 + CO_2$$

Further hydrolysis of ammonia leads to formation of NH_4^+ and hydroxide (OH^-) ions, thereby raising the pH to the requisite level over 7.2,

$$NH_3 + H_2O \longrightarrow NH_4^+ + OH^-$$

The high pH > 7 brought about by urealysis is also ideal for precipitation of calcium carbonate apatite, and explains the typical coexistence of struvite and calcium carbonate apatite in staghorns. The relative decrease in stone inhibitors may also play a role in struvite physicochemistry. For example, the potent stone inhibitor citrate normally complexes with urinary calcium and magnesium, but is depleted by bacterial metabolism during active infection.(8) It is hypothesized that the decreased concentration of citrate in the urine leaves a greater concentration of free calcium and magnesium to form struvite/calcium carbonate apatite crystals.

Other factors such as alteration in urothelial mucosal physiology have been implicated in struvite stone crystallization. Glycosaminoglycans (GAGs) normally cover the outermost layer of umbrella cells of the urothelium, forming a natural barrier against bacterial adherence and infection.(9, 10) *In vitro* studies on rats have demonstrated that removal of this GAG layer from rat bladder urothelium increases adherence of struvite crystals to the mucosa five- to six-fold, compared to intact rat urothelium.

Parsons demonstrated that ammonium (formed by urealysis) interferes with the defensive function of the GAG layer by binding with their sulfate groups, allowing bacterial adherence to, and invasion of the urothelial surface.(11) Once the bacteria have invaded the urothelial lining, an inflammatory response follows, leading to accumulation of matrix and other mucoproteins.(12) Ultrastructural studies of struvite stones have shown that these macromolecules form fibrous organic matrices, serving as the lattice for bacterial colony growth and struvite crystal aggregation and growth.(13)

Staghorns have traditionally been classified as borderline, partial, or complete.(14) Borderline staghorns involve the pelvis and one calyx, partial staghorns involve the pelvis and two or more calyces, whereas complete staghorns encompass the entire pelvicaliceal system. Others prefer to describe staghorn stone surface area (SSA) as a more informative measure of stone burden. SSA has been shown to be an accurate and reproducible measure with close correlation to actual stone volume as measured by three-dimensional CT techniques.(15, 16)

MICROBIOLOGY OF STRUVITE CALCULI

The requirements for struvite calculi precipitation include a urinary pH > 7.2 and the presence of urease-producing organisms. Urease has been found in numerous bacterial, fungal,

Table 10.1 Urease-producing organisms.(62)

Organisms	Usually (>90% of isolates)	Occasionally (5–30% of isolates)
Gram-negative Bacteria	*Proteus rettgeri*	*Klebsiella pneumonia*
	Proteus vulgaris	Klebsiella oxytoca
	Proteus mirabilis	Serratia marcescens
	Proteus morgani	Hemophilus parainfluenzae
	Providencia stuartii	Bordetella bronchiseptica
	Hemophilus influenza	Aeromonas hydrophila
	Bordetella pertussis	Pseudomonas aeruginosa
	Bacteroides corrodens	*Pasteurella* spp.
	Yersinia enterocolitica	
	Brucella spp.	
	Flavobacterium spp.	
Gram-positive bacteria	Staphylococcus aureus	*Staphylococcus epidermidis*
	Micrococcus varions	*Bacillus* spp.
	Corynebacterium ulcerans	Corynebacterium murium
	Corynebacterium renale	Corynebacterium equi
	Corynebacterium ovis	Peptococcus asacharolyticus
	Corynebacterium hofmannii	Clostridium tetani
		Mycobacterium rhodochrous
Mycoplasma	T strain *Mycoplasma*	
	Ureaplasma urealyticum	
Yeasts	*Cryptococcus*	
	Rhodotorula	
	Sporobolmyces	
	Candida humicola	
	Trichosporon cutaneum	

and parasitic organisms, but most commonly in gram negative bacteria. Silverman and Stamey reported that 87% of infection related calculi were caused by *Proteus mirabilis*.(17) The alkalinity requirement is met by hydrolysis of urea to ammonium. The most common diagnostic test for identifying urease-producing organisms is growing them on urea agar and detecting the plate change color as the pH rises with urealysis. Table 10.1 summarizes the most common causative organisms in struvite stone pathogenesis.

In some cases, special culture techniques are required to isolate the causative organism. For example, the urease-producing *Ureaplasma urealyticum* is a fastidious organism which cannot be grown by conventional bacterial culture techniques, and requires special cultures.(18, 19) Mobarak et al. studied 30 patients with urinary infection stones and cultured both the mid-stream urine and infection stones retrieved surgically. Bacterial cultures using conventional methods and also *Ureaplasma*-specific cultures (A7 agar and U9 broth) were performed. Cultures revealed that 86.7% of patients had aerobic organisms (*E. coli* in 46.7%, *Klebsiella* in 30%, *Proteus* in 6.7% and *Pseudomonas* in 3.3%) and 26.7% showed *U. urealyticum* in mid-stream urine. The stone cultures revealed aerobic organisms in 76.7%, and *U. urealyticum* in 20%. Sensitivity tests for *U. urealyticum* showed that minocycline was the most effective antimicrobial followed by tetracycline and ciprofloxacin. These data indicate that special culture requests to the microbiology laboratory are prudent, particularly in the setting of struvite crystals with sterile pyuria.

EPIDEMIOLOGY

The incidence and prevalence of infection stones varies with geographic location, patient gender, and presence or absence of associated physiological or anatomic anomalies. In one study from the Mineral and Metabolism Clinic at the University of Texas, Southwestern Medical Center in Dallas, USA, infection stones accounted for 1–5% of patients presenting for metabolic evaluation for recurrent urolithiasis.(2)

In a similar Italian study on 2,086 consecutive patients examined over 15 years in a mineral metabolism clinic, the incidence of infection stones was 22%.(20) In patients with a history of struvite stones, persistent infection was present in 46% (*Proteus* 18%), underlying anatomic urinary tract anomaly was diagnosed in 18.8%, and a urinary risk factor for metabolic stone disease was detected in 42% upon 24-hour urine collection. In another study on 1,354 stones derived from numerous urology departments in the northern African nation of Algeria, the reported incidence of struvite stones was 3.7% in men and 6.7% in women.(21)

This wide range of struvite calculi incidence (from 1 to 22%) likely reflects differences in referral patterns, data reporting, and true geographic variation. For example, some authors combine struvite and calcium carbonate apatite calculi in their reports, whereas others report them separately. Some studies report the incidence of struvite stone only in patients seen at a single stone clinic, whereas other authors have reported the incidence of struvite among stones sent for analysis to national laboratories with a wider catchment area.

Several risk factors for infection stones have been established. Women are afflicted with infection stones more frequently than men. In the abovementioned Italian study, although 57% of the patients in the study group were men, women accounted for 62% of patients presenting with infection stones, for a relative risk of 1.6:1 for female gender and struvite stones.(20) In a different report on 27,980 urinary stones sent for analysis to the National French "Laboratoire Cristal" from 1976 to 2001, women had a 2.9-fold higher risk for infection calculi.(22)

It is also accepted that those with spinal cord injuries (SCI) and neurogenic bladder from various causes are at increased risk for infection calculi. In particular, those with poor bladder compliance, an upper motoneuron syndrome or complete spinal injury with detrusor hyper-reflexia are at highest risk. In some of these patients managed with indwelling urethral catheters or suprapubic cystostomies, struvite stones may form more readily due to retrograde renal infection with urease-producing organisms.

In an Australian study on 1,669 patients with SCI treated from 1982 and 1996, 58 patients (3.5% of the SCI population) were treated for 144 episodes of struvite calculi in their upper tracts.(23) 30% of these stones were complete or partial staghorns and the majority (53%) of struvite stone formers developed their first stone over 10 years after injury. The development of recurrent urinary tract infections was the most common mode of presentation, and risk factors for upper tract struvite calculus formation were use of indwelling catheters (49%), history of bladder stones (52%), and presence of vesicoureteral reflux (28%) on videourodynamic studies. With appropriate surgical treatment, their stone-free rate was 87% and renal function was preserved in 72%. The authors suggest the implementation of preventive measures such as early intermittent catheterization, sphincterotomy and bladder augmentation where possible, to create a catheter-free, low-pressure reservoir.

CLINICAL FINDINGS

Struvite stone patients present in a variety of ways, and most will report a history of chronic flank pain, malaise, fever, dysuria, and intermittent hematuria. They will not usually present with acute renal colic like patients with other stone types, because struvite stones are rarely found in the ureter. This is because struvite calculi are able to grow quite rapidly, and are capable of filling the entire renal collecting system in a matter of weeks to months. Thus, they are most commonly found in the kidney or bladder, and rarely during ureteral transit.

If an infection stone is suspected in a patient, a complete history and physical examination helps lead to a prompt diagnosis. The physician should inquire about a history of recurrent urinary tract infections, immunosuppressed state (diabetes mellitus, steroid intake, etc.), or history of previous stone disease. The past surgical history should screen for urological procedures that could be complicated by renal or ureteral obstruction, or a history of operations to correct anatomic obstruction in the urinary tract.

Medications have not been causally implicated in struvite stone pathophysiology, but a patient who gives a history of using multiple, alternating antibiotics can point further to this diagnosis. There have been no studies suggesting a familial tendency for struvite stones.

The physical examination may demonstrate a chronically ill-appearing patient with signs of chronic infection. In acute pyelonephritis or pyonephrosis, a more toxic appearance may be characteristic, with frequent findings of costovertebral angle tenderness. The examination should be used as an opportunity for the surgeon to think about the optimal surgical options should a staghorn calculus be found. Body habitus, presence of vertebral kyphoscoliosis,

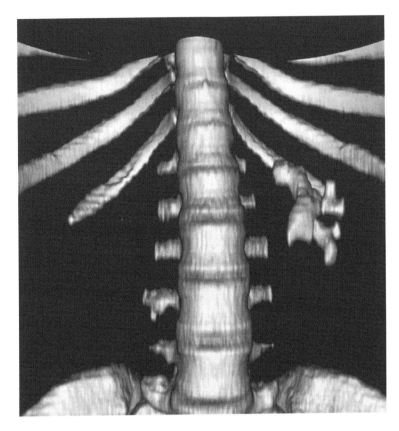

Figure 10.1 Three dimensional computed tomography reconstruction of complete left staghorn calculus. Calyceal anatomy and relationship to bony landmarks are appreciable

organomegaly, bleeding diathesis, and other factors must be considered in choosing the optimal treatment strategy on a case-by-case approach.

Laboratory studies should include a complete blood count and basic metabolic panel, as chronic infection and hydronephrosis can progress to pyonephrosis, abscess formation, and xanthogranulomatous pyelonephritis. Urinalysis will often demonstrate microscopic hematuria, leukocytosis, and presence of coffin-lid struvite crystals. Routine bacterial and fungal urine culture are critical before proceeding with definitive surgery, and on some occasions, special culture techniques may be necessary for organisms such as *Ureaplasma urealyticum*, particularly in the setting of struvite crystals with sterile pyuria.

Different imaging modalities have different strengths and weaknesses in the diagnosis, operative planning and follow-up of patients with struvite stones. Renal sonography may be used for diagnosis because large branched renal calculi can be easily detected. However, sonography is inadequate for surgical planning and for follow-up because small residual calculi (<5mm) can be missed. Plain films and traditional intravenous urography (IVU) can be used for diagnosis because most infection stones are at least faintly radioopaque. Although IVU is no longer widely available, it can be invaluable for planning PCNL.

Noncontrast and contrast enhanced computed tomography (CT) urography are the most commonly used and most versatile radiographic tests for struvite stone diagnosis, surgical planning, and follow-up. All struvite stones and stone fragments can be detected on CT, and detailed intrarenal and perirenal anatomy can be appreciated for surgical planning purposes. With routine use of three-dimensional reconstructions (3-D CT), CT urograms can be studied for PCNL planning (Figure 10.1).

Nuclear renography is also useful for determining differential renal function and subsequent surgical planning. Magnetic resonance urography on the other hand does not have a role in struvite stone management.

NATURAL HISTORY OF INFECTION STAGHORN CALCULI

The natural history of nonoperative management of struvite calculi has been studied by several groups. Vargas et al. reported on 95 patients with infectious stones followed for one to six years.(24) Only 1% was truly asymptomatic and clinical complications occurred in 77 percent of patients. Of these patients, renal tissue was pathologically analyzed in 84 cases, and pyonephrosis was found in 20 percent, xanthogranulomatous pyelonephritis in 8 percent, end stage hydronephrotic kidney in 7 percent, severe pyelonephritic changes in 7 percent, and perinephric abscess in 5 percent.

In a different study, Blandy and Singh described the 10-year mortality and complication rate in patients undergoing active treatment vs. conservative management for infection related staghorn calculi.(25) Sixty patients were managed conservatively, compared to operative removal in 125 cases. The overall mortality rate in patients treated conservatively was 28%, carcinoma developing in 4 cases and life-threatening pyonephrosis in 16 (27%). In contrast, in the surgically treated group, the 10-year mortality rate was 7.2%, with a stone recurrence rate of 17%.

Similarly dismal results were observed during conservative management of infectious staghorn calculi in Japan. Koga et al. treated 167 patients with staghorn calculi, 61 of whom were followed conservatively for 1–18 years (average 7.8).(26) Among those managed nonsurgically, chronic renal failure occurred in 22 patients (36%) and 7 died from uremia. The causes of chronic renal failure were bilateral staghorn calculi, staghorn calculi and contralateral urinary calculi, and chronic pyelonephritis of the contralateral kidney. These morbidity and mortality rates were significantly higher than in the 106 patients who underwent surgical management. A total of 47 patients underwent nephrectomy and pathologic analysis revealed severe hydronephrosis, renal abscess, and xanthogranulomatous pyelonephritis.

Teichman et al. also reported on 177 consecutive staghorn calculus patients in Minnesota to determine risk factors for ultimate renal deterioration and renal cause specific death.(27) After a mean follow-up of 7.7 years, the overall rate of renal deterioration was 28%. Renal deterioration was associated more frequently among patients with solitary vs. nonsolitary kidneys (77% vs. 21%, $p < 0.001$), previous vs. initial stones (39% vs. 14%, $p = 0.03$), recurrent vs. nonrecurrent calculi (39% vs. 22%, $p = 0.07$), hypertension vs. normotension (50% vs. 22%, $p = 0.006$), complete vs. partial staghorn calculi (34% vs. 13%, $p = 0.02$), diversion vs. no diversion (58% vs. 19%, $p < 0.001$) and neurogenic bladder vs. normal voiding (47% vs. 21%, $p = 0.006$), as well as those who refused treatment vs. treated patients (100% vs. 28%, $p < 0.001$). No patient with complete clearance of fragments died of renal-related causes compared to 3% of those without clearance of fragments and 67% of those who refused treatment ($p < 0.001$).

Thus, nonoperative management should be reserved for only the most debilitated patients who cannot undergo an operation. In all other cases, the initial goal is to surgically clear all visible calculi and then medically prevent recurrent stones and infections. Fortunately, there are data showing that end-stage renal disease is not inevitable for struvite stone formers, underscoring the importance of aggressive surgical therapy in this group. Gupta et al. reviewed their last 2,000 urinary stone patients and identified 33 (1.65%) with serum creatinine levels of 2.0 mg/dL or greater at presentation.(28) Complete or partial staghorn calculi were found in 21 of the 33 patients (64%), including 8 with bilateral staghorn calculi. The mean serum creatinine level before surgical intervention was 3.2 mg/dL (range 2.0 to 7.5), and after appropriate surgical therapy (PCNL, SWL, URS), the mean decrease in serum creatinine was 1.2 mg/dL ($p < 0.001$), independent of relief of obstruction.

TREATMENT

The primary goal of staghorn stone management is complete stone eradication in order to prevent stone regrowth, renal deterioration, and persistent infection. The safety and efficacy of endourological techniques have been widely demonstrated, such that open surgery and chemolysis have fallen out of common use.

In 2005, the American Urological Association (AUA) published their Guidelines on the Management of Staghorn Calculi in order to standardize the myriad therapies used.(29) Four major surgical options were recommended in these guidelines, namely, PCNL monotherapy,

SWL monotherapy, open surgery, and combined PCNL and SWL. After extracting the primary literature on staghorn calculi from 1992 to 2003, 32 articles were determined to have adequate information to include in the analysis. The Panel defined a standard "index patient" as one who is "an adult with a staghorn stone (non-cystine, non uric acid) who has two functioning kidneys (function of both kidneys is relatively equal) or a solitary kidney with normal function, and whose overall medical condition, body habitus, and anatomy permit performance of any of the four accepted active treatment modalities, including the use of anesthesia." The reader is referred to the full report for further details on the methodology and their comprehensive review of the available data.(29) Based on their review of the available data, their recommendations for the index patient were summarized as follows:

1   A newly diagnosed patient should be actively treated. Nonsurgical treatments is not considered a viable alternative except in those patients otherwise too ill to tolerate stone removal,
2   Percutaneous nephrolithotomy should be the first treatment utilized for most patients,
3   If combination therapy is undertaken, percutaneous nephroscopy should be the last procedure for most patients,
4   Shock-wave lithotripsy monotherapy should not be used for most patients; however, if it is undertaken, adequate drainage of the treated renal unit should be established before treatment,
5   Open surgery (nephrolithotomy by any method) should not be used for most patients.

Percutaneous Nephrostolithotomy (PCNL)

Percutaneous stone removal became popular in the 1980s as the primary means for stone removal when stone burden exceeds 2cm. It has emerged as the treatment of choice because of superior stone-free outcomes with acceptably low morbidity. In particular, advances in instrumentation and technique such as use of flexible nephroscopy with Holmium laser lithotripsy, improved basket retrieval devices, and the safe implementation of multiple percutaneous access tracts (as needed) have combined to make PCNL monotherapy the preferred approach. Further technical details on PCNL are available in other chapters of this text.

In the 2005 AUA guidelines, the stone-free rate as determined using meta-analysis methods was 78%, with a 95% confidence interval (95% C.I.) of 74–83%.(29) A median 1.9 procedures were required to achieve this stone-free rate. The overall risk of transfusion was 18% (95% C.I. of 14–24%), and risk of serious complications was 15% (95% C.I. 7–27%). Risks included injury to adjacent organs (colon, spleen, liver), hydropneumothorax, collecting system perforations, sepsis, vascular injury, and renal loss.

While PCNL has become increasingly popular over the past 20 years, only two prospective, randomized trials have been conducted to evaluate outcomes. Meretyk and colleagues from Hadassah Medical Center in Israel prospectively randomized 50 kidneys with complete staghorn calculi.(30) Twenty-seven renal units were treated with SWL monotherapy (group 1) and 23 were treated with PCNL and SWL (group 2) if residual stones were present. Stone-free rates were significantly higher in group 2 compared with group 1 (74% vs. 22%, $P = 0.0005$). Furthermore, the complication rate was higher in group 1 despite placement of indwelling ureteral stents before SWL in all cases. Persistent steinstrasse occurred in 3 patients in group 1, and septic complications occurred in 10 patients in group 1 compared to 2 episodes in group 2 ($p = 0.007$). The incidence of secondary unplanned procedures was greater in group 1 compared to group 2. Eight unplanned procedures were required in group 1 compared to only one in group 2 ($p = 0.03$). The only major complication in group 2 was an infected pleural effusion in one patient, which resolved with tube thoracostomy and antibiotics. The investigators concluded that PCNL-based therapy was superior to SWL monotherapy in the treatment of staghorn calculi.

After publication of the 2005 AUA Guidelines, Al-Kohlany et al. from Mansoura University, Egypt, published another prospective randomized trial comparing PCNL and open surgery for complete staghorn calculi.(31) A total of 79 patients with 88 complete staghorn stones (occupying more than 80% of the collecting system) were randomized to PCNL ($n = 43$) or open surgery ($n=45$). Patients in either group with residual stones underwent SWL, and the mean follow-up was relatively short at 4.9 months (range 3–14 months). They found no statistically significantly different stone-free rates at the time of discharge (49% vs. 66%) and at >3 months follow-up (74% vs. 82%). Renal function was also stable or showed improvement in 91% of the PCNL group, compared to 87% of the open surgery group ($p > 0.05$). While stone-free rates and renal functional preservation were similar between the two groups, the PCNL group experienced a significantly lower complication rate (16% vs. 38%, $p < 0.05$), shorter operative time (127 minutes vs. 204 minutes, $p < 0.001$), shorter hospital stay (6.4 vs. 10 days, $p < 0.001$), and earlier return to work (2.5 vs. 4.1 weeks, $p < 0.001$). The authors concluded that PCNL is preferred to open surgery for complete staghorn calculi because comparable stone-free rates can be achieved, with lower morbidity and shorter convalescence time.

Several important technical advances in PCNL deserve mention in the management of staghorn calculi. Firstly, flexible nephroscopy is mandatory after debulking the dominant stone using ultrasonic or pneumatic lithotripsy. This is because branches of struvite stones can hide beyond some of the sharp angles in the pelvicaliceal system that cannot be safely negotiated with the rigid nephroscope. Wong and Leveillee demonstrated the importance and safety of this technique in 45 patients with a mean stone burden of 6.7 cm (range 5.0–10.0 cm).(32) The authors achieved a remarkable 95% stone-free rate after a mean 1.6 procedures, by complementing rigid nephroscopy with flexible nephroscopy/holmium:YAG lithotripsy and nitinol basket stone extraction.

Secondly, in the most complex branched staghorn calculi, the surgeon must be prepared to establish multiple percutaneous tracts in order to achieve maximal stone clearance. This can be performed at the time of initial PCNL if there is clearly visible large radioopaque fragments, or at the time of second look nephroscopy in the situation where residual fragments cannot be reached using the flexible nephrsocope. Aron et al. illustrated its utility and safety in a large group of patients with massive staghorn stones.(33) In the 121 renal units in their series, the mean stone surface area was 4,800 mm^2, mean dimensions of 6.9 x 6.9 cm, with a range of 3,089 mm^2 to 6,012 mm^2. More than 70% of patients required three or more percutaneous tracts, of which 92 (76%) were supracostal. The authors reported an 84% complete clearance rate that improved to 94% with SWL in 8 renal units with small residual fragments. Complications included blood transfusion ($n = 18$), pseudoaneurysm ($n = 2$), fever ($n = 22$), septic shock ($n = 1$), and hydrothorax ($n = 3$), for an overall minor and major complication rate of 38%. Interestingly, calcium oxalate stones accounted for 91% of these staghorns, and the authors also failed to comment on renal functional status before and after surgery. Based on these observations, the authors advocated aggressive multitract approach to large staghorns to maximize stone-free rates.

In another very similar study from India, 164 renal units with staghorns were treated with multitract PCNL.(34) A total of 420 tracts were used (mean 2.6 tracts per kidney), ranging from 2 to 6 tracts per kidney. PCNL monotherapy was successful in complete stone clearance in 71%, and improved to 89% after second look nephroscopy in 30 patients and SWL in 16 patients. There was a 31% transfusion rate and 3.4% required angioembolization for persistent postoperative bleeding. Other complications included urosepsis in 5%, hydrothorax in 4% and perinephric urinoma in one patient. These authors also advocated the multitract approach for the largest staghorns in order to maximize stone free rates.

The abovementioned studies also underscore the importance of second-look nephroscopy. Singla et al. were able to increase the stone-free rate by 18% by performing second look nephroscopy.(34).Traditionally, KUB and/or plain nephro-tomograms were used to identify residual stones post-PCNL and determine the need for second look flexible nephroscopy. Although these modalities are inexpensive and quick, their sensitivity in detecting residual calculi is marginal. Denstedt and colleagues compared the sensitivity of KUB and plain nephrotomograms in detecting residual calculi in 29 patients with large renal calculi undergoing PCNL.(35) Using second-look flexible nephroscopy as the gold standard for identifying residual stones, they found that KUB and nephrotomograms overestimated stone-free rates by 35% and 17%, respectively. Consequently, they encouraged the liberal use of flexible nephroscopy to achieve a stone free state after PCNL, regardless of the results of the imaging studies.

With the widespread use of nonenhanced helical CT to identify renal and ureteral calculi, recent investigators compared the sensitivity of noncontrast CT with flexible nephroscopy in detecting residual stones after PCNL. Along with accurate identification of residual stones, CT has the additional advantage of precisely pinpointing the location of residual fragments and their relation to the nephrostomy tract, further facilitating retrieval of residual stones. Pearle and co-workers prospectively compared KUB, noncontrast CT, and flexible nephroscopy for their ability to detect residual stones in 36 patients with 41 renal units undergoing PCNL for large or complex renal calculi.(36) Using flexible nephroscopy as the gold standard, CT had a sensitivity of 100% and specificity of 62%, compared with 46% and 82%, respectively, for KUB. Thus, in their series, selective use of flexible nephroscopy based on CT findings resulted in only 12% of patients undergoing an unnecessary operation compared with 32% of patients if flexible nephroscopy was performed in all patients, as was their routine.

Extracorporeal Shockwave Lithotripsy Monotherapy

Among the four major treatment modalities used for staghorns, the AUA Guidelines Panel found that SWL monotherapy had the lowest success rate.(29) Detailed descriptions on the operative technique are discussed elsewhere in this text. The stone-free rate was determined using meta-analysis methods and calculated to be 54%, with a 95% confidence interval (95% C.I.) of 45–64%. The overall risk of transfusion was indeterminable due to insufficient data and risk of serious complications was 19% (95% C.I. 11–30%). Risks included colic requiring admission, significant perirenal hematoma, obstruction including steinstrasse, pyelonephritis, and renal loss.

Meretyk et al.'s randomized study on PCNL and SWL monotherapy illustrates the problems with the latter approach.(30) In that study, the stone-free rate was a dismal 22%, and this approach was marred with a high complication rate, despite placement of indwelling ureteral stents before SWL. Persistent steinstrasse occurred in 3 patients (11%), and septic complications occurred in 10 patients (37%). Eight unplanned procedures (30%) were required after SWL, to treat sepsis and steinstrasse. Therefore, while SWL is the least invasive of the operative approaches, it should be not be used alone, but rather in combination with PCNL.

Combination PCNL and SWL

The combined use of PCNL and SWL has been practiced since its introduction in 1987 by Streem et al.(37) This combination, or "sandwich therapy" consists of PCNL followed by SWL and PCNL, in order to treat residual inaccessible infundibulocaliceal stone extensions or fragments. In their systematic review of the literature, the AUA Guidelines Panel found that the median stone-free rate after combination PCNL and SWL was 66% (95% C.I. 60–72%).(29) The overall risk of significant complications was 14% (95% C.I. 9–20%). The guidelines Panel emphasized that percutaneous nephroscopy should be the last procedure for patients undergoing combination therapy because several authors have demonstrated a remarkably low stone-free rate of 23% when SWL was the last combination procedure.(38) Although the original intent of "sandwich therapy" was debulking with PCNL followed by SWL and PCNL of residual fragments, the final percutaneous nephroscopy step was often abandoned in favor of spontaneous passage of fragments, and this may explain the poor stone-free rates after combination therapy.

In contrast, current PCNL monotherapy with more aggressive multitract access, second-look nephroscopy and use of intraoperative flexible nephroscopy have led to higher stone-free rates. Historical studies such as those from Streem et al. reported a stone-free rate of only 63%, with a hospital stay of 12.2 days and transfusion rate of 14%.(39) These results are inferior to currently available studies where stone-free rates of more than 80% can be expected. In one large series of 343 cases of staghorn calculi PCNL alone achieved a stone-free rate of 91% compared with 78.1% to 79.1% with the combination approach.(16) In the 2005 AUA Guidelines, when PCNL monotherapy was compared to combination therapy, a higher stone-free rate (78% vs. 66%, respectively), lower total procedures (1.9 vs. 3.3, respectively), and similar transfusion rates (18% vs. 17%, respectively) were observed.

Ureteroscopy

To date, there have been no published series of flexible ureteroscopy (URS) as monotherapy for staghorn calculi. In their guidelines, the Panel concluded there was insufficient evidence to support the use of URS in staghorn stone management. However, flexible ureteroscopy has been used in combination with PCNL to avoid multiple access tracts and to access calyces that would be difficult to access in an antegrade manner. Marguet et al. tested this method in seven patients who had staghorns and multiple satellite caliceal stones that would have required second and third percutaneous access tracts.(40) After targeting the problematic satellite calices, patients underwent Holmium laser lithotripsy using a 14French ureteral access sheath in the supine position. Patients were then repositioned prone for standard PCNL, and only one tract was used. Their stone-free rate was 70%, and when this group from Duke University compared this group to those who underwent multiple-access PNCL, there was no difference in operative time (142 vs. 166 minutes, $p = 0.36$) but less blood loss among patients treated with the combined approach (79 vs. 345 mL, $p < 0.05$).

In a similar study, Landman et al. reported on nine staghorn calculi managed using a combination of URS and PCNL via a single lower-pole access.(41) In this case, patients were prone for the entire procedure, and flexible URS (using an access sheath) and PCNL were performed simultaneously. They reported a stone-free rate of 78% using a single nephrostomy tract, and no major and four (44%) minor complications occurred.

Laparoscopic Surgery

Laparoscopic anatrophic nephrolithotomy for staghorn calculi has been described in the literature.(42–44) However, these cases are very rare and not enough follow-up data are available to compare this method to the preferred PCNL approach. With the proven safety and efficacy of multitract PCNL, second-look and flexible nephroscopy, the laparoscopic anatrophic approach should be viewed cautiously.

Laparoscopic stone surgery may a reasonable alternative in patients who require concomitant heminephrectomy, pyeloplasty or in those with ectopic kidneys that cannot be safely accessed percutaneously. However, for the index patient, the AUA Panel stated that there were insufficient data to include laparoscopy in their 2005 Guidelines.

Open Surgery

Anatrophic nephrolithotomy and pyelolithotomy operations are becoming exceedingly rare operations because of the efficacy and lower morbidity after endourological surgery. In 2000, only 2% of Medicare patients undergoing a stone-removing procedure were treated with open surgery.(45) In tertiary referral centers, this number dips below 1% of currently used operative techniques. The AUA Guidelines Panel suggests that: "open surgery is an appropriate treatment alternative in unusual situations when a struvite staghorn calculus is not expected to be removable by a reasonable number of percutaneous lithotripsy and/or SWL procedures".

Although open surgery is rarely indicated, Matlaga et al. demonstrated that it can be performed safely and effectively in the select patient who cannot be safely rendered stone free using endoscopic methods.(46) At Wake Forest University where anatrophic nephrolithotomy was popularized by Boyce and Smith, they observed that open surgery was performed in 4.1% cases in 1989. With the advent of SWL and PCNL, these authors reviewed 986 cases performed between 1998 and 2001, and found that only 0.7% were done open. Their indications for open surgery in these seven patients were morbid obesity, large symptomatic anterior caliceal diverticular stones, large stone volume with infundibular stenosis and massive collecting system dilation. All patients were rendered stone free.

Nonsurgical therapies

Infection stones resulting from urease-producing bacteria are best managed with complete surgical removal of the stones. Nonsurgical treatment is appropriate in two scenarios; namely, in patients with significant comorbidities who cannot tolerate endourological stone removal procedures, and to prevent stone recurrence after successful stone eradication.

In the former case, the 2005 AUA Guidelines Panel stated emphatically that nonsurgical treatment (antibiotics, urease inhibitors and other supportive measures) is not standard of care, except in those otherwise too ill to tolerate stone removal.(29) Strategies for prevention of stone recurrence can be categorized into dissolution therapy (chemolysis), antibiotics, urease inhibitors, urinary acidification, and dietary modification.

Dissolution therapy

Due to the prolonged hospital stay, cost and risk of complications, chemolysis has a very limited role in the contemporary management of infection related staghorn stones. Furthermore, with the high stone-free rate that can be attained by PCNL, second look and flexible nephroscopy, this labor intensive therapy has fallen out of favor.

From a historic standpoint, in 1938 Hellstrom first dissolved a struvite stone using boric acid and permanganate. In 1943, Suby and Albright developed Suby's solution G, which could be instilled into the kidney via a nephrostomy tube or ureteral catheter. In their initial report, 6 patients had partial or complete stone dissolution. Mulvaney then modified this solution by adding D-gluconic acid (Hemiacidrin or Renacidin®) and published the first report dissolving infection stones in 9 of 13 patients, either partially or completely. However, a report of four deaths during intrarenal irrigation led to an FDA ban on renal Renacidin® use. Because chemolysis is risky, the following precautions must be exercised during intrarenal chemolysis:

1   Low intrarenal pressures must be maintained (<30 cm water),
2   Serum magnesium and phosphate must be monitored closely,
3   The urine must be sterile. Broad-spectrum antibiotics are given for 14 days in the perioperative period,
4   The collecting system must be unobstructed and there must be no extravasation.

In one of the few contemporary series on chemolysis as active treatment, Tiselius et al. from Sweden reported their results on 118 patients with staghorn stones who underwent combined SWL and percutaneous chemolysis.(47) Interestingly, this is the approach used for all patients with struvite staghorns referred to their tertiary referral center. After placement of two 7Fr pigtail nephrostomy tubes and 7Fr double J stents under intravenous sedation alone, each patient was treated with repeated shock-wave lithotripsy (SWL) sessions (unmodified Dornier HM3 lithotripter) and percutaneous chemolysis with Renacidin®. After a 32-day mean duration of hospital stay (range 5–82), a stone-free rate of 77% was recorded, and no patient required percutaneous, ureteroscopic or open surgery. The mean number of SWL required was 3.4, and the mean number of days of Renacidin® irrigation was 21. The most common complication was nephrostomy tube dislodgment in 15 patients, followed by 3 patients with sepsis which resolved with antibiotics. The authors concluded that the long period necessary for completing the treatment in the most complicated cases might render the procedure less attractive as a standard method, but it is nevertheless an excellent option in high-risk patients and in all those patients in whom other procedures are impossible.

Another indication for Renacidin® irrigation is in those with residual apatite or struvite calculi after percutaneous renal surgery. In two studies, residual calculi were eradicated in 71–80% of patients after 5 to 7 days of irrigation of the renal collecting system using Renacidin®. (48, 49) However, the rare use of chemolysis and the paucity of data led the AUA Guidelines Panel to state that there was insufficient information available for the role of dissolution therapy in their 2005 Guidelines on staghorn calculi.(29)

Antibiotics

Culture-specific preoperative and perioperative antibiotics are critical to prevent sepsis during endourological surgery for struvite calculi. Furthermore, there are data that suggest that long-term, low-dose, culture specific antimicrobials are important to prevent new stone growth and progression after surgery. Firstly, there are *in vitro* data that a reduction in the colony count from 10^7 to 10^5 per cc reduces the urease concentration by 99% in the urine.(50) Thus, while long-term culture-specific antimicrobials may not render the urine completely sterile, the reduction in urease may limit ammoniagenesis and stone progression. Furthermore, by minimizing urease concentrations, small fragments after surgery may even be eradicated because *in vitro* and *in vivo* studies have demonstrated that struvite calculi may dissolve in sterile urine.(51)

The importance of antibiotics was illustrated by Martinez-Pineiro et al., who reported on 99 patients surgically treated for staghorn calculi.(52) 71.7% of the calculi were infection stones, of which 50.7% harbored *Proteus* species bacteria. 17% of patients were noted to have residual stones after surgery, and during follow-up, 46.7% of these cases had recurrent infections and 33.3% had regrowth of staghorn stone. When stratified by presence or absence of infection on follow-up, progressive growth of the recurrent stone occurred in 61.5% of the infected cases, while only 12.5% of patients with sterile urine had recurrent stone growth. These data demonstrate the critical need to treat urinary infection to prevent struvite stone progression, and the authors emphasized the importance of long-term antibiotic therapy on follow-up after staghorn surgery. While antibiotics are important adjuncts to surgery, the 2005 AUA Guidelines Panel stated emphatically that treatment with antibiotics alone is not standard of care.(29)

Urease Inhibitors

Acetohydroxamic acid (AHA) is the only FDA-approved urease inhibitor and most widely used oral medication that irreversibly inhibits bacterial urease.(53, 54) AHA has a high renal clearance, can penetrate the bacterial cell wall, and acts synergistically with several antibiotics. Three randomized, placebo-controlled studies demonstrated significant reduction in stone growth with AHA compared with placebo.

In one randomized double-blind study, 18 patients receiving AHA (15 mg per kilogram of body weight per day, in divided oral doses) for a mean of 15.8 months, were compared to 19 patients who received placebo for a mean of 19.6 months.(55) Seven patients given placebo reached a pre-determined end point: a 100% increase in the two-dimensional surface area of their stones. No patient who received AHA had a doubling of stone size ($p < 0.01$). Nine patients receiving the drug and one patient receiving placebo required a decrease in dosage or cessation of treatment because of adverse effects ($p < 0.01$). Episodes of tremulousness (n = 5, $p < 0.05$), which reversed with a decrease in drug dose, and thrombophlebitis (n = 3, $p > 0.05$) were limited to the group given AHA.

This study demonstrated that AHA effectively inhibits the growth of struvite stones in the short term in patients infected with urea-splitting bacteria, but the prevalence of adverse reactions appears was high. Similar results on effectiveness were noted in two other randomized trials on AHA, but serious neurologic, hematologic, and dermatologic side effects led to more than 20% of patients discontinuing AHA, thereby limiting its usefulness.(53, 54) Lastly, AHA is contraindicated in patients with serum creatinine greater than 2.5 mg/dL because of increased toxicity and poor urinary concentration, further limiting its utility because many patients with struvite stones have pre-existing renal insufficiency.

Urinary acidification

Alkaline urine of pH>7.19, which occurs as a result of urealysis, is necessary for the urine to become supersaturated with struvite and carbonate apatite. Therefore, urinary acidification has been tested as a means to reverse or limit struvite stone growth. Jacobs et al. tested the ability of L-methionine to acidify urine in an *in vitro* model using artificial stones made of struvite (BON(N)-STONES).(56) L-methionine was added to artificial urine to achieve four different pH-values (pH 5.75, pH 6.0, pH 6.25, pH 6.5). The authors found that the dissolution rate of struvite stones in artificial urine increased with a decreasing pH. The diminution of pH from 6.5 to 5.75 led to an increase of the dissolution rate of more than 35%. The authors suggested that oral intake of 1,500–3,000 mg daily of L-methionine may lead to a sufficient acidification for a good dissolution of struvite stones, but this has not been tested in humans.

In a different approach, Donnellan et al. from Australia performed gastric patch pyeloplasty in the rabbit in order to lower urinary pH.(57) A gastric segment was harvested based on branches of the left gastro-epiploic artery and urine culture, serum gastrin and electrolytes were assessed at regular intervals. Sustained urinary acidification was produced in 7 animals (47%) with a mean pH decrease of 2.27. In another 2 rabbits (13%) the urine was initially acidic but subsequently became alkaline due to ureteral obstruction. Electrolytes and gastrin were unchanged in these rabbits and urine culture was positive in 2. Histological testing revealed nonspecific inflammatory changes of the renal pelvis. Anastomotic complications were the most common surgical complication and the most common cause of failed acidification and those animals treated without stents and H-2 blockade were at significantly greater risk for anastomotic leakage. While urinary acidification was achieved, the authors stated that further study is required to assess the ^# effect of this procedure for treating and preventing upper tract struvite calculi.

Dietary modification

Dietary modification aims to deplete the substrates of struvite calculi, including urinary phosphate, magnesium, and ammonia. Most papers in the literature are from veterinary sources, as feline struvite stones are a significant problem. In humans, the only studied diet was proposed by Shorr.(58) This included a regimen of a low-phosphorous, low-calcium diet with oral estrogens and aluminum hydroxide gel. The rationale was that aluminum hydroxide gel would bind phosphate in the gut and become eliminated in the stool. The estrogens could decrease hypercalciuria by enhancing bone mineralization. This diet was actually tested in a

3.5-year follow-up study by Lavengood et al.(59) Patients maintained on the Shorr regimen had a 10% struvite stone recurrence rate compared to 30% in patients who did not follow the regimen. However, the authors stated that dietary compliance was difficult because many patients developed constipation, anorexia, lethargy, bone pain, and hypercalciuria. Another significant limitation is that unopposed oral estrogen has been associated with increased risk of breast and uterine cancers.(60, 61)

CONCLUSIONS

Although struvite calculi represent less than ten percent of urolithiasis cases, their potential for causing renal demise and patient morbidity make them important for physicians to recognize and treat appropriately. The newly diagnosed patient should be actively treated with an endoscopic approach, if possible. PCNL monotherapy in conjunction with flexible nephroscopy, Holmium laser lithotripsy, and multitract access will give the patient the best chance to be stone free. SWL monotherapy and open surgery should not be used as primary treatment in contemporary practice because of the associated morbidity and lower stone free rates. Long-term, culture-specific suppressive antibiotics should be strongly considered in patients after struvite stone surgery to decrease recurrence and progression rates. Other adjunctive medical therapies such as chemolysis, oral urease inhibitors, urinary acidification and dietary modification are not well tolerated and not well-studied, but may be recommended in appropriate clinical situations.

REFERENCES

1. Segura JW. Staghorn calculi. Urol Clin North Am 1997; 24(1): 71–80.
2. Pak CY. Medical management of nephrolithiasis in Dallas: update 1987. J Urol 1988; 140(3): 461–7.
3. Jungers P, Joly D, Barbey F, Choukroun G, Daudon M. ESRD caused by nephrolithiasis: prevalence, mechanisms, and prevention. Am J Kidney Dis 2004; 44(5): 799–805.
4. Beck EM, Riehle RA Jr. The fate of residual fragments after extracorporeal shock wave lithotripsy monotherapy of infection stones. J Urol 1991; 145(1): 6–9.
5. Streem SB. Long-term incidence and risk factors for recurrent stones following percutaneous nephrostolithotomy or percutaneous nephrostolithotomy/extracorporeal shock wave lithotripsy for infection related calculi. J Urol 1995; 153: 584–7.
6. McAleer IM, Kaplan GW, Bradley JS, Carroll SF. Staghorn calculus endotoxin expression in sepsis. Urology 2002; 59(4): 601.
7. Bichler KH, Eipper E, Naber K et al. Urinary infection stones. Int J Antimicrob Agents 2002; 19(6): 488–98.
8. Edin-Liljegren A, Rodin L, Grenabo L, Hedelin H. The importance of glucose for the Escherichia coli mediated citrate depletion in synthetic and human urine. Scand J Urol Nephrol 2001; 35(2): 106–11.
9. Parsons CL, Greenspan C, Moore SW, Mulholland SG. Role of surface mucin in primary antibacterial defense of bladder. Urology 1977; 9(1): 48–52.
10. Parsons CL, Greenspan C, Mulholland SG. The primary antibacterial defense mechanism of the bladder. Invest Urol 1975; 13(1): 72–8.
11. Parsons CL, Stauffer C, Mulholland SG, Griffith DP. Effect of ammonium on bacterial adherence to bladder transitional epithelium. J Urol 1984; 132(2): 365–6.
12. Grenabo L, Hedelin H, Hugosson J, Pettersson S. Adherence of urease-induced crystals to rat bladder epithelium following acute infection with different uropathogenic microorganisms. J Urol 1988; 140(2): 428–30.
13. Dumanski AJ, Hedelin H, Edin-Liljegren A, Beauchemin D, McLean RJ. Unique ability of the Proteus mirabilis capsule to enhance mineral growth in infectious urinary calculi. Infect Immun 1994; 62(7): 2998–3003.
14. Griffith DP, Valiquette L. PICA/burden: a staging system for upper tract urinary stones. J Urol 1987; 138(2): 253–7.
15. Leder RA, Nelson RC. Three-dimensional CT of the genitourinary tract. J Endourol 2001; 15(1): 37–46.
16. Lam HS, Lingeman JE, Russo R, Chua GT. Stone surface area determination techniques: a unifying concept of staghorn stone burden assessment. J Urol 1992; 148: 1026–9.
17. Silverman DE, Stamey TA. Management of infection stones: the Stanford experience. Medicine (Baltimore) 1983; 62(1): 44–51.
18. Pettersson S, Brorson JE, Grenabo L, Hedelin H. Ureaplasma urealyticum in infectious urinary tract stones. Lancet 1983; 1(8323): 526–7.
19. Mobarak A, Tharwat A. Ureaplasma urealyticum as a causative organism of urinary tract infection stones. J Egypt Public Health Assoc 1996; 71(3–4): 309–19.

20. Trinchieri A, Rovera F, Nespoli R, Curro A. Clinical observations on 2086 patients with upper urinary tract stone. Arch Ital Urol Androl 1996; 68(4): 251–62.

21. Djelloul Z, Djelloul A, Bedjaoui A et al. [Urinary stones in Western Algeria: study of the composition of 1,354 urinary stones in relation to their anatomical site and the age and gender of the patients]. Prog Urol 2006; 16(3): 328–35.

22. Daudon M, Dore JC, Jungers P, Lacour B. Changes in stone composition according to age and gender of patients: a multivariate epidemiological approach. Urol Res 2004; 32(3): 241–7.

23. Donnellan SM, Bolton DM. The impact of contemporary bladder management techniques on struvite calculi associated with spinal cord injury. BJU Int 1999; 84(3): 280–5.

24. Vargas AD, Bragin SD, Mendez R. Staghorn calculis: its clinical presentation, complications and management. J Urol 1982; 127(5): 860–2.

25. Blandy JP, Singh M. The case for a more aggressive approach to staghorn stones. J Urol 1976; 115(5): 505–6.

26. Koga S, Arakaki Y, Matsuoka M, Ohyama C. Staghorn calculi–long-term results of management. Br J Urol 1991; 68(2): 122–4.

27. Teichman JM, Long RD, Hulbert JC. Long-term renal fate and prognosis after staghorn calculus management. J Urol 1995; 153(5): 1403–7.

28. Gupta M, Bolton DM, Gupta PN, Stoller ML. Improved renal function following aggressive treatment of urolithiasis and concurrent mild to moderate renal insufficiency. J Urol 1994; 152(4): 1086–90.

29. Preminger GM, Assimos DG, Lingeman JE et al. Chapter 1: AUA guideline on management of staghorn calculi: diagnosis and treatment recommendations. J Urol 2005; 173(6): 1991–2000.

30. Meretyk S, Gofrit ON, Gafni O et al. Complete staghorn calculi: random prospective comparison between extracorporeal shock wave lithotripsy monotherapy and combined with percutaneous nephrostolithotomy. J Urol 1997; 157(3): 780–6.

31. Al-Kohlany KM, Shokeir AA, Mosbah A et al. Treatment of complete staghorn stones: a prospective randomized comparison of open surgery vs. percutaneous nephrolithotomy. J Urol 2005; 173(2): 469–73.

32. Wong C, Leveillee RJ. Single upper-pole percutaneous access for treatment of > or = 5-cm complex branched staghorn calculi: is shockwave lithotripsy necessary? J Endourol 2002; 16(7): 477–81.

33. Aron M, Yadav R, Goel R et al. Multi-tract percutaneous nephrolithotomy for large complete staghorn calculi. Urol Int 2005; 75(4): 327–32.

34. Singla M, Srivastava A, Kapoor R et al. Aggressive Approach to Staghorn Calculi-Safety and Efficacy of Multiple Tracts Percutaneous Nephrolithotomy. Urology 2008; 71: 1039–42.

35. Denstedt JD, Clayman RV, Picus DD. Comparison of endoscopic and radiological residual fragment rate following percutaneous nephrolithotripsy. J Urol 1991; 145(4): 703–5.

36. Pearle MS, Watamull LM, Mullican MA. Sensitivity of noncontrast helical computerized tomography and plain film radiography compared to flexible nephroscopy for detecting residual fragments after percutaneous nephrostolithotomy. J Urol 1999; 162(1): 23–6.

37. Streem SB, Lammert G. Long-term efficacy of combination therapy for struvite staghorn calculi. J Urol 1992; 147(3): 563–6.

38. Leroy AJ, Segura JW, Williams HJ Jr, Patterson DE. Percutaneous renal calculus removal in an extracorporeal shock wave lithotripsy practice. J Urol 1987; 138(4): 703–6.

39. Streem SB, Yost A, Dolmatch B. Combination "sandwich" therapy for extensive renal calculi in 100 consecutive patients: immediate, long-term and stratified results from a 10-year experience. J Urol 1997; 158(2): 342–5.

40. Marguet CG, Springhart WP, Tan YH et al. Simultaneous combined use of flexible ureteroscopy and percutaneous nephrolithotomy to reduce the number of access tracts in the management of complex renal calculi. BJU Int 2005; 96(7): 1097–100.

41. Landman J, Venkatesh R, Lee DI et al. Combined percutaneous and retrograde approach to staghorn calculi with application of the ureteral access sheath to facilitate percutaneous nephrolithotomy. J Urol 2003; 169(1): 64–7.

42. Simforoosh N, Aminsharifi A, Tabibi A et al. Laparoscopic anatrophic nephrolithotomy for managing large staghorn calculi. BJU Int 2008; 101(10): 1293–6.

43. Deger S, Tuellmann M, Schoenberger B et al. Laparoscopic anatrophic nephrolithotomy. Scand J Urol Nephrol 2004; 38(3): 263–5.

44. Kaouk JH, Gill IS, Desai MM et al. Laparoscopic anatrophic nephrolithotomy: feasibility study in a chronic porcine model. J Urol 2003; 169(2): 691–6.

45. Kerbl K, Rehman J, Landman J et al. Current management of urolithiasis: progress or regress? J Endourol 2002; 16(5): 281–8.

46. Matlaga BR, Assimos DG. Changing indications of open stone surgery. Urology 2002; 59(4): 490–3.

47. Tiselius HG, Hellgren E, Andersson A, Borrud-Ohlsson A, Eriksson I. Minimally invasive treatment of infection staghorn stones with shock wave lithotripsy and chemolysis. Scand J Urol Nephrol 1999; 33(5): 286–90.

48. Wall I, Tiselius HG, Larsson L. Hemiacidrin: a useful component in the treatment of infectious renal stones. Eur Urol 1988; 15(1–2): 26–30.

49. Angermeier K, Streem SB, Yost A. Simplified infusion method for 10% hemiacidrin irrigation of renal pelvis. Urology 1993; 41(3): 243–6.
50. Griffith DP, Osborne CA. Infection (urease) stones. Miner Electrolyte Metab 1987; 13(4): 278–85.
51. Griffith DP, Moskowitz PA, Carlton CE Jr. Adjunctive chemotherapy of infection-induced staghorn calculi. J Urol 1979; 121(6): 711–5.
52. Martinez-Pineiro JA, de Iriarte EG, Armero AH. The problem of recurrences and infection after surgical removal of staghorn calculi. Eur Urol 1982; 8(2): 94–101.
53. Griffith DP, Gleeson MJ, Lee H et al. Randomized, double-blind trial of Lithostat (acetohydroxamic acid) in the palliative treatment of infection-induced urinary calculi. Eur Urol 1991; 20(3): 243–7.
54. Griffith DP, Khonsari F, Skurnick JH, James KE. A randomized trial of acetohydroxamic acid for the treatment and prevention of infection-induced urinary stones in spinal cord injury patients. J Urol 1988; 140(2): 318–24.
55. Williams JJ, Rodman JS, Peterson CM. A randomized double-blind study of acetohydroxamic acid in struvite nephrolithiasis. N Engl J Med 1984; 311(12): 760–4.
56. Jacobs D, Heimbach D, Hesse A. Chemolysis of struvite stones by acidification of artificial urine--an in vitro study. Scand J Urol Nephrol 2001; 35(5): 345–9.
57. Donnellan SM, Ryan AJ, Bolton DM. Gastric patch pyeloplasty: development of an animal model to produce upper tract urinary acidification for treating struvite urinary calculi. J Urol 2001; 166(2): 684–7.
58. Shorr E, Carter AC. Aluminum gels in the management of renal phosphatic calculi. J Am Med Assoc 1950; 144(18): 1549–56.
59. Lavengood RW Jr, Marshall VF. The prevention of renal phosphatic calculi in the presence of infection by the Shorr regimen. J Urol 1972; 108(3): 368–71.
60. Opatrny L, Dell'Aniello S, Assouline S, Suissa S. Hormone replacement therapy use and variations in the risk of breast cancer. Bjog 2008; 115(2): 169–75.
61. Boruban MC, Altundag K, Kilic GS, Blankstein J. From endometrial hyperplasia to endometrial cancer: insight into the biology and possible medical preventive measures. Eur J Cancer Prev 2008; 17(2): 133–8.
62. Griffith Ga. Infection stones. In: Pak R, editor. Urolithiasis. A Medical and Surgical Reference. Philadelphia PA: W.B. Saunders & Co, 1990: 113–32.

11 | Shock-wave lithotripsy: Indications and technique

Amy E Krambeck and James E Lingeman

INTRODUCTION

Shock-wave lithotripsy (SWL) was first performed by Chaussy and colleagues in Munich in 1980 utilizing a prototype device that was created by Dornier, a West German aerospace firm, as a spin-off of military research.(1) The first widely distributed clinical lithotriptor, the Dornier HM3, was introduced in 1983 and continues to be in use today, 25 years after its introduction. (2) The first SWL treatment in the United States was performed by Dr. James E. Lingeman at Methodist Hospital in Indianapolis in February, 1984.(3) The initial results for treatment of renal calculi with SWL were very encouraging and thus resulted in the rapid acceptance of this noninvasive technology as a treatment alternative for renal and ureteral calculi.(3)

Following its introduction into clinical use, SWL was applied to a broad spectrum of upper urinary tract stone problems. With growing experience, urologists realized that there was a limit to the ability of the kidney and ureter to discharge stone fragments and, thus, the concept of stone burden (stone size and number) became important in selecting appropriate patients for SWL. Other factors such as stone composition and variations in renal anatomy have also become appreciated as important factors influencing SWL outcomes. Unfortunately, the assessment of the merits of SWL relative to other minimally invasive treatment modalities such as ureteroscopy and percutaneous stone removal have been hindered by the lack of high-quality data. The vast majority of data published on SWL outcomes arise from single institution case series. There is very little level 1 evidence available to help guide decision making for most clinical and stone parameters. Furthermore, decisions about SWL indications are distorted by a common treatment philosophy around the world which is since SWL in noninvasive multiple treatments can be applied without damage to the patient.

Although SWL has revolutionized the treatment of stone disease it does have limitations and poses potential clinical complications. Today, the concept of SWL has become deceptively simple with only a few parameters to be controlled such as patient selection, number of shock waves, power settings, shock wave rate, and protocol of treatment. Unfortunately, to ensure safe treatment practices further parameters should be evaluated. The focus of this chapter is on appropriate patient selection for SWL, which is determined by both patient and stone characteristics. We will also focus on techniques to optimize SWL outcomes by maximizing stone comminution and limiting tissue damage.

INDICATIONS FOR SHOCK-WAVE LITHOTRIPSY

The primary goal of any surgical treatment for stone disease is to achieve maximal stone clearance with minimal patient morbidity. SWL can provide a safe and effective stone treatment when applied to the appropriately selected patient and clinical scenario. Early SWL reports indicated that 80–85% of patients harboring uncomplicated renal calculi could be treated successfully.(4–6) Despite the high early success rates of SWL, certain factors have been identified as predictors of poor stone clearance rates: stones greater than 2 cm in size, stones within dependent or obstructed portions of the kidney, certain stone compositions, body habitus, and unsatisfactory targeting of the stone.(7) Before choosing SWL the physician must consider certain factors including: stone characteristics (size, number, location, composition), renal anatomy (obstruction, hydronephrosis, diverticulum, ectopia, horseshoe), and patient conditions (infection, obesity, body habitus, coagulopathy, age, renal function, hypertension).(8) The simplest tool to determine if SWL should be utilized is "Lingeman's Law" **(Figure 11.1)** for the management of renal lithiasis, which states, "if the stone problem is simple, do SWL; if the

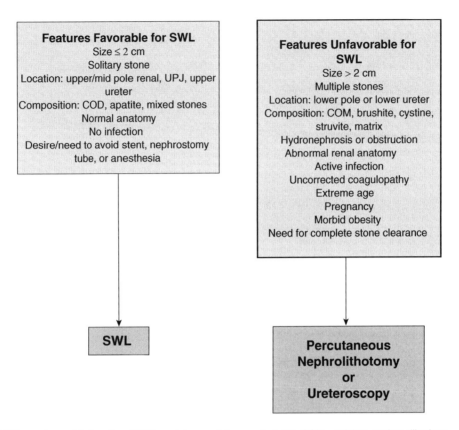

UPJ = ureteropelvic junction, COM = calcium oxalate monohydrate, COD = calcium oxalate dihydrate

Figure 11.1 "Lingeman's Law" for the management of nephrolithiasis, which states, "if the stone problem is simple, do SWL; if the stone problem is not simple do percutaneous nephrolithotomy or ureteroscopy

stone problem is not simple do percutaneous nephrolithotomy or ureteroscopy." To expand on this principal we address certain calculus, anatomic and patient characteristics which help predict SWL success.

Stone Size and Number

Stone burden is potentially the most significant factor in determining if SWL is the appropriate surgical intervention.(9) Multiple authors have demonstrated as the stone burden increases, the stone-free rate declines and the need for ancillary procedures and re-treatment rises **(Figure 11.2)**.(3, 10–12) Larger stone burdens are associated with a higher rate of residuals stones, which can be particularly problematic for patients with struvite calculi who require complete stone clearance to prevent continued infection.(13) Additionally, regardless of the individual stone sizes the presence of multiple stones has been shown to adversely affects the results of SWL.(10, 14, 15)

The mean overall stone-free rates of SWL for the treatment of patients with solitary stones stratified by size are 79.9% (range 63%–90%), 64.1% (range 50%–82.7%), and 53.7% (range 33.3%–81.4%) for stones 10 mm or less, 11 to 20 mm, and larger than 20 mm respectively.(8) Fortunately, the majority (60%) of stones fall within the high SWL success category of less than 10 mm.(8, 14, 16) In general, stones less than 10 mm respond well to SWL regardless of composition or location and should be considered ideal for this treatment modality. SWL results for calculi between 10 to 20 mm in size depend more on stone composition and location. Although SWL is often the initial treatment for stones in this size category, consideration should be given to other more invasive treatments, such as ureteroscopy or percutaneous nephrolithotomy, if the patient has factors associated with decreased SWL success (i.e., cystine or brushite stones, lower pole location, or abnormal anatomy).(8)

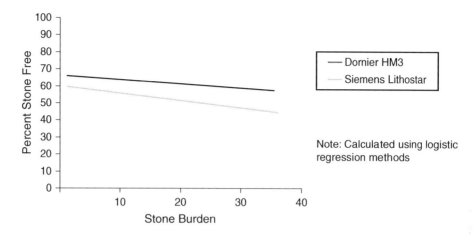

Figure 11.2 Comparison of stone-free rates of two different lithotriptors, the Dornier HM3 and the Siemens Lithostar, related to stone burden. Stone-free rates decrease as stone burden increases.

Stones greater than 20 mm in size are poorly suited for SWL. The frequency of multiple SWL treatments has been shown to increase from 10% to 33% when stone size increased from 1 to 2 cm to 2 to 3 cm.(17) Stone-free rates for stones of this size treated with SWL monotherapy have been reported to be as low as 33 to 65%.(17–19) Based on the need for ancillary procedures and retreatment rates the National Institutes of Health Consensus Conference recommends patients with stones larger than 2 cm initially be treated with percutaneous nephrolithotomy, not SWL. SWL can be used as an adjunct only, to treat any residual fragments if needed. (20) If the patient desires to proceed with SWL despite appropriate counseling regarding the high retreatment rate and potential complications, then ureteral stenting is recommended.(20) Based on the 2005 AUA Nephrolithiasis Guideline Committee SWL should not be considered a monotherapy for Staghorn calculi.(21) If SWL is used in combination with percutaneous nephrolithotomy it should be used as an adjunct with percutaneous nephrolithotomy being the primary procedure.(8, 21)

Stone Location

The treatment of lower pole calculi with SWL is an area of significant controversy.(22) Lingeman and colleagues first noted the limitations of SWL for lower calculi when he reported a 60% stone-free rate for lower pole stones treated with SWL compared to a 90% rate for similar stones treated with percutaneous nephrolithotomy.(23) In this study, increasing stone burden was associated with progressively less successful stone-free outcomes with SWL; stones smaller than 10 mm demonstrated a stone-free rate of 74% compared to 56% for stones 10 to 20 mm.(23) Analysis of several studies have demonstrated mean stone-free rates of 67.8%, 54.6%, and 28.8% for lower pole stones less than 10 mm, 10 to 20 mm, and greater than 20 mm treated with SWL.(23–28) Interestingly, since the mid 1980s there has been an increase in the number of SWLs performed for lower pole stones with 2% performed in 1984 compared to 48% in 1991.(23)It has been proposed that the change in distribution is the result of small, radiolucent fragments gravitating to more dependent calyces after SWL therapy. These fragments act as a nidus for further stone growth, ultimately resulting in a greater incidence of lower pole stones.(29)

Reasons for poor clearance of fragments after SWL from the lower pole could be purely gravity dependent (30); however, other investigators have also evaluated such aspects as infundibulopelvic angle, infundibular length, infundibular width, infundibular height, and complex calyx.(8) Sampaio and colleagues found that 72% of patients were rendered stone free after SWL of a lower pole stone if the infundibulopelvic angles was greater than 90 degrees, but only 23% were stone free when the angle was less than 90 degrees.(31) Other authors have found similar correlations between infundibulopelvic angle and stone-free results.(30, 32) Infundibular width has also been evaluated as a factor for lower pole SWL success, with investigators noting an infundibular width less than 5 mm as a risk factor for residual fragments compared to a width greater than 5 mm.(30, 32–35) Keeley went on to report an association between the combination of infundibulopelvic angle of less than 90 degrees, infundibular length of more than 3 cm and infundibular width of 5 mm or less with treatment failure.(28) In an analysis of 11 mm to 20 mm lower pole stones treated with SWL he found that when all of these unfavorable factors were present in the same patient the stone-free rate was only 9% compared to 71% if all three factors were absent.(28)

Despite these compelling data other significant studies have found no association between renal anatomy and lower pole SWL failure.(36–38) One possible reason for the confounding results is the low reproducibility of lower pole anatomic measurements. Infundibular width can vary based on the phase of the pyelogram, degree of external compression, and ureteral peristalsis.(28, 39) Furthermore, many of the studies focusing on renal anatomy as a function of SWL success failed to factor in stone composition or type of lithotriptor as possible confounding factors.(28, 39) Tuckey and associates have suggested a simpler anatomic measurement that is easily reproducible.(34) They found the calyceal pelvic height (vertical distance from the lowermost point of the calyx to highest point of the lower lip of the pelvis) was a reproducible measurement predictive of SWL failure. A calyceal pelvic height less than 15 mm was associated with a 92% stone clearance rate, but a height of greater than 15 mm was associated with only a 52% clearance rate.(34)

Although it is widely accepted that lower pole stone-free rates after SWL are poor several authors support SWL as a primary monotherapy for lower pole stones. Comparison of SWL with percutaneous nephrolithotomy for lower pole stones have demonstrated inferior stone-free results of 63% vs. 100%, 23% vs. 93%, and 14% vs. 86% for stones less than 10 mm, 11 mm to 20 mm, and greater than 20 mm respective.(38) Elbahnasy found similar results with an overall SWL stone-free rate of 56% compared to 85% for percutaneous nephrolithotomy for lower pole calculi; however, the investigator noted similar clinical stone recurrence rates between the two groups at 20 months (10% vs. 11%).(30) Cass also noted similar low stone clearance rates and minimal recurrence rates for lower pole stones treated with SWL compared to percutaneous nephrolithotomy, but also noted decreased complication rates, lower secondary and repeat procedures, and shorter hospital stays with SWL.(40) Others have noted poor stone clearance rates of less than 65% after SWL of lower pole calculi, but a minimal need for secondary intervention.(41, 42) These findings have lead several investigators to consider SWL as primary therapy for lower pole stones less than 2 cm. A comparison of SWL to ureteroscopy for stones less than 10 mm reported no significant difference in stone-free rates between the two techniques (35% SWL vs. 50% ureteroscopy).(43) Based on these data we believe SWL can be considered primary therapy for lower pole calculi after appropriate patient counseling regarding the risk of significant residual fragments. If complete stone clearance is necessary (i.e. infected stones), percutaneous nephrolithotomy should be considered for stones greater than 10 mm.

The 2007 AUA guidelines on ureteral calculi suggest both ureteroscopy and SWL are appropriate treatment for ureteral calculi greater than 10 mm regardless of location.(44) Uncomplicated stones less than 10 mm should be allowed an appropriate time interval for spontaneous passage before SWL or ureteroscopy is employed. Patients should be counseled of the higher stone-free rate noted with ureteroscopy over SWL, but also of the higher concomitant complications rate of ureteroscopy over SWL.(44) This meta-analysis noted a SWL stone-free rate of 82%, 73%, and 74% for proximal, mid, and distal ureteral stones, respectively.(44) These data is a change from the previous 1997 guidelines, which recommended SWL as first-line therapy for proximal ureteral stones. The current guidelines also revealed a significant decline in the SWL distal ureteral stone-free rate compared to 1997. This decline most likely reflects changes in lithotriptor design from first to current generation machines. The guidelines also noted a decrease in SWL stone-free rates with ureteral stones greater than 10 mm compared to stones less than 10 cm, but strongly state routine stenting is not necessary for uncomplicated ureteral stone SWL.

Stone Composition

The readiness with which a stone is fragmented by SWL is variable among stones of different composition. Even stones of the same composition may fragment differently.(45–49) Adjusted for size, cystine, and brushite calculi are the most resistant to SWL, followed by calcium oxalate monohydrate.(50) Following in order of descending fragility are struvite, calcium oxalate dihydrate, and uric acid stones.(49–50) Stone composition not only predicts how easily a stone will fragment with SWL, but also can predict how it fragments. Cystine and calcium oxalate mono-hydrate tend to fragment into large pieces after SWL that are difficult to clear from the collecting system.(49, 51) In general any patient with brushite, cystine, or calcium oxalate monohydrate stones should not be treated with SWL unless the stone burden is small.(8) Unfortunately, aside from cystine stones which can easily be diagnosed by identifying cystine crystals in the urine, it is not currently possible to predict calcium oxalate monohydrate or brushite stone compositions preoperatively.

When SWL is used unselectively for the treatment of cystine stones results are poor, with stone-free rates of approximately 70% for stones 20 mm or less and 40% for stones greater than 20 mm.(8) The higher rate of stone fragmentation noted with small stones may be a result of molecular structure. Cystine can produce rough or smooth appearing crystalline structures. Bhatta and associates demonstrated that smooth cystine stones are more resistant to SWL com-pared to the rough appearing stones.(45) An *in vitro* study by Kim and associates confirmed that rough cystine stones more easily fragmented with SWL compared to smooth stones. They also demonstrated that homogenous appearing cystine stones on helical CT required more than 60% more shock waves to fragment compared to inhomogenous cystine stones.(52) Unfortunately, with current imaging techniques we are unable to accurately distinguish between resistant and fragmentable cystine stones preoperatively and therefore do not routinely use SWL for the treatment of cystine calculi.

Brushite calculi should follow a similar treatment algorithm to that for cystine stones. Overall SWL treatment success rate for brushite stones has been reported at 65%, but only 11% of patients were stone free with a mean of 1.5 SWL sessions per stone.(53) There are some con-cerns that SWL is actually associated with the development of brushite stones. The occurrence of brushite stones is increasing and retrospective evaluation has demonstrated SWL use is more fre-quent among brushite stone formers than among a similar cohort of calcium stone formers.(51)

SWL may be ineffective at treating other stone types due to their soft nature or relative radiolucent appearance. Matrix calculi are composed of as much as 75% organic matter and are radiolucent. They are often associated with urea-splitting bacteriuria. SWL is usually ineffec-tive because of the gelatinous nature of the stone and they are usually best treated by percuta-neous nephrolithotomy not SWL or ureteroscopy.(54) The protease inhibitor drug indinavir is another soft, radiolucent stone. These stones cannot be appreciated with standard radiography or computed tomography (CT). In rare instances they can have a calcium component making them radiographically visible.(55) The incidence of symptomatic stones in treated patients is approximately 12.4% at a mean of 21.5 weeks after initiation of the drug.(56) In general these stones resolve with conservative management and discontinuation of the drug, no surgical intervention is necessary.(55–57)

Collecting System Obstruction and Hydronephrosis

Stone-free rates after SWL for patients with hydronephrosis and/or obstruction are poor.(10, 58) A retrospective study of 161 patients followed for 20 months identified a significant associa-tion of hydronephrosis with the failure to clear residual fragments.(15) In multivariate analysis hydronephrosis was the single most significant factor for stone passage, greater than multiple stones at time of treatment.(15) Any patient with obstruction distal to the stone is unlikely to clear stone fragments unless the obstruction is alleviated before SWL. If both obstruction and infection are present, SWL should not be performed as it can result in life-threatening urosepsis.(59)

Abnormal Renal Anatomy

Several renal anatomic anomalies have been found to be associated with an increased risk of stone formation and deserve special consideration if SWL is to be used as the primary treat-ment for renal calculi. These conditions include ureteropelvic junction obstruction, horseshoe kidney, ectopic or fusion anomalies, and calyceal diverticula. Although not a congenital abnor-mality, the transplanted kidney also creates a unique treatment scenario and will be covered in this segment.

Adult ureteropelvic junction obstruction is frequently associated with urinary calculi. A stone at the ureteropelvic junction can exacerbate the degree of obstruction and further com-promise renal function.(60) Stone formation in these patients is not only a function of urinary stasis and outlet obstruction, but also underlying metabolic abnormalities, which are present in the majority of patients.(61) Due to outlet obstruction, SWL is generally ineffective for these patients and concomitant definitive treatment of the obstruction should be performed before or at time of stone treatment either by percutaneous endopyelotomy, ureteroscopic endopyelotomy, open or laparoscopic pyeloplasty.(8)

Horseshoe kidneys are malrotated and reside lower in the abdomen than normal kidneys due to halting of renal assent by the inferior mesenteric artery. The ureteropelvic junction is often anomalous because of the high ureteral insertion into an elongated renal pelvis, which can result in impaired urine drainage.(8) Up to two-thirds of horseshoe kidney patients are found to have hydronephrosis, infection, or urolithiasis.(62) Despite these conditions SWL can achieve satisfactory results in the properly selected patient with a stone burden less than 1.5 cm and a nonobstructed system.(8) The kidney malrotation can make localization of the calyces and calculi more difficult, especially for stones in the anteromedial location. By placing the patient in the prone positioning localization of the stone is facilitated.(63) Others have described a "blast path" technique, which works on the premise that sufficient acoustic pressure for stone fragmentation exists beyond F2 along the shock-wave axis and thus allows for positioning distal to F2.(64) Results of SWL for calculi in the horseshoe kidney vary widely with stone-free rates ranging from 28% to 78%.(62, 65–69) When success is stratified by location stone-free rate is inferior for lower calyceal stones (53.8%) compared to middle or upper calyceal locations (100%) in the horseshoe kidney.(67) In addition to stone location, size appears to play a critical role. Patients with stones greater than 1 cm in a horseshoe kidney treated with SWL have a stone-free rate of less than 30%.(68) Furthermore, patients with renal calculi in a horseshoe kidney treated with SWL require a higher number of shock waves per treatment and experience a higher re-treatment rate than patients with similar stones in normal renal units.(3, 4, 10) If SWL is to be used, achievement of a stone-free collecting system is important for patients with horseshoe kidneys, as recurrences rates as high as 86% has been reported for these patients left with residual fragments compared to 14% if rendered stone free.(62)

Ectopic kidneys can be found in approximately 1 in 2,200 to 1 in 3,000 patients and can be located in almost any abdominal or thoracic location, but the most common site is in the pelvis.(8) SWL should be considered the primary therapy for calculi 2 cm or less in these kidneys if technically feasible.(70, 71) Treatment can be administered as for an anatomically normal kidney; however, a prone position may be necessary if the bony pelvis shields the targeted stone from the shock waves.

Similar in location to the ectopic pelvic kidney, calculi in the allograft kidney can present special challenges. The reported incidence of stones in an allograft kidney ranges from 0.4% to 1.76%.(72–75) SWL has been reported to be successful in the treatment of allograft urolithiasis, but ancillary procedures are common and multiple sessions may be required. Challacombe and colleagues report on 13 renal transplant patients with allograft calculi treated with SWL, of which 62% required multiple treatment session. Additionally, eight patients required ureteral stent placement and four required percutaneous nephrostomy tube placement to relieve obstruction.(73) Others have reported success rates of 87–100% with SWL for these patients but have cited multiple calculi and stones greater than 15 mm as risk factors for ancillary procedures or repeat treatment for complete stone clearance.(74, 75) Since the risk of complications are significant in the transplant patient population and the goal should be complete stone clearance, strong consideration should be given to more definitive therapy such as percutaneous nephrolithotomy. Percutaneous nephrolithotomy has been found to be safe and effective at preserving renal function while obtaining complete stone clearance in this cohort.(76) If SWL is to be used for allograft nephrolithiasis it is important that urinary tract infections are appropriately treated and all obstruction is relieved to avoid sepsis and further renal function compromise. Like the pelvic kidney a prone position may be necessary to perform SWL if the bony pelvis shields the stone.

The use of SWL for the treatment of patients with calculi in calyceal diverticulum is controversial. Although SWL may adequately fragment the stone it does not eradicate the diverticulum, which should be performed at time of stone removal to prevent stone recurrence.(77) The stone-free rate for diverticular calculi treated with SWL averages only 21% (range 4%–58%).(19) Initial symptom-free rates range from 36% to 86% on short-term follow-up.(19, 78) However, on extended follow-up some of the patients initially rendered symptom free will become symptomatic and require re-treatment.(79) We therefore do not recommend SWL for calyceal diverticula except under exceptional circumstances.

Infection and Inflammation

History of urinary tract infection is not a contraindication to SWL; however, careful consideration must be given to this clinical scenario. The incidence of sepsis after uncomplicated SWL is less than 1%, but increases to 2.7%–56% if staghorn calculi are treated.(59, 80) The risk of sepsis after SWL also increases if the urine culture demonstrates bacterial growth before SWL or if there is presence of obstruction.(8, 59) For this reason SWL should only be performed if the urine is sterile at time of treatment or no distal obstruction is noted. For high-risk patient consideration should be given to prophylactic antibiotic therapy peri-procedurally.(81) Moreover, urinary tract infections in the presence of renal calculi can be difficult to eradicate unless all the offending stones are completely removed. If the patient appears to have an infected stone, consideration should be given to percutaneous nephrolithotomy or ureteroscopy as treatment options over SWL after appropriate antibiotic therapy. Both of these procedures, unlike SWL, can assure complete stone removal.

Obesity and Body Habitus

Obesity is not a contraindication to SWL, but can limit effectiveness. Morbid obesity (defined as more than 100 lbs overweight, >200% of ideal body weight, or BMI greater than 40) may make SWL impractical or technically impossible due to weight limitations on the lithotriptor gantry/table and inability to target the stone radiographically. Thomas and Cass reported successful treatment of 81 obese patients, weighing more than 300 lbs, with SWL using high-energy settings. Overall stone-free rate for this study was 68% at 3 months postoperatively and retreatment rates were 11%.(82) Despite these promising results, body mass index has been found to be a significant negative predictor of a stone-free outcome after SWL.(83, 84) Skin-to-stone distance greater than 10 cm has also been shown to decrease SWL stone-free outcomes regardless of overall patient size.(85)Therefore, if SWL is to be used for the morbidly obese patient the lithotriptor with the greatest focal length and highest peak pressure should be selected.(86) Pediatric patients or those with spine or limb deformities may also be difficult to position for SWL. If severe deformities that would preclude appropriate coupling or radiographic localization are encountered, consideration should be given to other treatment modalities.(8)

Patient Comorbidities

Several patient comorbidities can make SWL technically difficulty or even unsafe. We attempt to cover the major recognized conditions. Treatment of patients with uncorrected coagulopathies can result in life-threatening retroperitoneal hemorrhage. However, SWL can be used safely once the bleeding diathesis has been corrected.(87, 88) If the coagulopathy is medically induced and cannot safely be discontinued due to other patient comorbidities, such has mechanical heart valve or drug-eluting cardiac stents, then ureteroscopy should be considered the appropriate treatment as it has proven safe in patients with uncorrected bleeding diatheses.(89, 90)

Cardiac arrhythmias have been shown to occur with spark gap and piezoelectric generators when not synchronized to the electrocardiogram; however, these arrhythmias are usually minor and not life threatening.(91–93) With newer generation lithotriptors synchronization is not necessary and patients with cardiac arrhythmias can safely be treated. Patients with pacemakers can also be treated safely with SWL. Before SWL, dual-chamber pacemakers should be reprogrammed to single-chamber mode and rate-responsive pacemakers should be reprogrammed to non-rate-responsive mode.(94)

Although there have been reports of inadvertent treatment of pregnant patients with SWL with no adverse sequelae to the fetus, pregnancy remains a contraindication to this treatment modality.(95, 96) Only ureteroscopy with holmium laser stone ablation or basket extraction has been proven safe during pregnancy.(8) If SWL is to be considered the treatment of choice, then the patient should be temporized with ureteral stenting until after the fetus is delivered and then SWL administered. Although no studies have demonstrated adverse effects of SWL on reproductive organs (88), some physicians choose to not perform SWL of distal ureteral stones in women of reproductive age to limit injury.

SWL treatment of patients with calcified abdominal aortic aneurysms may be hazardous and bears special mention. Several case reports of abdominal aortic aneurysm rupture after SWL are present in the literature (97, 98); however, further studies have demonstrated safety of

SWL in this clinical scenario. In an *in vitro* study with a maximum of only 1,000 shock waves administered, Vasavada et al. demonstrated no significant pathologic difference in aneurismal tissue after SWL treatment.(99) Several reports of safe treatment of patients with both aortic and renal aneurysms without complications have also been made.(88, 100–103) Carey and Streem have previously published guidelines for the use of SWL in the presence of a calcified aneurysm. (104) They suggest the aneurysm should be asymptomatic, and the diameter less than 2 cm if renal or 5 cm if abdominal aortic. To ensure that minimal pressure is generated at the aneurysm the stone to aneurysm distance should be 5 cm or more on CT and the aneurysm should not lie along the parallel axis of the shock wave. Additionally, the energy setting should not be greater than or the equivalent of 18 kV.(104) Despite these recommendations, due to the potential devastating effects of thromboembolic events or aneurysm rupture we suggest consideration be given to ureteroscopy or percutaneous nephrolithotomy if abdominal aneurysm is present.

The most common and widely accepted complication of SWL is acute subcapsular hematoma formation. Reports focusing on electrohydraulic lithotriptors have noted an incidence of symptomatic post SWL perirenal hematoma in 0.2 to 1.5% of treated patients. (105–109) However, the actual rate of subclinical hematoma formation is much higher. Routine screening with CT or magnetic resonance imaging (MRI) has demonstrated the rate of perirenal hematoma formation post-SWL to be as high as 20 to 25%.(110–112) Most resolve without lasting adverse effects and only rarely will they persist.(113) Although a rare event, large hematomas can lead to the need for blood transfusions and even acute renal failure.(106, 107, 114–118) Risk factors for hematoma using electrohydraulic lithotriptors have been identified and include pretreatment UTI, bilateral SWL procedures, and hypertension.(106) The degree of hypertension appeared to be a significant risk factor, as poorly controlled hypertension was found to further increase the rate of post-SWL hematoma formation from 2.5% to 3.8%.(106) Other small studies have noted an association between post-electrohydraulic SWL subcapsular hematoma formation and pre-existing hypertension, diabetes mellitus, coronary artery disease, and obesity.(107, 119) The development of a subcapsular hematoma appears to also depend on age. A study of 415 SWL procedures using an electromagnetic lithotriptor demonstrated a subcapsular hematoma rate of 4.1%. Hypertension and number of shocks administered were not associated with hematoma formation. However, excluding individuals with clotting abnormalities, the probability of developing an SWL-induced hematoma was nearly two-fold per decade in multivariate analysis.(120) Thus, advanced age appears to be a significant risk factor associated with post-SWL complications.

Certain patient populations require special consideration if SWL is to be implemented and include: children, elderly patients, those with hypertension and renal insufficiency. These patient populations have been associated with the enhancement of possible SWL adverse effects and care should be taken to limit the number and energy of shock wave administered in these circumstances. Although no studies have definitively associated SWL with the long-term development of renal failure, several studies have demonstrated significant acute renal injury post SWL in the animal and human model (110, 121–123) and concerns exist of the potential to exacerbate underlying renal insufficiency. Extreme age appear to be a particular risk factor. Although SWL is considered overall safe in children, a 9-year follow-up of children treated with SWL noted a decrease in overall renal size not only in the treated kidney but also the contralateral normal kidney.(124) These findings have lead to concerns of long-term renal function compromise. Janetschek and colleagues identified age of 60 years as a risk factor for SWL-induced elevated resistive indices. In their 26 month follow-up study elevated resistive indices (45% of patients) were noted almost exclusively in patients over the age of 60 years with a rate of new onset hypertension was 17.5%.(125)This study has lead to concerns of injury to the aged kidney with SWL.

Patient Expectations

The patient's expectations must be taken into account before recommending SWL. Patients should be informed of the risks and benefits of all available treatment modalities, including spontaneous passage, percutaneous nephrolithotomy, ureteroscopy, and SWL. Although SWL is the least invasive method second to spontaneous passage, it often requires lengthy follow-up until all fragments clears. It also carries the risk of unplanned additional invasive procedures and re-treatment.(126) If the patient is looking for immediate or near immediate stone-free status with a single procedure then they may be better suited for ureteroscopy or percutaneous nephrolithotomy. However, patients may choose SWL due to apprehension of the anesthesia associated with ureteroscopy and percutaneous nephrolithotomy. A major benefit of SWL is that it can be performed under light sedation or even anesthesia free. Additionally, ureteroscopy and percutaneous nephrolithotomy carry the possibility of a temporary ureteral stent or nephrostomy tube, which most patients prefer to avoid.

SHOCK-WAVE LITHOTRIPSY TECHNIQUES

Since the clinical introduction of SWL over 25 years ago, much knowledge has been gained into the physics behind stone comminution. Recent research has identified several factors that can improve not only the overall safety of SWL but also the technical and overall success. These factors include: lithotriptor characteristics, treatment rate, pretreatment protocols, coupling, and imaging. We will briefly review each topic.

Lithotriptor Characteristics
The first clinical lithotriptor, the HM3, was highly effective and obtained unchallenged stone-free rates above 70%.(3) However, the large water bath, one-time use electrodes, and the need for general anesthesia lead to the development of newer generations of lithotriptors. Newer lithotriptors are dry-head devices with the treatment head enclosed by a water-filled cushion. Electromagnetic lithotriptors now have shock sources with a lifetime of close to one million shock waves, and some lithotriptors are even "anesthesia free."

To limit pain during SWL the aperture of the shock source was widened to spread the energy of the shock pulse over a broader area of the body. This allowed for the production of higher acoustic pressures within the focal volume but also narrowed the focal zone.(127) The narrower the focal zone, the harder it is to keep shock waves on the targeted stone as it moves during respiratory excursion.(128) Narrow focal zone, high-pressure machines tend to have lower stone-free rates, require more retreatments, and show an increased occurrence of adverse effects.(84, 129–137) Thus, the strategy to make lithotripsy anesthesia free while producing powerful shock waves reduced both the efficiency and the safety of the lithotriptors. It is possible for some patients to be treated effectively without general or regional anesthesia, but stone-free rates are improved if the patient is anesthetized, and treatment under anesthesia in the United States is common with most centers using intravenous sedation regardless of the type of lithotriptor.(8, 138)

In an attempt to reproduce some of the effectiveness of the original HM3, some manufacturers have introduced lithotriptors with wider focal zones or adjustable width focal zones. There is now a lithotriptor that produces shock waves at low peak positive pressures (<20 MPa) delivered to a focal zone of ~18 mm.(139) Recent studies indicate that the shear stress within the stone is enhanced when the focal width is broader than the stone and thus width of focal zone is critical for successful stone breakage.(140–142)

Shock-Wave Rate
It has recently been shown that shock-wave rate has a significant effect on the efficiency of stone breakage and limitation of renal vascular injury, with slower rate being better. Tissue injury in the experimental porcine model has shown to dramatically decrease when shock-wave rate is slowed to 30 shock waves per minutes **(Figure 11.3)**. (143, 144) By slowing the firing rate of the lithotriptor to 30 shock waves per minute the lesion size in the porcine kidney was decreased to less than 0.1% of the functional renal volume (FRV) compared to approximately 6% FRV at 120 shock waves per minutes.(143) Similar human studies have yet to be performed.

A number of clinical studies report that slowing the firing rate of the lithotriptor to 60 shock waves per minute gives better outcomes than treatment at the typical rate of 120 shock waves per minutes.(145–150) This effect is seen with both electrohydraulic and electromagnetic lithotriptors. One advantage of slowing the shock-wave rate is that fewer shock waves are needed for treatment, but this also increases the overall treatment time. Lengthening treatment time has the potential to produce practicality and administrative obstacles for high volume centers and therefore, may be slow to gain acceptance.

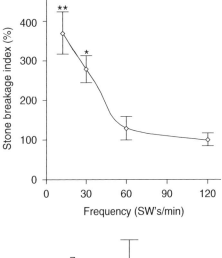

Figure 11.3 The efficiency of stone fragmentation in vitro is inversely related to the rate of shock waves (SW) administration. Similar findings have been documented in clinical trials.

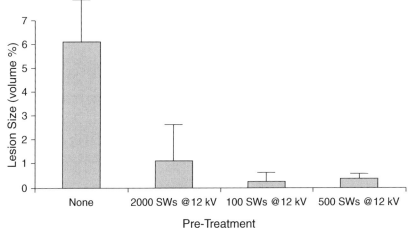

Figure 11.4 Effects of SWL pretreatment protocols on renal hemorrhagic lesion in the porcine model. Pretreatment of the kidney with low-dose SWL demonstrates a decrease in the size of the renal hemorrhagic lesion.

One possible explanation for the benefits of slow rate may be its effect on the negative pressure wave of the shock wave. Cavitation bubbles generated by passage of the shock wave grow, collapse, and produce micro bubbles that can persist between pulses acting to seed more cavitation initiated by subsequent shock waves.(144) The shorter the interval between shock waves, the more cavitation nuclei survive. The leading positive pressure phase of the shock pulse is unaffected by the very small persistent cavitation bubbles, but the trailing tensile phase of the shock wave is reduced.(144, 151) *In vitro* studies using high-speed imaging show a reduction in bubble interactions with stone phantoms at fast rate (120 shock waves per minute) compared to a slower shock wave rate (60 shock waves per minute).(152) This may begin to explain why stone breakage is less efficient as the firing rate increases.

Pretreatment and Treatment Protocols

Certain treatment or "priming" protocols have been shown to decrease shock wave-induced renal tissue damage in the animal model.(153) Using the HM3 lithotriptor a standard clinical dose of 2,000 shock waves at 24 kV (120 shock waves per minute) created a lesion in the porcine model measuring approximately 6% of the FRV. The lesion size was reduced to 0.3% of the FRV by simply pretreating the kidney with as few as 100 shock waves at 12 kV before completion of the dose with the higher amplitude pulses **(Figure 11.4)**.(153) Further studies have suggested that it is not the low volume priming dose that is protective but rather the interruption of

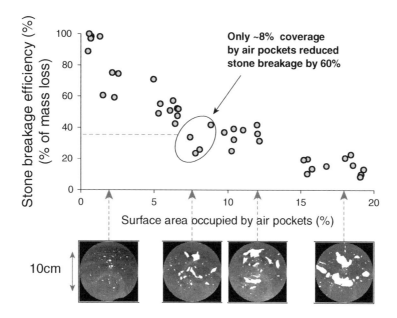

Figure 11.5   Effects of lithotriptor coupling on stone breakage. As the amount of air pockets between the treatment head and the patient's skin increase, the efficiency of stone breakage decreases.

shock-wave delivery. In a similar study the renal lesion was the same size when the priming dose was delivered at 12, 18, 24 kV.(154) However, only when a 3–4 minute pause was instituted following the priming dosing before resuming the clinical shock-wave treatment was renal protection observed. Thus, the priming dose was only protective when followed by a brief delay.

With early lithotriptors, radiologic imaging of the stone could be challenging and it was difficult to determine when adequate stone fragmentation had occurred. This couple with the misperception that shock waves cause little-to-no injury has led some centers to adopt the use of predetermined set doses for most standard stone cases. Stone fragility is variable and it is likely that in most cases fewer shock waves are needed than are used. We recommend frequent imaging of stones during SWL and discontinuation of the treatment once stone comminution is noted on imaging to limit potential injury.

Acoustic Coupling

Coupling of the patient skin to the lithotriptor interface is essential in the propagation of shock waves to the targeted stone. Although an excellent form of coupling, the ~950 liter water bath of the HM3 was cumbersome, requiring a large surgical facility not only for the bath itself, but also the gantry. The development of the dry treatment head eliminated the large space requirements and made lithotriptors transportable; thus making this technology available to every urologist. Unfortunately, achieving adequate coupling with these machines is difficult. Air pockets can be created at the interface between the cushion of the treatment head and the patient's skin. *In vitro* studies have demonstrated that a 20–40% reduction in stone breakage can be observed if just 2% of the coupling interface is covered by air pockets **Figure 11.5)**.(155) Thus, variability in coupling can produce variability in outcomes for the same machine.

Inadequate coupling may also contribute to adverse effects. When coupling is poor, more shock waves are needed to break a stone, thus exposing the patient to a higher dose of shock-wave energy. Although this shock-wave energy is attenuated by the poor coupling, negative pressure above the cavitation threshold is still delivered.(155)

Currently there is no way to assess the quality of coupling; however, *in vitro* studies have found a few simple steps that can be taken to improve dry-head device coupling.(156) In a recent study coupling was enhanced if the gel was applied as a large bolus to the lithotriptor cushion directly from the stock jug and not a tube. Squeezing the gel from the tube introduced more air bubbles. Spreading the gel over the cushion also introduced air bubbles and the investigators found that better results were observed if the gel was placed as a large bolus on the treatment head and allowed to spread upon contact between the treatment head and the skin. (156) In short, minimize the handling of the gel. Inflation of the water cushion also collapses air pockets but is not a substitute for good gel application.

Stone Imaging

Certain stone types including cystine, brushite, and calcium oxalate monohydrate are relatively resistant to SWL. However, knowledge of patient stone type is not readily available unless the stone analysis was performed on previous stone events or if the patient has a medical/family history suggestive of the above stone types. Advancements are being made in the area of preoperative imaging in an attempt to gain preoperative knowledge of stone type, which would limit unnecessary SWL treatment. It has long been suggested that X-ray attenuation values may be useful in predicting fragility. However, recent studies have demonstrated that Hounsfield units correlate best with stone size, not fragility.(157, 158) When stones were graded on the basis of having internal structures visible by helical CT, those "heterogeneous" stones required half the number of shock waves to break to completion than stones that had "homogeneous" structure. (158) Kim and associates noted cystine stone fragility was associated with CT heterogeneity in an *in vitro* model; finding the more heterogeneous the stone the more easily it fragmented with SWL.(52) Thus, although Hounsfield unit measurements do not accurately predict stone fragility, it may be possible to determine the shock-wave susceptibility of a stone based on CT-imaged heterogeneity. This information has the potential to be used for stone-tailored shock-wave dosing.

CONCLUSIONS

SWL is a safe and appropriate treatment option for most urinary tract calculi when appropriately employed. When evaluating SWL as a treatment option, consideration of certain patient and stone characteristics should be made. SWL is highly successful when used for solitary stones less than 2 cm in size. However, outcomes are decreased when the stone is in a lower pole location or a hydronephrotic system. Certain stone compositions including cystine, brushite, calcium oxalate monohydrate, and matrix are relatively resistant to SWL and consideration should be given to other treatment modalities when these compositions are present. Regardless of stone size, location, or composition, SWL should not be used in the following circumstances: acute infection, urinary tract obstruction, uncorrected coagulopathies, and extreme ages. Patient expectations should also be assessed and counseling regarding realistic outcomes should be provided to insure patient satisfaction.

Once SWL is determined to be the appropriate treatment option, certain variables can be modified to increase its effectiveness. Lithotriptors with wide focal zones and decreased peak pressures appear to have improved outcomes over the "anesthesia-free" high peak pressure machines. Administration of anesthesia regardless of type of lithotriptor can also improve stone fragmentation rates. By slowing the shock-wave rate treatment efficacy is increased while limiting tissue injury. Pretreatment protocols have also demonstrated tissue protective effects, specifically when a 3–4 minute pause is instituted. SWL should also be tailored to the patient by administering only the number and intensity of shocks needed to break the stone and by avoiding set treatment protocols. Finally, every attempt at maximal coupling should be made to ensure efficient shock-wave delivery. By appropriate patient selection and minor treatment modifications we can help to ensure patient safety and limit retreatment rates of SWL.

REFERENCES

1. Chaussy C, Brendel W, Schmiedt E. Extracorporeally induced destruction of kidney stones by shock waves. Lancet 1980; 2: 1265–8.
2. Chaussy C, Schmiedt G. Shock wave treatment of stones in the upper urinary tract. Urol Clin North Am 1983; 10: 743–50.

3. Lingeman JE, Newman D, Mertz JH et al. Extracorporeal shock wave lithotripsy: the Methodist Hospital of Indiana experience. J Urol 1986; 135: 1134–7.

4. Chaussy C, Schmiedt E, Extracorporeal shock wave lithotripsy (ESWL) for kidney stones. An alternative to surgery? Urol Radiol 1984; 6: 80–7.

5. Krings F, Tuerk C, Steinkogler I, Marberger M. Extracorporeal shock wave lithotripsy retreatment ("stir-up") promotes discharge of persistent caliceal stone fragments after primary extracorporeal shock wave lithotripsy. J Urol 1992; 148: 1040–1.

6. Wickham JE. Treatment of urinary tract stones [Review]. BMJ 1993; 307: 1414–7.

7. Grasso M, Loisides P, Beaghler M, Bagley D. The case for primary endoscopic management of upper urinary tract calculi: I. a critical review of 121 extracorporeal shock-wave lithotripsy failures. Urology 1995; 45: 363–71.

8. Lingeman JE, Matlaga BR, Evan AP. Surgical management of upper urinary tract calculi. In: Kavoussi LR, Novick AC, Partin AW, Peters CA, Wein AJ eds, Campbell-Walsh Urology, 9th edn (Saunders-Elsevier: Philadelphia, 2007: 1431–507.

9. Motola JA, Smith AD. Therapeutic options for the management of upper tract calculi. Urol Clin North Am 1990; 17: 191–206.

10. Drach GW, Dretler S, Fair W et al. Report of the United States cooperative study of extracorporeal shock wave lithotripsy. J Urol 1986; 135: 1127–33.

11. Politis G, Griffith D. Ureteroscopy in management of ureteral calculi. Urology 1987; 30: 39–42.

12. el Damanhoury H, Scharfe T, Ruth J, Roos S, Hohenfellner R. Extracorporeal shock wave lithotripsy of urinary calculi: experience in treatment of 3,270 patients using the Siemens Lithostar and Lithostar Plus. J Urol 1991; 145: 484–8.

13. Segura JW. The role of percutaneous surgery in renal and ureteral stone removal. J Urol 1989; 141: 780–1.

14. Cass AS. Comparison of first generation (Dornier HM3) and second generation (Medston STS) lithotriptors: treatment results with 13,864 renal and ureteral calculi. J Urol 1995; 153: 588–92.

15. Shigeta M, Kasaoka Y, Yasumoto H et al. Fate of residual fragments after successful extracorporeal shock wave lithotripsy. Int J Urol 1999; 6: 169–72.

16. Logarakis NF, Jewett MA, Luvmes J, Honey RJ. Variation in clinical outcome following shock wave lithotripsy. J Urol 2000; 163: 721–5.

17. Lingeman JE, Coury TA, Newman DM et al. Comparison of results and morbidity of percutaneous nephrostolithotomy and extracorporeal shock wave lithotripsy. J Urol 1987; 138: 485–90.

18. Psihramis KE, Jewett MA, Bombardier C, Caron D, Ryan M. Lithostar extracorporeal shock wave lithotripsy: the first 1,000 patients. Toronto Lithotripsy Associates. J Urol 1992; 147: 1006–9.

19. Renner C, Rassweiler J. Treatment of renal stones by extracorporeal shock wave lithotripsy. Nephron 1999; 81(suppl 1): 71–81.

20. Consensus conference. Prevention and treatment of kidney stones. JAMA 1988; 260: 977–81.

21. Preminger GM, Assimos DG, Lingeman JE et al. Chapter 1: AUA guideline on management of Staghorn calculi: diagnosis and treatment recommendations. J Urol 2005; 173: 1991–2000.

22. Tolley DA, Downey P. Current advances in shock wave lithotripsy. Curr Opin Urol 1999; 9: 319–23.

23. Lingeman JE, Siegel YI, Steele B, Nyhuis AW, Woods JR. Management of lower pole nephrolithiasis: a critical analysis. J Urol 1994; 151: 663–7.

24. Havel D, Saussine C, Fath C et al. Single stones of the lower pole of the kidney. Comparative results of extracorporeal shock wave lithotripsy and percutaneous nephrolithotomy. Eur Urol 1998; 33: 396–400.

25. Kupeli B, Biri H, Sinik Z et al. Extracorporeal shock wave lithotripsy for lower caliceal calculi. Eur Urol 1998; 34: 203–6.

26. May DJ, Chandhoke PS, Efficacy and cost-effectiveness of extracorporeal shock wave lithotripsy for solitary lower pole renal calculi. J Urol 1998; 159: 24–7.

27. Talic RF, El Faqih SR. Extracorporeal shock wave lithotripsy for lower pole nephrolithiasis: efficacy and variables that influence treatment outcome. Urology 1998; 51: 544–7.

28. Keeley FX Jr, Moussa SA, Smith G, Tolley DA. Clearance of lower-pole stones following shock wave lithotripsy: effect of the infundibulopelvic angle. Eur Urol 1999; 36: 371–5.

29. Carr LK, D'A Honey J, Jewett MA et al. New stone formation: a comparison of extracorporeal shock wave lithotripsy and percutaneous nephrolithotomy. J Urol 1996; 155: 1565–7.

30. Elbahnasy AM, Shalhav AL, Hoenig DM et al. Lower caliceal stone clearance after shock wave lithotripsy or ureteroscopy: the impact of lower pole radiographic anatomy. J Urol 1998; 159: 676–82.

31. Sampaio FJ, D'Anunciacao AL, Silva EC. Comparative follow-up of patients with acute and obtuse infundibulum-pelvic angle submitted to extracorporeal shockwave lithotripsy for lower caliceal stones: preliminary report and proposed study design. J Endourol 1997; 11: 157–61.

32. Sabnis RB, Naik K, Patel SH, Desai MR, Bapat SD. Extracorporeal shock wave lithotripsy for lower calyceal stones: can clearance be predicted? Br J Urol 1997; 80: 853–7.

33. Gupta NP, Singh DV, Hemal AK, Mandal S. Infundibulopelvic anatomy and clearance of inferior caliceal calculi with shock wave lithotripsy. J Urol 2000; 163: 24–7.

34. Tuckey J, Devasia A, Murthy L, Ramsden P, Thomas D. Is there a simpler method for predicting lower pole stone clearance after shock wave lithotripsy than measuring infundibulopelvic angle? J Endourol 2000; 14: 475–8.

35. Sumino Y, Mimata H, Tasaki Y et al. Predictors of lower pole renal stone clearance after extracorporeal shock wave lithotripsy. J Urol 2002; 168: 1344–7.

36. Madbouly K, Sheir KZ, Elsobky E. Impact of lower pole renal anatomy on stone clearance after shock wave lithotripsy: fact or fiction? J Urol 2001; 165: 1415–8.

37. Sorensen CM, Chandhoke PS. Is lower pole caliceal anatomy predictive of extracorporeal shock wave lithotripsy success for primary lower pole kidney stones? J Urol 2002; 168: 2377–82.

38. Albala DM, Assimos DG, Clayman RV et al. Lower pole I: a prospective randomized trial of extracorporeal shock wave lithotripsy and percutaneous nephrostolithotomy for lower pole nephrolithiasis-initial results. J Urol 2001; 166: 2072–80.

39. Pace KT, Weir MJ, Tariq N, Honey RJ. Low success rate of repeated shock wave lithotripsy for ureteral stones after failed initial treatment. J Urol 2000; 164: 1905–7.

40. Cass AS. Extracorporeal shockwave lithotripsy or percutaneous nephrolithotomy for lower pole nephrolithiasis? J Endourol. 1996; 10: 17–20.

41. Obek C, Onal B, Kantay K et al. The efficacy of extracorporeal shock wave lithotripsy for isolated lower pole calculi compared with isolated middle and upper caliceal calculi. J Urol 2001; 166: 2081–4.

42. Chen RN, Streem SB. Extracorporeal shock wave lithotripsy for lower pole calculi: long-term radiographic and clinical outcome. J Urol 1996; 156: 1572–5.

43. Pearle MS, Lingeman JE, Leveillee R et al. Prospective, randomized trial comparing shock wave lithotripsy and ureteroscopy for lower pole caliceal calculi 1 cm or less. J Urol 2005; 173: 2005–9.

44. Preminger GM, Tiselius HG, Assimos DG et al. American Urological Association Education and Research, Inc. European Association of Urology. 2007 Guideline for the management of ureteral calculi. Eur Urol 2007; 52: 1610–31.

45. Bhatta KM, Prien EL Jr, Dretler SP. Cystine calculi-rough and smooth: a new clinical distinction. J Urol 1989: 142: 937–40.

46. Sakamoto W, Kishimoto T, Takegaki Y et al. Stone fragility – measurement of stone mineral content by dual photon absorptiometry. Eur Urol 1991; 20: 150–3.

47. Wang YH, Grenabo L, Hedelin H et al. Analysis of stone fragility in vitro and in vivo with piezoelectric shock waves using the EDAP LT-01. J Urol 1993; 149: 699–702.

48. Wu TT, Hsu TH, Chen MT, Chang LS. Efficacy of in vitro stone fragmentation by extracorporeal, electrohydraulic, and pulsed-dye laser lithotripsy. J Endourol 1993; 7: 391–3.

49. Pittomvils G, Vandeursen H, Hellemans J et al. Stone geometry and structure dependence on extracorporeal shock wave lithotripsy. J Endourol 1993; 7: 357–62.

50. Saw KC, McAteer JA, Monga AG et al. Helical CT of urinary calculi: effect of stone composition, stone size, and scan collimation. AJR Am J Roentgenol 2000; 175: 329–32.

51. Parks JH, Worcester EM, Coe FL, Evan AP, Lingeman JE. Clinical implications of abundant calcium phosphate in routinely analyzed kidney stones, Kidney Int 2004; 66: 777–85.

52. Kim SC, Burns EK, Lingeman JE et al. Cystine calculi: correlation of CT-visible structure, CT number, and stone morphology with fragmentation by shock wave lithotripsy. Urol Res 2007; 35: 319–24.

53. Klee LW, Brito CG, Lingeman JE, The clinical implications of brushite calculi. J Urol 1991; 145: 715–8.

54. Bani-Hani AH, Segura JW, LeRoy AJ. Urinary matrix calculi: our experience at a single institution. J Urol 2005; 173: 120–3.

55. Sundaram CP, Saltzman B. Urolithiasis associated with protease inhibitors. J Endourol 1999; 13: 309–12.

56. Reiter WJ, Schon-Pernerstorfer H, Dorfinger K, Hofbauer J, Marberger M. Frequency of urolithiasis in individuals seropositive for human immunodeficiency virus treated with indinavir is higher than previously assumed. J Urol 1999; 161: 1082–4.

57. Kohan AD, Armenakas NA, Fracchia JA. Indinavir urolithiasis: an emerging cause of renal colic in patients with human immunodeficiency virus. J Urol 1999; 161: 1765–8.

58. Winfield HN, Clayman RV, Chaussy CG et al. Monotherapy of staghorn renal calculi: a comparative study between percutaneous nephrolithotomy and extracorporeal shock wave lithotripsy. J Urol 1988; 139: 895–9.

59. Meretyk S, Gofrit ON, Gafnio O et al. Complete staghorn calculi: random prospective comparison between extracorporeal shock wave lithotripsy monotherapy and combined with percutaneous nephrostolithotomy. J Urol 1997; 157: 780–6.

60. Rutchik SD, Resnick MI. Ureteropelvic junction obstruction and renal calculi. Pathophysiology and implications for management. Urol Clin North Am 1998; 25: 317–21.

61. Husmann DA, Milliner DS, Segura JW. Ureteropelvic junction obstruction with a simultaneous renal calculus: long-term followup. J Urol 1995; 153: 1399–402.

62. Lampel A, Hohenfellner M, Schultz-Lampel D et al. Urolithiasis in horseshoe kidneys: therapeutic management. Urology 1996; 47: 182–6.

63. Jenkins AD, Gillenwater JY. Extracorporeal shock wave lithotripsy in the prone position: treatment of stones in the distal ureter or anomalous kidney. J Urol 1988; 139: 911–5.

64. Locke DR, Newman RC, Steinbock GS, Finlayson B. Extracorporeal shock-wave lithotripsy in horseshoe kidneys. Urology 1990; 35: 407–11.

65. Esuvaranathan K, Tan EC, Tung KH, Foo KT. Stones in horseshoe kidneys: results of treatment by extracorporeal shock wave lithotripsy and endourology. 1991; 146: 1213–5.

66. Vandeursen H, Baert L. Electromagnetic extracorporeal shock wave lithotripsy for calculi in horseshoe kidneys. J Urol 1992; 148: 1120–2.

67. Theiss M, Wirth MP, Frohmuller HG. Extracorporeal shock wave lithotripsy in patients with renal malformations. Br J Urol 1993; 72: 534–8.

68. Kirkali Z, Esen AA, Mungan MU. Effectiveness of extracorporeal shockwave lithotripsy in the management of stone-bearing horseshoe kidneys. J Endourol 1996; 10: 13–5.

69. Kupeli B, Isen K, Biri H et al. Extracorporeal shockwave lithotripsy in anomalous kidneys. J Endourol 1999; 13: 349–52.

70. Zafar FS, Lingeman JE. Value of laparoscopy in the management of calculi complicating renal malformations. J Endourol 1996; 10: 379–83.

71. Harmon WJ, Kleer E, Segura JW. Laparoscopic pyelolithotomy for calculus removal in a pelvic kidney. J Urol 1996; 155: 2019–20.

72. Rhee BK, Bretan PN Jr, Stoller ML. Urolithiasis in renal and combined pancreas-renal transplant recipients. J Urol 1999; 161: 1458–62.

73. Challacombe B, Dasgupta P, Tiptaft R et al. Multimodal management of urolithiasis in renal transplantation. BJU Int 2005; 96: 385–9.

74. Millan Rodriguez F, Gonzalez de Chaves E, Rousaud Baron F, Izquierdo Latorre F, and Rousaud Baron A. Treatment of urinary calculi in transplanted kidney with extracorporeal shock wave lithotripsy. Arch Esp Urol 2003; 56: 793–8.

75. Klingler HC, Kramer G, Lodde M, Marberger M. Urolithiasis in allograft kidneys. Urology 2002; 59: 344–8.

76. Krambeck AE, LeRoy AJ, Patterson DE, Gettman MT. Percutaneous nephrolithotomy success in the transplant kidney. J Urol Publication pending December 2008.

77. Cohen TD, Preminger GM. Management of calyceal calculi. Urol Clin North Am 1997; 24: 81–96.

78. Streem SB, Yost A. Treatment of caliceal diverticular calculi with extracorporeal shock wave lithotripsy: patient selection and extended followup. J Urol 1992; 148: 1043–6.

79. Jones JA, Lingeman JE, Steidle CP. The roles of extracorporeal shock wave lithotripsy and percutaneous nephrostolithotomy in the management of pyelocaliceal diverticula. J Urol 1991; 146: 724–7.

80. Lam HS, Lingeman JE, Mosbaugh PG et al. Evolution of the technique of combination treatment for staghorn calculi: a decreasing role for extracorporeal shock wave lithotripsy. J Urol 1992; 148: 1058–62.

81. Bierkens AF, Hendrikx AJ, Ezz el Din KE et al. The value of antibiotic prophylaxis during extracorporeal shock wave lithotripsy in the prevention of urinary tract infections in patients with urine proven sterile prior to treatment. Eur Urol 1997; 31: 30–5.

82. Thomas R, Cass A. Extracorporeal shock wave lithotripsy in morbidly obese patients. J Urol 1993; 150: 30–2.

83. Ackermann DK, Fuhrimann R, Pfluger D, Studer UE, Zingg EJ. Prognosis after extracorporeal shock wave lithotripsy of radiopaque renal calculi: a multivariate analysis. Eur Urol 1994; 25: 105–9.

84. Portis AJ, Yan Y, Pattaras JG et al. Matched pair analysis of shock wave lithotripsy effectiveness for comparison of lithotriptors. J Urol 2003; 169: 58–62.

85. Pareek G, Hedican SP, Lee Jr FT, Nakada SY. Shock wave lithotripsy success determined by skin-to-stone distance on computed tomography. Urology 2005: 66: 941–4.

86. Hofmann R, Stoller ML. Endoscopic and open stone surgery in morbidly obese patients. J Urol 1992; 148: 1108–11.

87. Streem SB, Yost A. Extracorporeal shock wave lithotripsy in patients with bleeding diatheses. J Urol 1991; 144: 1347–8.

88. Streem SB. Contemporary clinical practice of shock wave lithotripsy: a reevaluation of contraindications. J Urol 1997; 157: 1197–203.

89. Grass M, Chalik Y. Principles and applications of laser lithotripsy: experience with the holmium laser lithotrite. J Clin Laser Med Surg 1998; 16: 3–7.

90. Watterson JD, Girvan AR, Cook AJ et al. Safety and efficacy of holmium:YAG laser lithotripsy in patients with bleeding diatheses. J Urol 2002; 168: 442–5.

91. Ector H, Janssens L, Baert L, De Geest H. Extracorporeal shock wave lithotripsy and cardiac arrhythmias, Pacing Clin Electrophysiol 1989; 12: 1910–7.

92. Greenstein A, Kaver I, Lechtman V, Braf Z. Cardiac arrhythmias during nonsynchronized extracorporeal shock wave lithotripsy. J Urol 1995; 154: 1321–2.

93. Kataoka H, Cardiac dysrhythmias related to extracorporeal shock wave lithotripsy using a piezoelectric lithotriptor in patients with kidney stones. J Urol 1995; 153: 1390–4.
94. Albers DD, Lybrand FE III, Axton JC, Wendelken JR. Shockwave lithotripsy and pacemakers: experience with 20 cases. J Endourol 1995; 9: 301–3.
95. Chaussy C, Fuchs G. Extracorporeal shock wave lithotripsy: the evolution of the revolution. Urologe A 1989; 28: 126–9.
96. Frankenschmidt A, Sommerkamp H. Shock wave lithotripsy during pregnancy: a successful clinical experiment. J Urol 1998; 159: 501–2.
97. Lazarides MK, Drista H, Arvanitas DP, Dayantas JN. Aortic aneurysm rupture after extracorporeal shock wave lithotripsy, Surgery 1996; 122: 112–3.
98. Taylor JD, McLoughlin GA, Parsons KF. Extracorporeal shock wave lithotripsy induced rupture of abdominal aortic aneurysm. Br J Urol 1995; 76: 262–3.
99. Vasavada SP, Streem SB, Kottke-Marchant K, Novick AC. Pathological effects of extracorporeally generated shock waves on calcified aortic aneurysm tissue. J Urol 1994; 152: 45–8.
100. Carey SW, Streem SB. Extracorporeal shock wave lithotripsy for patients with calcified ipsilateral renal arterial or abdominal artic aneurysms. J Urol 1992; 148: 18–20.
101. Deliveliotis C, Kostakopoulos A, Stavropoulos N et al. Extracorporeal shock wave lithotripsy in 5 patients with aortic aneurysm. J Urol 1995; 154: 1671–2.
102. Ignatoff JM, Nelson J B. Use of extracorporeal shock wave lithotripsy in a solitary kidney with renal artery aneurysm. J Urol 1993; 149: 359–60.
103. Thomas R, Cherry R, Neal DW Jr. The use of extracorporeal shock wave lithotripsy in patients with aortic aneurysms. J Urol 1991; 146: 409–10.
104. Carey SW, Streem SB. Extracorporeal shock wave lithotripsy for patients with calcified ipsilateral renal arterial or abdominal aortic aneurysms. J Urol 1992; 148: 18–20.
105. Roth RA, Beckmann CF. Complications of extracorporeal shock-wave lithotripsy and percutaneous nephrolithotomy. Urol Clin North Am 1988; 15: 155–66.
106. Knapp PM, Kulb TB, Lingeman JE et al. Extracorporeal shock wave lithotripsy-induced peri-renal hematomas. J Urol 1988; 139: 700–3.
107. Newman LH, Saltzman B. Identifying risk factors in development of clinically significant post-shock-wave lithotripsy subcapsular hematomas. Urology 1991; 38: 35–8.
108. Chaussy C, Schuller J, Schmiedt E et al. Extracorporeal shock-wave lithotripsy (ESWL) for treatment of urolithiasis. Urology 1984; 23: 59–66.
109. Tillotson CL, Deluca SA. Complications of extracorporeal shock wave lithotripsy. Am Fam Physician 1988; 38: 161–3.
110. Kaude JV, Williams CM, Millner MR, Scott KN, Finlayson B. Renal morphology and function immediately after extracorporeal shock-wave lithotripsy. Am J Roentgenol 1985; 145: 305–13.
111. Rubin JI, Arger PH, Pollack HM et al. Kidney changes after extracorporeal shock wave lithotripsy: CT evaluation. Radiology 1987; 162: 21–4.
112. Baumgartner BR, Dickey KW, Ambrose SS et al. Kidney changes after extracorporeal shock wave lithotripsy: appearance on MR imaging. Radiology 1987; 163: 531–4.
113. Krishnamurthi V, Steeem SB. Long-term radiographic and functional outcome of extracorporeal shock wave lithotripsy induced perirenal hematomas. J Urol 1995; 154: 1673–5.
114. Treglia A, Moscoloni M. Irreversible acute renal failure after bilateral extracorporeal shock wave lithotripsy. J Nephrol 1999; 12: 190–2.
115. Liguori G, Trombetta C, Bucci S et al. Reversible acute renal failure after unilateral extracorporeal shock-wave lithotripsy. Urol Res 2004; 32: 25–7.
116. Tuteja AK, Pulliam JP, Lehman TH, Elzinga LW. Anuric renal failure from massive bilateral renal hematoma following extracorporeal shock wave lithotripsy. Urology 1997; 50: 606–8.
117. Baskin LS, Stoller ML. Severe haemorrhage after extracorporeal shock wave lithotripsy; radiological evaluation. Br J Urol 1992; 69: 214–5.
118. Maziak DE, Ralph-Edwards A, Deitel M et al. Massive perirenal and intra-abdominal bleeding after sock-wave lithotripsy: case report. Can J Surg 1994; 37: 329–32.
119. Coptcoat MJ, Webb DR, Kellett MJ et al. The complications of extracorporeal shockwave lithotripsy: management and prevention. Br J Urol 1987; 58: 578–80.
120. Dhar NB, Thornton J, Karafa MT, Streem SB. A multivariate analysis of risk factors associated with subcapsular hematoma formation following electromagnetic shock wave lithotripsy. J Urol 2004; 172: 2271–4.
121. Evan AP, Willis LR, Lingeman JE, McAteer JA. Renal trauma and the risk of long-term complications in shock wave lithotripsy. Nephron 1998; 78: 1–8.
122. Lechevallier E, Siles S, Ortega JC, Coulange C. Comparison by SPECT of renal scars after extracorporeal shock wave lithotripsy and percutaneous nephrolithotomy. J Endourol 1993; 7: 465–7.
123. Umekawa T, Kohri K, Yoshioka K, Iguchi M, Kurita T. Production of anti-glomerular basement membrane antibody after extracorporeal shock wave lithotripsy. Urol Int 1994; 52: 106–8.

124. Lifshitz DA, Lingeman JE, Zafar FS et al. Alterations in predicted growth rates of pediatric kidneys treated with extracorporeal shockwave lithotripsy. J Endurol 1998; 12: 469–75.

125. Janetschek G, Frauscher F, Knapp R et al. New onset hypertension after extracorporeal shock wave lithotripsy: age related incidence and prediction by intrarenal resistive index. J Urol 1997; 158: 346–51.

126. Peschel R, Janetschek G, Bartsch G. Extracorporeal shock wave lithotripsy vs. ureteroscopy for distal ureteral calculi: a prospective randomized study. J Urol 1999; 162: 1909–12.

127. Cleveland RO, McAteer JA. The physics of shock wave lithotripsy. In: Smith's Textbook on Endourology. Edited by AD smith, GH Badlani, DH Bagley, RV Clayman, SG Docimo, GH Jordan et al. Hamilton, Ontario, Canada: BC Decker, Inc, 2007: 317–32.

128. Cleveland RO, Anglade R, Babayan RK. Effect of stone motion on in vitro comminution efficiency of Storz Modulith SLX. J Endourol 2004; 18: 629–33.

129. Lingeman JE, Lithotripsy systems. In: Smith's Textbook on Endourology. Edited by AD Smith, GH Badlani, DH Bagley, RV Clayman, SG Docimo, GH Jordan et al. Hamilton, Ontario, Canada: BC Decker, Inc, 2007: 333–42.

130. Bierkens AF, Hendrikx AJ, de Kort JV et al, Efficacy of second generation lithotriptors: a milticenter comparative study of 2,206 extracorporeal shock wave lithotripsy treatments with the Siemens Lithostar, Dornier HM4, Wolf Piezolith 2300, Direx Tripter X-1 and Breakstone lithotriptors. J Urol 1992; 148: 1052–6.

131. Chan SL, Stothers L, Rowley A et al. A prospective trial comparing the efficacy and complications of the modified Dornier HM3 and MFL 5000 lithotriptors for solitary renal calculi. J Urol 1995; 153: 1794–7.

132. Hoag CC, Taylor WN, Rowley VA. The efficacy of the Dornier Doli S lithotripter for renal stones. Can J Urol 2006; 13: 3358–63.

133. Tan EC, Tung KH, Foo KT. Comparative studies of extracorporeal shock wave lithotripsy by Dornier HM3, EDAP LT 01 and Sonolith 2000 devices. J Urol 1991; 146: 294–7.

134. Ueda S, Matsuoka K, Yamashita T et al. Perirenal hematomas caused by SWL with EDAP LT-01 lithotripter. J Endourol 1993; 7: 11–5.

135. Ng CF, Thompson TJ, McLornan L, Tolley DA. Single-center experience using three shock wave lithotripters with different generator designs in management of urinary calculi. J Endourol 2006; 20: 1–8.

136. Graber SF, Danuser H, Hochreiter WW, Studer UE. A prospective randomized trial comparing 2 lithotriptors for stone disintegration and induced renal trauma. J Urol 2003; 169: 54–7.

137. Gerber R, Studer UE, Danuser H. Is newer always better? A comparative study of 3 lithotriptor generations. J Urol 2005; 173: 2013–6.

138. Eichel L, Batzold P, Erturk E. Operator experience and adequate anesthesia improve treatment outcome with third-generation lithotripters. J Endourol 2001; 15: 671–3.

139. Eisenmenger W, Du XX, Tang C et al. The first clinical results of "wide-focus and low-pressure" ESWL. Ultrasound Med Biol 2002; 28: 769–74.

140. Cleveland RO, Sapozhnikov OA. Modeling elastic wave propagation in kidney stones with application to shock wave lithotripsy. J Acoust Soc Am 2005; 118: 2667–76.

141. Sapozhnikov OA, Maxwell AD, MacConaghy B, Bailey MR. A mechanistic analysis of stone fracture in lithotripsy. J Acoust Soc Am 2007; 112: 1190–02.

142. Cleveland RO, Luo H, Williams JC Jr. Stress waves in human kidney stones: shear dominates spall in shock wave lithotripsy. J Urol 2007; 177: 415 (abstract 1258).

143. Evan AP, McAteer JA, Connors BA, Blomgren PM and Lingeman JE. Renal injury during shock wave lithotripsy is significantly reduced by slowing the rate of shock wave delivery. BJU Int 2007; 100: 624–8.

144. Pishchalnikov YA, McAteer JA, Williams Jr JC, Pishchalnikova IV, Vonderhaar RJ. Why stones break better at slow shock wave rates than at fast rates: in vitro study with a research electrohydraulic lithotripter. J Endourol 2006; 20: 537–41.

145. Pace KT, Ghiculete D, Harju M, Honey RJ. Shock wave lithotripsy at 60 or 120 shocks per minute: a randomized, double-blind trial. J Urol 2005; 174: 595–9.

146. Yilmaz E, Batislam E, Basar M et al. Optimal frequency in extracorporeal shock wave lithotripsy: prospective randomized study. Urology 2005; 66: 1160–4.

147. Madbouly K, El-Tiraifi AM, Seida et al. Slow vs. fast shock wave lithotripsy rate for urolithiasis: a prospective randomized study. J Urol 2005; 173: 127–30.

148. Chacko J, Moore M, Sankey N, Chandhoke PS. Does a slower treatment rate impact the efficacy of extracorporeal shock wave lithotripsy for solitary kidney or ureteral stones? J Urol 2006; 175: 1370–3.

149. Kato Y, Yamaguchi S, Hori J, Okuyama M, Kakizaki H. Improvement of stone comminution by slow delivery rate of shock waves in extracorporeal lithotripsy. Intl J Urol 2006; 13: 1461–5.

150. Semins MJ, Trock BJ, Matlaga BR. The effect of shock wave rate on the outcome of shock wave lithotripsy: a meta-analysis. J Urol 2008; 179: 194–7.

151. Pishchalnikov YA, Sapozhnikov OA, Bailey M et al. Cavitation selectively reduces the negative-pressure phase of lithotripter shock waves. Acoust Res Let Online 2005; 6: 280–x.
152. Pishchalnikov YA, Kaehr MM, McAteer JA. Influence of pulse repetition rate on cavitation oat the surface of an object targeted by lithotripter shock waves. Proc IMECE 2007; 41387.
153. Willis LR, Evan AP, Connors BA et al. Prevention of lithotripsy-induced renal injury by pretreating kidneys with low-energy shock waves. J Am Soc Nephrol 2006; 17: 663–73.
154. Connors BA, Evan AP, Blomgren PM et al. Effect of initial shock wave voltage on SWL-induced lesion size during step-wise voltage ramping, BJU Int 2008 (In-press).
155. Pishchalnikov YA, Neucks JS, VonDerHaar RJ et al. Air pockets trapped during routine coupling in dry-head lithotripsy can significantly reduce the delivery of shock wave energy. J Urol 2006; 176: 2706–10.
156. Neucks JS, Pishchalnikov YA, Zancanaro AJ et al. Improved acoustic coupling for shock wave lithotripsy. Urol Res 2008; 36: 61–6.
157. Williams JC Jr, Zarse CA, Jackson ME, Lingeman JE, McAteer JA. Using helical CT to predict stone fragility in shock wave lithotripsy (SWL). In: Renal Stone Disease: Proceedings of the First International Urolithiasis Research Symposium. Edited by AP Evan, JE Lingeman and JC Williams. Melville: American Institute of Physics, 2007: 326–39.
158. Zarse CA, Hameed TA, Jackson ME et al. CT visible internal stone structure, but not Hounsfield unit value, of calcium oxalate monohydrate (COM) calculi predicts lithotripsy fragility in vitro. Urol Res 2007; 35: 201–6.

12 | Percutaneous nephrolithotomy: Indications and technique

Reem Al-Bareeq, Geoffrey R Wignall, and John D Denstedt

Percutaneous nephrolithotomy (PCNL) has evolved considerably since Rupel and Brown (1) first removed a renal stone through a nephrostomy tract in 1941. Fernstrom and Johansson established PCNL as an accepted surgical technique performing a nephrostomy tract strictly for removing a stone in 1976.(2) It was only after 1979, that Smith, Alken, and Clayman popularized the technique and became pioneers in the field of endourology.(3–5)

As the percutaneous era continued, the indications for this advanced technique began to expand and could be utilized for more complex renal stones along with the growing experience. The advent of effective intracorporeal lithotripsy devices such as ultrasound also contributed to this expanding role. Extracorporeal shock wave lithotripsy (ESWL) developed concurrently to PCNL. Lingeman and Newman in 1986 reported stone-free rates of 95% for stones less than 1 cm, 87% for stones between 1 and 2 cm, 48% for stones between 2 and 3 cm and 35% for stones larger than 3 cm with shock wave lithotripsy.(6)

Percutaneous nephrolithotomy demonstrated obvious advantages when compared to ESWL in regards to stone-free status for complex stone problems (7, 8) and proving its superiority in removal of larger stones with minimal morbidity.(9)

The indications for PCNL have evolved to include (10, 11):

- Stone size >2 cm
- Hard stones such as cystine stones
- Lower pole stones >1 cm
- Infection stones and staghorns
- Failure of contraindications to shock wave lithotripsy
- Patients with renal anatomic variations
- Certainty of final result

This chapter will examine in detail the current indications for percutaneous nephrolithotomy and outline the technique of PCNL.

STONE SIZE

Stone size is an essential factor in determining the effectiveness of any stone removal modality. Success rate decreases as stone volume increases when shock wave lithotripsy is utilized.(6, 8, 12) Most authors consider the upper practical limit for ESWL to be the largest stone diameter of 20 mm to obtain the greatest benefit from this procedure.(13, 14) As such, the EUA guidelines for urolithiasis updated in 2008 recommended PCNL as the first-line treatment for renal stones with the largest stone diameter more than 20 mm.(15)

Staghorn stones have always represented a challenging surgical problem for urologists. It is necessary to completely remove all stones to eradicate any causative organisms, relieve obstruction and prevent further stone growth, infection and renal deterioration. An untreated staghorn calculi can result in destruction of the kidney and/or life-threatening sepsis.(16)

However, complete or partial staghorn calculi may require multiple tracts or combination procedures such as sandwich therapy. "Sandwich therapy" entails PCNL followed by ESWL then PCNL which can be used for standard staghorn calculi patients.(17, 18) The overall stone-free rates comparing the different modalities in studies from July 92 through to July 2003 reviewed by AUA Nephrolithiasis guideline panel were highest for PCNL (78%) and lowest for ESWL (54%). Combination therapy had an estimated stone-free rate of 66%. An estimate of the total number of procedures performed revealed PCNL requires 1.9 total procedures while combination therapy and ESWL require 3.3 and 3.6 procedures respectively. (17) AUA guidelines recommend PCNL as the first line treatment option for most staghorn calculi patients which was supported by the only randomized prospective trial comparing PCNL to ESWL for staghorn stones.(17) This study demonstrated that PCNL-based therapy had more than three times greater stone-free rates than ESWL monotherapy.(19)

STONE COMPOSITION

Stone composition dictates the hardness of renal calculi and the fragmentation ability of shock wave lithotripsy. The hardest stones are typically composed of cytine, calcium oxalate mono-hydrate, and brushite.(20) PCNL is the most suitable option for hard stones that are resistant to fracture using SWL.(10) However, predicting stone composition pre-treatment is difficult. The presence of certain crystals in urine, recurrent urinary infections or radiolucent stone on plain imaging may indicate a cystine, struvite, or uric acid composition respectively. Advanced imaging may also provide an indication of stone hardness and fragmentation ability. In 1996, Dretler et al. described four distinct radiographic classes for calcium oxalate stones but lacked clinical correlation to be used in clinical decision making.(21)

CT scan has evolved to be the imaging modality of choice for most patients with renal and ureteral stones. Hounsfield unit density on noncontrast CT scan has been demonstrated to have some utility in differentiating hard vs. soft stones and possibly predicting outcomes with extracorporeal shock wave lithotripsy. *In vitro* studies demonstrated the level of attenuation of various stone compositions differentiating uric acid stones (below 1,000 HU), calcium oxalate monohydrate, and phosphate stones (above 1,000 HU).(22–24) However, there was an overlap in hounsfield units for calcium oxalate monohydrate and struvites stones which to an extent limits the discernment of exact stone composition using CT..(22, 24) *In vivo* studies that have been undertaken to correlate SWL success rates according to CT Hounsfield units showed a higher stone clearance rate with lower HU density of the stone.(25) Joseph et al. performed SWL in 30 patients and found that those with stones <500 HU had 100% stone clearance and required a median of 2,500 shocks. Patients with stones ranging between 500 and 1,000 HU had a clearance rate of 86% and median shocks of 3,390. However, calculi >1,000 HU had a clearance rate of 56% and required a median of 7,300 shock waves.(25)

LOWER POLE STONES

Lower pole renal stones treated with extracorporeal shock wave lithotripsy have been documented to have lower stone free rates due to reduced clearance of stone fragments. A number of studies have examined the relationship of anatomic configurations including infundibulopelvic angle, lower pole infundibular length, and lower pole infundibular width on outcomes of shock wave lithotripsy. Sampaio and Aragao described anatomical features from endocasts of the collecting systems of cavaderic kidneys, which could be correlated to stone clearance.(26) These include the angle between the lower pole infundibulum and renal pelvis, the diameter of the lower pole infundibulum, and the spatial distribution of the calices. The authors concluded that a lower pole infundibulopelvic angle less than 90 degrees, lower pole infundibulum diameter less than 4 mm and multiple lower pole calices may decrease stone clearance.(27) They studied the influence of the lower infundibulum-pelvic angle on fragment retention in 74 patients undergoing ESWL therapy for the treatment of lower-pole calculi. At a mean follow-up of 9 months, 75% of the patients presenting with an angle of greater than 90 degrees between the lower infundibulum where the stone was located and the renal pelvis became stone-free within 3 months. However, only 23% of the patients presenting with an angle less than 90 degrees between the lower infundibulum and the renal pelvis became stone-free during the follow-up.(27) Elbahnasy et al. have determined the parameters of renal spatial anatomy that contribute to stone passage. Unfavorable factors are an infundibulopelvic angle less than 70 degrees, infundibular length greater than 3 cm, and an infundibular width less than 5 mm.(28)

A meta-analysis by Lingeman demonstrated a stone-free rate of 90% for lower pole stones treated by PCNL as compared to a 59% stone-free rate after treatment with ESWL.(29) A multicenter randomized prospective trial comparing PCNL to ESWL for treatment of lower pole stones revealed significantly higher overall stone-free rates with PCNL (95%) compared to ESWL (37%). Re-treatment rates were also higher for ESWL (16% vs. 9%) as were ancillary treatments (14% vs. 2%) compared to PCNL. The study group recommended that stones under 1.0 cm be managed with ESWL while stones 1.0 cm or larger should undergo PCNL.(8)

Preminger reiterated these findings in reporting results of a randomized, prospective multi-institutional trial comparing the stone-free rates between SWL and PCNL for lower pole stones in 112 patients. He suggested that SWL is less effective for lower pole calculi especially stones greater than 1 cm in diameter and PCNL had higher overall stone-free rates (96%).(30)

INFECTION STONES

Infection-related stones are characterized by their large size and rapid growth often in a staghorn configuration.(31) Struvite renal calculi are associated with urease-producing bacteria in a patient population characterized clinically by recurrent urinary tract infections. Patients must be rendered completely stone-free to minimize the risk of recurrent stone formation.(10) Bacteria which reside in the interstices of the stone may represent a nidus for further stone formation. The AUA Nephrolithiasis Guideline panel again recommends complete stone removal to "eradicate any causative organisms, relieve obstruction, prevent further stone growth and any associated infection and preserve renal function."(17) Percutaneous nephrolithotripsy represents the procedure of choice for most struvite urinary calculi which may commonly occur in patients with renal anatomic abnormalities or urinary diversions. As much as possible, urinary infection must be cleared before the procedure to reduce the risk of postoperative sepsis due to surgical manipulation. Preserving renal function is one of the main goals in the management of staghorn stones. A suitable therapy to maintain or improve the renal function of patients with large staghorn stones is combination therapy of PCNL followed by ESWL or secondary nephroscopy. This improvement in renal function was demonstrated by Streem and Lammert who performed "sandwich therapy" for 28 patients with extensive struvite staghorn calculi. After 12–55 months of followup with antibiotic prophylaxis, renal function remained stable or improved in 93% of the patients. However, 30% of patients had persistent infection and there was a recurrence of staghorn stones in 22%.(32)

FAILURE OR CONTRAINDICATIONS TO ESWL

With the initial conception of ESWL by Chaussey in the early 1980s there were numerous contraindications to ESWL. Most of the initial contraindications have subsequently been resolved.

Pregnancy and uncorrectable bleeding diathesis remain amongst the only absolute contraindications to ESWL therapy. Retrograde ureteroscopy and laser lithotripsy have emerged as a very viable treatment alternative for these populations of patients.

Percutaneous nephrolithotripsy is also contraindicated in those with bleeding diathesis and is only very rarely the preferred option in pregnant patients. Extracorporeal shock wave lithotripsy may not be an option in patients with unusual body habitus who cannot be properly positioned on the shock wave device and percutaneous surgery is often an option in these patients.

Surgery in obese patients is, for the most part, technically more challenging than in non-obese patients. While it would be reasonable to assume that PCNL would be more challenging in this patient population, the reality is that with appropriate skill and adequate instrumentation PCNL may be successfully performed in obese individuals. Several studies have demonstrated that PCNL is a safe and effective treatment in obese patients.(33–35) Stone-free rate, length of hospital stay, and transfusion rate are similar in obese patients with no increase in the rate of complications.(33–35)

PCNL can be technically challenging in obese patients due to difficult patient positioning and technical limitations. In the prone position, obese individuals may have difficulty with lung excursion due to the extra weight placed on the chest wall. Adequate padding under the upper chest as well as placing the operating table in a slight reverse Trendelenburg position will enhance the ease of ventilation. Standard PCNL instrumentation may be of insufficient length in morbidly obese patients limiting the surgeon's ability to access all areas of the renal collecting system. Extra long nephroscopic sheaths and nephroscopes are currently available and assist greatly for PCNL in this population.(36) Alternative techniques such as performing a cut-down to the muscle followed by renal access have been described, however are not routinely employed with the availability of long instruments.(37)

When shock wave lithotripsy fails, for intrarenal calculi an endoscopic procedure, either percutaneously or in a retrograde fashion via ureteroscopy, is the usual salvage procedure that must be considered. The appropriate endoscopic procedure when ESWL fails is often defined by stone volume with a larger stone volume being more appropriately managed by PCNL and a stone volume of 1 cm or less being best approached by way of retrograde ureteroscopy. Patients and physicians need to consider the various pros and cons including overall invasiveness of the procedure when deciding on which salvage therapy to undertake.

PATIENTS WITH RENAL ANATOMIC VARIATION

Anatomically variant kidneys have an increased susceptibility to stone disease due to stasis and infection. Horseshoe kidney is a common renal anomaly present in roughly 1 in 300 people and is twice as common in males as in females. As with many other renal anomalies, horseshoe kidneys are associated with abnormal position and malrotation resulting in varying degrees of obstruction and an increased risk of stone formation. Studies reporting results of SWL for calculi in horseshoe kidneys present a wide range of stone-free rates from as low as 28% to as high as 80%.(38–41) Stone-free rates decline sharply with increasing stone size, and stones greater than 1.5 cm are likely better managed with PCNL.(38) Several studies have reported excellent stone-free rates following PCNL ranging from 73 to 87% in patients with calculi in horseshoe kidneys.(42–44) Preoperative imaging should be reviewed to adequately assess the anatomy and to avoid complications such as colonic injury.

A multi-institutional study of a large group of patients with symptomatic calculi in a horseshoe kidney was done to evaluate the usefulness, safety, and efficacy of PCNL as the primary therapeutic approach.(44) Overall stone-free rate after PCNL was 87.5% at 3 months with overall incidence of major complications of 12.5%. There was a preference toward an upper pole caliceal access (15pts) due to the lower abdominal position of the horseshoe kidney. The malrotation of the kidney necessitates a more posterior puncture.(44, 45)

PCNL is ideally suited in the majority of cases of calyceal diverticular stones with superior stone free rates ranging from 80 to 100% and providing access through which obliteration of the diverticulum may be performed.(46–48) Direct puncture into the diverticulum provides the best access for treatment of the stone and diverticular obliteration. Options for management of the diverticulum following stone removal include fulguration of the diverticular lining, dilation of the communication between the diverticulum and the collecting system or creation of a neoinfundibulum.

Calculi in pelvic kidneys that cannot be successfully managed through less invasive means may be managed with PCNL although this is often more difficult due to the proximity of surrounding abdominal structures. Accurate visualization of abdominal viscera and vessels with imaging such as computed tomography is essential to minimize the risk during percutaneous access. Reports of successful laparoscopic-guided PCNL have been described.(49–56) The advantage of this approach is the ability to manipulate the bowel away from the kidney providing a clear path for percutaneous access under direct vision. Watterson et al. reported performing PCNL on a pelvic kidney via the greater sciatic foramen. In the prone position, access was achieved through the buttock and the stone was removed using standard PCNL techniques.(57)

PCNL has been successful in transplanted kidneys although urolithiasis is rare. The different configuration of the transplanted ureter may impede fragment passage after shock wave lithotripsy. The position of the transplanted kidney makes it easily accessible through the anterior abdomen and amenable to PCNL.(58–61) It is essential to obtain a CT scan preoperatively to assess for the possibility of intervening viscus.

CERTAINTY OF FINAL RESULTS

Social factors have always played a role in decision making surrounding the appropriate treatment for urolithiasis. Certain patient populations are required to be stone-free in order to perform their occupation. An example of such a group includes airline pilots who are required to be completely stone-free in order to undertake their profession. Choice of technique utilized must be practical and best suited to the individual patient's needs and stone problem. Zheng et al. reviewed records of aviation pilots that were treated in four tertiary stone centers to determine the treatment outcomes of this population and the best-suited treatment options. Stone-free rates for ESWL, PCNL and ureteroscopy were 35%, 100%, and 100%, respectively. The mean time lost from work for ESWL, PCNL, and ureteroscopy was 4.7, 2.6, and 1.6weeks, respectively. The authors concluded that endoscopic management should be undertaken for this population for stone-free rates to be maximized and time lost from work is minimized.(62) Repeated ineffective treatments which do not render the patient completely stone-free lead to prolonged time off of work and in many situations PCNL provides the most efficient means by which to achieve a stone-free rate in a single procedure.

OPERATIVE TECHNIQUES

In this section of the chapter we will discuss techniques for percutaneous nephrolithotomy from the renal access through the post-operative management of the PCNL patient. We present our preferred techniques recognizing that there are variations of each part of the procedure. Where relevant, we address alternative approaches such as the choice of who will perform the access (i.e. radiologist vs. urologist), the technique of access, and the choice of intracorporeal lithotriptor.

Preoperative Preparation and Positioning

Adequate treatment of documented urinary tract infection is required before surgery. Consent is obtained after the risks and benefits of the procedure have been discussed including infection, bleeding requiring embolization and/or transfusion and injury to associated organs (i.e. liver, bowel). Broad-spectrum antibiotics are administered on the day of surgery. Blood transfusion is required in less than 1% of patients undergoing PCNL at our institution and we do not routinely cross-match patients for blood products prior to surgery.

Following induction of general anesthesia, the patient is placed in the prone position and all pressure points are carefully inspected and supported to avoid injury. A pillow is placed under the chest as a support to allow for optimal ventilation. If there is a significant curvature of the lumbar spine, particularly in thin patients a 1L irrigation bag may be placed beneath the lower abdomen for support. The flank and perineum are widely prepped and draped to allow exposure for cystoscopy as well as percutaneous renal access.

Renal Access

Of prime importance to a successful PCNL is an appropriately planned and acquired percutaneous renal access. Ideally the access should be placed at the tip of the selected entry calyx rather than into the infundibulum or renal pelvis. We routinely acquire our own percutaneous access as we feel this provides the greatest likelihood of entry into the desired calyx as well as the ability to obtain additional access points as required during the procedure. Several studies have addressed the issue of percutaneous renal access by a urologist vs. that by interventional radiologists.(63–65) Urologist-acquired renal access has been shown to be safe and, in many cases, more effective than radiologist-acquired access.(64, 65) That said, most percutaneous renal access in the United States is performed by radiologists rather than urologists.

Our preferred technique is an antegrade approach under fluoroscopic guidance; however, retrograde access has been described.(66) Hosking and Reid reported their experience with over 200 cases of retrograde nephrostomy.(66) The authors reported successful establishment of a nephrostomy tract in 98% of cases with a mean time of 27.9 minutes to establish the tract. As with any technique of percutaneous access, retrograde access should not be attempted without a suitable period of mentoring under an urologist skilled in the technique.

In our technique, flexible cystoscopy is performed in the prone position and an open-ended ureteral catheter is passed in a retrograde fashion. Retrograde pyelography via the ureteral catheter defines the calyceal anatomy. When possible we enter the collecting system via a posterior calyx, as this gives the most direct route to the renal pelvis and ureter and reduces

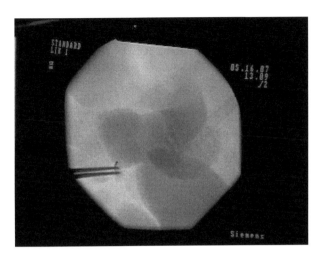

Figure 12.1 Advancement of access needle into the tip of a dilated calyx.

unnecessary torquing of the nephroscope during the procedure. Access below the 12th rib is preferred; however, certain instances require access above the 11th or 12th ribs which may be accomplished with a slight increase in thoracic complications such as hydrothorax. Situations where intercostal access might be required include large, branched calculi and those cases where access to the ureteropelvic junction is necessary (i.e. concomitant endopyelotomy or antegrade ureteroscopy). In the setting of an isolated calyceal or diverticular stone, access is best acquired directly into the stone-bearing calyx or diverticulum. The gentle injection of a small amount of air through the ureteral catheter is often helpful in identifying posterior calyces as these will preferentially fill with air in the prone position. With the C-arm in the AP plane, an 18G Chiba needle is positioned over the tip of the desired entry calyx. The needle is advanced along the AP plane in a controlled fashion until the tip of the needle begins to deflect with the respiratory movement of the kidney (Figure 12.1). The C-arm is rotated 30degeres laterally and the needle is carefully advanced until the tip penetrates the entry calyx. The needle should not be advanced further into the calyx once the stylet has been removed. Urine may be seen flowing from the hub of the needle; however, the absence of urine does not necessarily mean that the needle is outside of the calyx. We confirm positioning in the collecting system by the gentle passage of a 0.035-inch hydrophilic guidewire that should pass easily and follow the contour of the calyx. If the initial passage of the wire is not into the collecting system, the needle is gently withdrawn roughly 1–2 mm and passage of the wire is reattempted. This maneuver is repeated until the guidewire is clearly into the collecting system or the needle has been withdrawn from the calyx. In the event that calyceal puncture is unsuccessful the needle should be withdrawn and access reattempted with the stylet replaced.

Once correct placement of the needle has been confirmed, the 0.035-inch hydrophilic wire is advanced into the collecting system. Ideally the wire is passed into the ureter and down to the bladder. We find that a 5F Kumpe angled catheter is invaluable in the passage of the wire down the ureter. We then advance the Kumpe catheter down the ureter and exchange the hydrophilic wire for a 0.038-inch superstiff guidewire with an adequate curl in the bladder. Care should be taken when advancing the stiff wire through the intramural ureter as a flap of mucosa may be raised inadvertently. Occasionally, when it is not possible to pass the hydrophilic wire into the ureter (i.e. large impacted UPJ stone or grossly hydronephrotic kidney), we will curl a Bentson wire in the renal pelvis or into an upper pole calyx and proceed with tract dilation. Once the nephrostomy tract has been established a wire can usually be passed down the ureter under direct vision. After the stiff guidewire has been passed we make a 2 cm skin incision and advance a one-step balloon dilator with the radio-opaque marker positioned in entry calyx or just into the renal pelvis. The tract is dilated and a 30F working sheath is advanced under fluoroscopy (Figure 12.2). It is important to avoid advancing either the balloon dilator or the working sheath beyond the renal pelvis and into the UPJ or proximal ureter. The guidewire is secured and rigid nephroscopy is performed.

Other options for tract dilation include introduction of progressively larger serial fascial dilators such as Amplatz renal dilators or metal coaxial dilators. We will occasionally advance

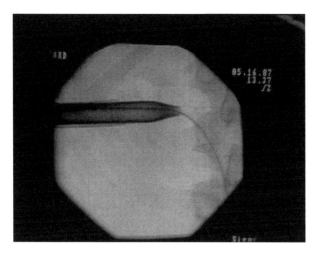

Figure 12.2 Advancement of the access sheath over a 30Fr Amplatz dilator.

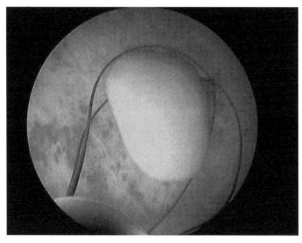

Figure 12.3 Basket manipulation of renal calculus using a rigid tipless stone basket.

a single 8/10F Amplatz coaxial dilator over the guidewire if resistance is met while passing the balloon dilator. This maneuver will usually allow for smooth passage of the balloon into the kidney.

Nephroscopy and Lithotripsy

Calculi measuring less than 1 cm in diameter may be extracted through the nephrostomy sheath without fragmentation. Stones may be removed using a variety of baskets, forceps, and graspers (Figure 12.3). Lithotripsy is performed for larger stones by using an appropriate intracorporeal lithotriptor such as pneumatic, laser or ultrasonic devices. We routinely use ultrasonic lithotripsy as this offers excellent stone fragmentation combined with suction to simultaneously evacuate stone debris (Figure 12.4). For hard stones that resist fragmentation with ultrasound, the ballistic lithotriptor is usually successful. Stones in the entry calyx and renal pelvis should be cleared initially to increase the working space. Often the nephroscope may be gently maneuvered to allow access to opposing calyces however excess torque should be avoided. Flexible nephroscopy should be performed to assess the remaining calyces for further stones. In the event that all stones cannot safely be reached with the rigid nephroscope we either place a second tract into the calyx containing the stone(s) or utilize the flexible nephroscope with either the holmium laser or electrohydraulic lithotripsy (EHL). Ureteral stent placement is not routinely required following uncomplicated PCNL; however in situations where the UPJ or proximal ureter has been manipulated we will consider passing a stent in an antegrade fashion. At the conclusion of the case we remove the sheath under direct vision with the rigid nephroscope as calculi may be concealed alongside the sheath. A nephrostomy tube is placed under fluoroscopic guidance. Our usual choice for a nephrostomy is a 16F Council-tipped urethral

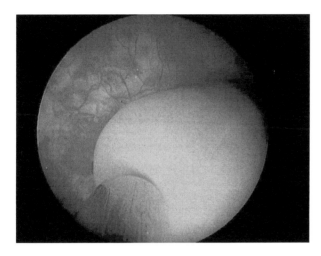

Figure 12.4 Ultrasonic lithotripsy.

catheter with 2–3cc of contrast in the balloon to confirm position in the renal pelvis. Other types of nephrostomy drainage (i.e. 8F pigtail) may be used as per surgeon preference.

We do not perform tubeless PCNL at our institution and prefer to maintain drainage and access in the immediate post-operative period. The nephrostomy is secured at the skin with a silk suture and the wound is cleaned and dressed. Active hemorrhage from the nephrostomy site is initially managed with pressure applied to the site. Persistent bleeding may often be controlled by passage of a larger caliber nephrostomy tube over a guidewire. In the event that this is not successful it may be necessary to utilize a Kaye tamponnade catheter to control bleeding. Finally, if bleeding persists or the patient becomes hemodynamically unstable, selective embolization may be required.

Postoperative Care

Our patients are routinely admitted for 24–48 hours postoperatively and imaging (KUB or CT) is obtained on the first postoperative day. If there is no further evidence of residual calculi the nephrostomy is clamped and the patient is observed for flank pain or signs of sepsis. An antegrade nephrostogram may be performed when there is a strong suspicion of distal obstruction. The nephrostomy may be removed and the patient discharged home provided they tolerate the trial of nephrostomy clamping. We will often take a "second look" with the flexible nephroscope in the clinic and basket residual stones through the nephrostomy tract which should be well established 1–2 days after surgery. Larger residual stone burdens might require a second PCNL under general anesthesia to render the patient stone-free. If a stent has been placed we evaluate the patient in the clinic the week after surgery and remove the stent with flexible cystoscopy. All patients are seen in the clinic 4–6 weeks post-operatively to be clinically assessed and to arrange further follow-up as required.

REFERENCES

1. Rupel E, Brow R. Nephroscopy with removal of stone following Nephrostomy for obstructive calculus anuria. J Urol 1941; 46: 177–82.
2. Ferntrom I, Johansson B. Percutaneous pyelolithotomy: a new extraction technique. Scan J Urol Nephrol 1976; 10: 257–59.
3. Clayman RV, Surya V, Miller RP et al. Percutaneous nephrolithotomy: an approach to branched and staghorn renal calculi. J Am Med Assoc 1983; 250: 73–5.
4. Badlani G, Smith AD, Cubelli V, Gnanasekaram G. Percutaneous stone extraction: institutional experience of 400 cases. J Urol 1985; 91: 52.
5. Alken P, Hutschenreiter G, Gunther R, Marberger M. Percutaneous stone manipulation. J Urol 1981; 125: 463–6.
6. Lingeman JE, Saywell RM Jr, Woods JR, Newman DM. Cost analysis of extracorporeal shock wave lithotripsy relative to other surgical and nonsurgical treatment alternatives for urolithiasis. Med Care 1986; 24: 1151–60.
7. Tiselius HG, Ackerman D, Alken P et al. Working Party on Lithiasis. European Association of Urology. Eur Urol 2001; 40(4): 363–71.

8. Albala DM, Assimos DG, Clayman RV et al. A prospective randomized trial of extracorporeal shock wave lithotripsy and percutaneous nephrostolithotomy for lower pole nephrolithiasis: initial results. J Urol 2001; 166: 2072–80.
9. Segura JW. Role of percutaneous procedures in management of renal calculi (review). Urol Clin North Am 1990; 17: 207–16.
10. Ramakumar S, Segura JW. Renal calculi: percutaneous management. Urol Clin North Am 2000; 27(4): 617–22.
11. Skolarikos A, Alivizatos G, De la Rosette J. Percutaneous nephrolithotomy and its legacy. Eur Urol 2005; 47: 22–8.
12. Segura JW, Patterson DE, LeRoy AJ et al. Percutaneous removal of kidney stones: review of 1000 cases. J Urol 1985; 134: 1077–81.
13. Coz F, Orvieto M, Bustos M et al. Extracorporeal shockwave lithotripsy of 2000 urinary calculi with the modulith SL-20: success and failure according to size and location of stones. J Endourol 2000; 14(3): 239–46
14. Rassweiler JJ, Renner C, Chaussy C, Thüroff S. Treatment of renal stones by extracorporeal shockwave lithotripsy: an update. Eur Urol 2001; 39(2): 187–99.
15. Tiselius HG, Alken P, Buck C et al. EUA guidelines for urolithiasis; 2008.
16. Koga S, Arakaki Y, Matsroka M, Ohyama C. Staghorn calculi-long term results of management. Br J Urol 1991; 68: 122.
17. Preminger Gm, Assimo Dg, Lingeman JE et al. AUA Nephrolithiasis Guideline Panel. Chapter 1: AUA guideline on management of staghorn calculi: diagnosis and treatment recommendations. J Urol 2005; 173(6): 1991–2000.
18. Streem SB. Sandwich therapy (review). Urol Clin North Am 1997; 24: 213–423.
19. Meretyk S, Gorfit O, Gafni O et al. Complete staghorn calculi: random prospective comparison between extracorporeal shock wave lithotripsy monotherapy and comined with percutaneous nephrostolithotomy. J Urol 1997; 157: 780.
20. Pittomvils F, Vandeurson H, Wevers M et al. The influence of internal stone structure upon the fracture behaviour of urinary calculi. Ultrasound Med Biol 1994; 20: 803–10.
21. Dretler SP, Polykoh G. Calcium oxalate stone morphology: fine-tuning our therapeutic distinctions. J Urol 1996; 155: 828–33.
22. Mostafavi MR, Ernst RD, Saltzman B. Accurate determination of chemical composition of urinary calculi by spiral computerized tomography. J Urol 1998; 159(3): 673–5.
23. Nakada SY, Hoff DG, Attai S et al. Determination of stone composition by noncontrast spiral computed tomography in clinical setting. Urology 2000; 55(6): 816–9.
24. Zarse CA, McAteer JA, Tann M et al. Helical computed tomography accurately reports urinary stone composition using attenuation values: in vitro verification using high-resolution micro-computed tomography calibrated to fourier transform infrared microspectroscopy. Urology 2004; 63: 828–33.
25. Joseph P, Mandal AK, Singh SK et al. Computerized tomography attenuation value of renal calculus: can it predict successful fragmentation of the calculus by extra-corporeal shock wave lithotripsy? A preliminary study. J Urol 2002; 167: 1968–71.
26. Sampaio FJ, Aragao AH. Limitations of extracorporeal shock wave lithotripsy for lower calyceal stones: anatomic insight. J Endourol 1994; 8: 241.
27. Sampaio FJ, D'Anunciacao AL, Silva EC. Comparative follow-up of patients with acute and obtuse infunibulum-pelvic angle submitted to extracorporeal shock wave lithotripsy for lower calyceal stones: preliminary report and proposed study design. J Endourol 1997; 11: 157.
28. Elbahnasy AM, Clayman R, Shalhav D et al. Lower pole caliceal stone clearance after shock wave lithotripsy, percutaneous nephrolithotomy and flexible ureteroscopy: impact of radiographic spatial anatomy. J Endourol 1998; 12: 113–9.
29. Lingeman JE, Siegel YI, Steele B et al. Managemnet of lower-pole nephrolithiasis: A critical analysis. J Urol 1994; 151: 663–7.
30. Preminger G. Management of lower pole renal calculi: shock wave lithotripsy vs. percutaneous nephrolithotomy vs. flexible ureteroscopy. Urol Res 2006; 34: 108–11.
31. Healy KA, Ogan K. Pathophysiology and Management of infectious staghorn calculi. Urol Clin North Am 2007; 34: 363–74.
32. Streem SB, Lammert G. Long-term efficacy of combination therapy for struvite staghorn calculi. J Urol 1992; 147: 563–6.
33. Pearle MS, Nakada SY, Womack JS et al. Outcomes of contemporary percutaneous nephrostolithotomy in morbidly obese patients. J Urol 1998; 160: 669–73.
34. El-Assmy AM, Shokeir AA, El-Nahas AR et al. Outcome of percutaneous nephrolithotomy: effect of body mass index. Eur Urol 2007; 52(1): 199–204.
35. Koo BC, Burtt G, Burgess NA. Percutaneous stone surgery in the obese: outcome stratified according to body mass index. BJU Int 2004; 93(9): 1296–9.
36. Giblin JG, Lossef S, Pahira JJ. A modification of standard percutaneous nephrolithotripsy technique for the morbidly obese patient. Urology 1995; 46(4): 491–3.

37. Curtis R, Thorpe AC, Marsh R. Modification of the technique of percutaneous nephrolithotomy in the morbidly obese patient. British journal of urology 1997; 79(1): 138–40.

38. Sheir KZ, Madbouly K, Elsobky E, Abdelkhalek M. Extracorporeal shock wave lithotripsy in anomalous kidneys: 11-year experience with two second-generation lithotripters. Urology 2003; 62(1): 10–5.

39. Tunc L, Tokgoz H, Tan MO et al. Stones in anomalous kidneys: results of treatment by shock wave lithotripsy in 150 patients. Int J Urol 2004; 11(10): 831–6.

40. Kirkali Z, Esen AA, Mungan MU. Effectiveness of extracorporeal shockwave lithotripsy in the management of stone-bearing horseshoe kidneys. J Endourol 1996; 10(1): 13–5.

41. Serrate R, Regue R, Prats J, Rius G. ESWL as the treatment for lithiasis in horseshoe kidney. Eur Urol 1991; 20(2): 122–5.

42. Al-Otaibi K, Hosking DH. Percutaneous stone removal in horseshoe kidneys. J Urol 1999; 162: 674–7.

43. Shokeir AA, El-Nahas AR, Shoma AM et al. Percutaneous nephrolithotomy in treatment of large stones within horseshoe kidneys. Urology 2004; 64(3): 426–9.

44. Raj GV, Auge BK, Weizer AZ et al. Percutaneous management of calculi within horseshoe kidneys. J Urol 2003; 170(1): 48–51.

45. Cussenot O, Desgrandchamps F, Ollier P et al. Anatomical bases of percutaneous surgery for calculi in horseshoe kidney. Surg Radiol Anat 1992; 14: 209.

46. Turna B, Raza A, Moussa S, Smith G, Tolley DA. Management of calyceal diverticular stones with extracorporeal shock wave lithotripsy and percutaneous nephrolithotomy: long-term outcome. BJU international 2007; 100(1): 151–6.

47. Monga M, Smith R, Ferral H, Thomas R. Percutaneous ablation of caliceal diverticulum: long-term followup. J Urol 2000; 163(1): 28–32.

48. Kim SC, Kuo RL, Tinmouth WW, Watkins S, Lingeman JE. Percutaneous nephrolithotomy for caliceal diverticular calculi: a novel single stage approach. J Urol 2005; 173(4): 1194–8.

49. Troxel SA, Low RK, Das S. Extraperitoneal laparoscopy-assisted percutaneous nephrolithotomy in a left pelvic kidney. J Endourol 2002; 16(9): 655–7.

50. Holman E, Toth C. Laparoscopically assisted percutaneous transperitoneal nephrolithotomy in pelvic dystopic kidneys: experience in 15 successful cases. J Laparoendosc Adv Surg Tech 1998; 8(6): 431–5.

51. Toth C, Holman E, Paszfor I et al. Laparoscopic controlled and assisted percutaneous transperitoneal nephrolithotomy in a pelvic dystrophic kidney. J Endourol 1993; 7: 303–5.

52. Hoenig DM, Shalhaw AL, Elbahnasy AM et al. Laparoscopic pyelolithotomy in a pelvic kidney: a case report and review of the literature. JSLS 1997; 1: 163–65

53. Figge M. Percutaneous transperitoneal nephrolithotomy. Eur Urol 1988; 14: 414–6.

54. Eshghi AM, Roth JS, Smith AD. Percutaneous transperitoneal approach to a pelvic kidney for endourological removal of staghorn calculi. J Urol 1985; 134: 525–7

55. Lee CK, Smith AD. Percutaneous transperitoneal approach to the pelvic kidney for endourologic removal of calculus: three cases with two successes. J Endourol 1992; 6: 133–5.

56. Zafar FS, Lingeman JE. Value of laparoscopy in the management of calculi complicating renal malformations. J Endourol 1996; 10: 379–83.

57. Watterson JD, Cook A, Sahajpal R et al. Percutaneous nephrolithotomy of a pelvic kidney: a posterior approach through the greater sciactic foramen. J Urol 2001; 166: 209–10.

58. Bailey IS, Griffin P, Evans C et al. Percutaneous surgery of the transplanted kidneys. Br J Urol 1989; 63: 327–28.

59. Fahlenkamp D, Oesterwitz H, Althaus P et al. Percutaneous management of urolithiasis after kidney transplantation: report of case and review of the literature review. Eur Urol 1988; 14: 330–2.

60. Minon CJ, Garcia TE, Garcia DE et al. Percutaneous nephrolithotomy in transplanted kidney. Urolgy 1991; 38: 232–4.

61. Lu HF, Shekarriz B, Stoller MI. Donor-gifted allograft urolithiasis: early percutaneous management. Urology 2002; 59(1): 25–7.

62. Zheng W, Beiko DT, Segura JW et al. Urinary calculi in aviation pilots: what is the best therapeutic approach? J Urol 2002; 168: 1341–3.

63. Lee CL, Anderson JK, Monga M. Residency training in percutaneous renal access: does it affect urological practice? J Urol 2004; 171: 592–5.

64. El-Assmy AM, Shokeir AA, Mohsen T et al. Renal access by urologist or radiologist for percutaneous nephrolithotomy--is it still an issue? J Urol 2007; 178: 916–20.

65. Watterson JD, Soon S, Jana K. Access related complications during percutaneous nephrolithotomy: urology vs. radiology at a single academic institution. J Urol 2006; 176(1): 142–5.

66. Hosking D, Reid R. The evaluation of retrograde nephrostomy in over 200 procedures. In: Walker V, Sutton R, Cameron E, eds. Urolithiasis: Proceedings of The Sixth International Symposium on Urolithiasis. New York: Plenium Press; 1989.

13 | Flexible ureterorenoscopy: Technique and indications

Olivier Traxer

INTRODUCTION

Flexible ureteropyeloscopy is rapidly becoming a major part of the urologist's therapeutic armamentarium. As with any sophisticated new technique, the operator must have a detailed knowledge of the features of the equipment, and perfect control of the instruments used. Over the past two decades flexible ureterorenoscope (F-URS) has continued to evolve and improve significantly including F-URS design, deflection capabilities, irrigation flow, imaging equipment, and durability. Due to these recent developments, endourologists have expanded the clinical indications for flexible ureterorenoscopy.

The purpose of this chapter is intended to thoroughly familiarize the prospective user with the technique and indications of flexible ureterorenoscopy, step by step, through the set-up for the procedure and the handling of the F-URS and describes the management of calculi, tumors of the upper urinary tract, caliceal diverticuli, and strictures.

ENDOSCOPES

Over the past 10 years, significant advances have been made in the management of upper urinary tract calculous disease, with the development of small-caliber F-URS that allows access to the entire collecting system with little or no effect on renal function. Advances in F-URS and the introduction of the Holmium-YAG laser have made ureterorenoscopy an alternative to SWL and percutaneous nephrolithotomy (PCNL) for treating renal calculi. F-URS today allows detailed calyceal examination and therapeutic interventions.(1)

Flexible ureterorenoscopy continues to be hindered by limited irrigation and small working channels, but newer F-URS offers much less limited deflection (Table 13.1). Most of the new generation of F-URS have a 0 degrees angle of visualization. Gyrus-ACMI DUR-8 Elite has a 9 degrees angle for earlier visualization of the instruments (essentially laser fibers) as they are advanced out of the working channel. Some of the flexible ureteroscopes have a beveled triangular tip to facilitate insertion into the ureteral orifice (Figure 13.1). All F-URS have a single 3.6 Fr working channel (Figure 13.2).(2) It is recommended to pass an instrument through the working channel when the F-URS is straight, otherwise the working channel can be damaged. The working channel is particularly vulnerable to damage from laser fibers, which are stiff and have a sharp tip. Once the instrument enters in the field of view, the F-URS can be deflected as needed. An instrument should never be forced through the channel of the F-URS. The 3.6 Fr working channel accept instruments up to 3–3.2 Fr (laser fibers, basket and graspers), but because the working channel is used also for irrigation an instrument in the channel will dramatically reduce the flow rate. Smaller (1.5–1.9 Fr) caliber nitinol basket and 200 μ laser fibers have the least deleterious effects on the flow rate and deflecting capabilities of the F-URS (3, 4) (Figure 13.3). The loss of flow may also be overcome by using automated pressure devices (Endoflow Socomed Promepla or EndoFMS).

Ureteroscope deflection

With the previous generation of F-URS, active deflection of the tip was controlled by a lever mechanism on the handle. Depending of the model, the tip could deflect from 130 to 180 degrees in either direction in the same plane.(5, 6) The Gyrus-ACMI DUR.-8 is the last F-URS from the previous generation with limited capabilities of deflection: combination of 180 degrees active primary downward deflection and 170 degrees active primary upward deflection. These two deflections are controlled by a deflection lever on the underside of the endoscope handle.

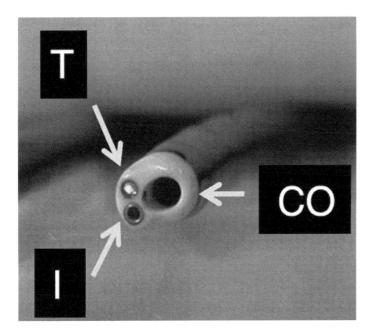

Figure 13.1 Distal Tip of a new generation flexible ureterorenoscope. Working channel 3,6 Fr (CO), optical fibers for light Transmission (T), optical fibers for Imaging (I).

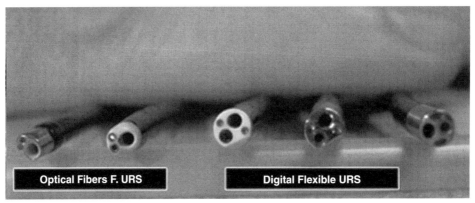

Figure 13.2 Comparison of external diameter of new generation of flexible ureterorenoscopes (optical fibers vs. digital). Constant working channel (3,6 Ch).

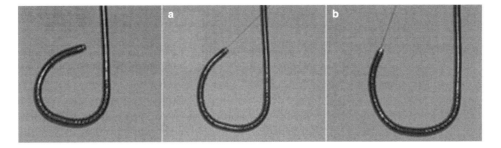

Figure 13.3 New generation of flexible ureterorenoscope with laser fiber in place. Minimal loss of deflection with a 200 µ laser fiber (A) and 365µ (B).

In 2001, ACMI was the first manufacturer to introduce a new generation of flexible URS with a double deflecting system: the DUR-8Elite (Figure 13.4). This specific ureteroscope presented an active 270 degrees deflection in the ventral direction allowing a complete exploration of renal cavities in more than 98% of cases.(7, 8)

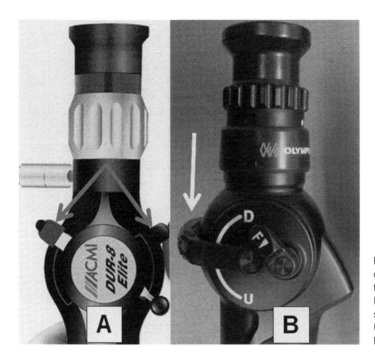

Figure 13.4 Comparison of handles of new generation flexible ureterorenoscopes. A : Gyrus-ACMI DUR 8 Elite with double deflecting system (blue arrows). B : Olympus URF-P5 with a single deflecting lever (white arrow).

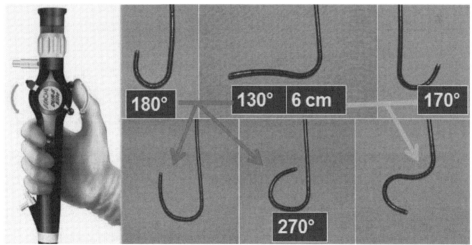

Figure 13.5   deflecting capabilities of the Gyrus-ACMI DUR 8 Elite.

Gyrus-ACMI introduced a new-generation F-URS (DUR-8 Elite) which combined 180 degrees active primary downward deflection and 170 degrees active primary upward deflection, as in the DUR.-8, but in addition to this primary deflection, the Elite provide a 130 degrees active secondary downward deflection. This secondary deflection is controlled by a second lever, on the top of the endoscope handle, and may be locked at any degree by means of a brake on the underside of the handle. The three deflections (primary down, primary up, and secondary down) offered by the DUR.-8 Elite may be used singly or together. When secondary downward deflection is used by itself, a 6-cm length at the distal end of the scope may be deflected 130 degrees. Primary downward deflection (180 degrees) followed by secondary downward deflection (130 degrees) gives 270 degrees in total downward deflection of the distal scope tip. The reverse-order sequence (secondary downward deflection followed by primary downward deflection) will produce a different pattern, with the deflected tip of the scope forming a curve with a much wider radius. If primary upward deflection is combined with secondary downward deflection (in either order) an S-shaped distal tip pattern will be obtained (9–11) (Figure 13.5).

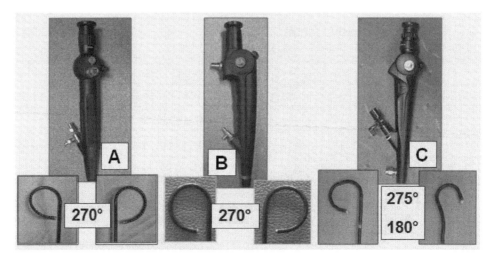

Figure 13.6   A: Flex-X2 Karl Storz. B: Viper Wolf. C: URF-P5 Olympus.

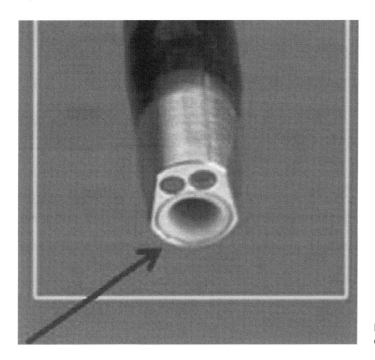

Figure 13.7   Flex-X2 Karl Storz endoscopy, with laserite.

One year after the introduction of the DUR-8 Elite, Karl Storz produced a new flexible URS, the Flex-X. This ureteroscope was the first to incorporate 270 degrees deflection in both directions (ventral and dorsal). By using this scope, complete exploration of renal cavities was also possible in more than 98% of cases (Figure 13.6). Two years later, Karl Storz improved the durability of the Flex-X by incorporating a new laser-resistant ceramic (Laserite) at the distal tip of the working channel (Flex-X2) (12) (Figure 13.7). The Viper from Wolf and recently the URF-P5 from Olympus completed the group of new generation of flexible URS. All these ureteroscopes present at least one active 270 degrees ventral deflection providing an optimal exploration of the collecting system including the lower pole (Figure 13.6).

For all these F-URS, the scope may be designed with intuitive or counterintuitive directions. Today, by using smaller caliber nitinol basket (1.5–1.9 Fr), the angle of active and passive deflection is no longer restricted even with a small laser fiber (200µ).(13) The deflection capabilities of these new F-URS are illustrated in Figure 13.8.

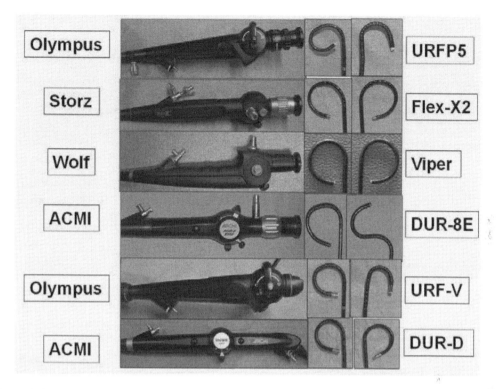

Figure 13.8 Handle and deflection capabilities of new flexible ureterorenoscope.

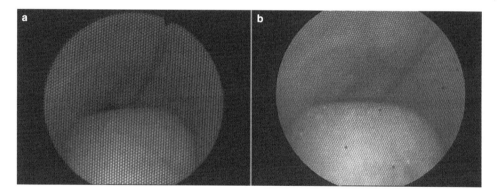

Figure 13.9 Moiré Effect. Constant improvements in the quality and number of optical fibers. Same patient: endoscopic view with F-URS containing 3500 optical fibers (A) and F-URS with 8000 optical fibers (B).

Until 2006, F-URS contains a coherent fiber optic bundle for image transmission and one or two noncoherent light transmitting fibre optic bundles. Optical properties of these new F-URS are sufficient and there are continued improvements in the quality and number of optical fibers (Figure 13.9). Advances in electro-optics continue to improve the urologist's ability to perform minimally invasive procedures. While the development of flexible fiberoptic ureteroscopes (URSs) has greatly facilitated upper tract procedures, distal sensor, digital technology may represent the next step in the evolution of endoscopy. Better image quality could translate into greater precision for diagnostic and treatment and shorter procedures. Thus, a new improvement has recently and dramatically improved image quality: a new digital F-URS was introduced in 2006 by Gyrus-ACMI (the DUR-D Invisio™) (Figure 13.10). This new flexible URS integrates a digital camera and light source in a single "plug and play" device. The digital camera is a CMOS imaging sensor and the light source is a light-emitting diode (LED). This digital F-URS is coupled to a digital control box that performs the equivalent functions

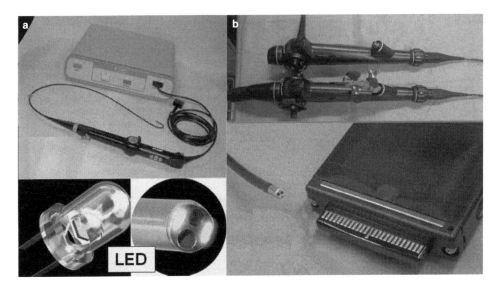

Figure 13.10 A Gyrus ACMI DUR-D Invisio. B : URF-V Olympus.

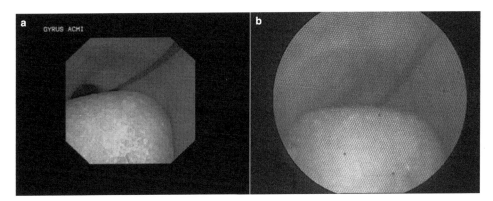

Figure 13.11 Same patient: endoscopic view with F-URS containing CMOS sensor (Gyrus ACMI DUR-D invisio) (A) vs. F-URS with 8000 optical fibers (B).

of the camera and light source for conventional system. White balancing is also unnecessary. Clayman et al. recently reported the superior *in vitro* resolution of the DUR-D over standard fiberoptic F-URS across different tests, including contrast discrimination and resolution with no pixilation or moiré effect (Figure 13.11) and this now represents now the current gold standard in image quality. However, the distal tip diameter of this digital scope is slightly greater (8.5F) than the equivalent standard nonvideo F-URS (7.5F) and the deflection unit is limited to 250 degrees in both directions (Figure 13.8). Future studies are still necessary to evaluate the manoeuvrability of this new digital URS in the renal collecting system to know if the "chip on the tip technology" will not compromise the deflection capabilities.

Olympus have introduced a new video-URS (URF-V) incorporating a charge coupled device (CCD) sensor (Figure 13.10). CCD, or Charge-Coupled Device image sensors, were developed at the end of the 1960s by scientists at Bell Labs, and were originally conceived not as a method of capturing photographic images, but as a way of storing computer data. This idea did not catch on; today we instead have RAM (Random Access Memory) chips in our computers which are, ironically enough, manufactured using the CMOS process. By 1975, CCDs were appearing in television cameras and flatbed scanners. The mid-80s saw CCDs appearing in the first "filmless" still cameras. CCDs rapidly attained great image quality but required a manufacturing process which was different from that used for manufacturing other computer chips such as processors and RAM. This means that specialized CCD fabs have to be constructed, and they cannot be used for making other components, thereby making CCDs more expensive.

Interline Transfer CCDs consist of many MOS (Metal Oxide Semiconductor) capacitors arranged in a pattern, usually in a square grid, which can capture and convert light photons into electrical charge, storing this charge before transferring it for processing by supporting chips. To record color information, colored filters are placed over each individual light receptor making it sensitive to only one light color (generally, Red, Green, and Blue filters are used, but this is not always the case). This gives a value for one color at each pixel, and the surrounding pixels can provide eight more values, four each of the two remaining colors from which they may be interpolated for our original pixel. After the exposure is complete, the charge is transferred row by row into a read-out register, and from there to an output amplifier, analog/digital converters and on for processing. This row-by-row processing of the CCD's light "data" is where the sensor gets the term "Charge-Coupled" in its name. One row of information is transferred to the read-out register, and the rows behind it are each shifted one row closer to the register. After being "read out", the charge is released and the register is empty again for the next charge.

CMOS, or Complementary Metal Oxide Semiconductor, is actually a generic term for the process used to create these image sensors, along with numerous other semiconductor items such as computer RAM, processors such as those from Intel and other manufacturers, and more. CMOS image sensors can be made in the same fabs as these other items, with the same equipment. This technology is, of necessity, very advanced given the amount of competition in processor and other markets contributing to new techniques in CMOS fabrication. The Active Pixel CMOS image sensors used in digital imaging are very similar to a CCD sensor, but with one major difference supporting circuitry is actually located alongside each light receptor, allowing noise at each pixel to be canceled out at the site. Other processes can be integrated right into the CMOS image sensor chip, eliminating the need for extra chips for things like analog/digital conversion, white balancing.

The new Olympus video-F-URS incorporates another new technology: the NBI Function. NBI function (Narrow Band Imaging) is an optical image enhancement technology which narrows the band width of the light output of the Olympus Exera II system from 415nm and 540 nm. This narrow band of light is strongly absorbed by haemoglobin and penetrates only the surface of tissue increasing the visibility of capillaries and other delicate tissue surface structures by enhancing contrast between the two. As a result, under NBI, capillaries on the surface are displayed in brown and veins in the sub-surface are displayed in cyan on the operating monitor (figure 13.12). This technology was recently evaluated with flexible cystoscopy in the detection or recurrent urothelial tumors of the bladder. Authors concluded that NBI has the potential to enhance the detection of recurrent urothelial tumors (p: 0.03). Olympus incorporates this NBI function on the video-URS. This function should be evaluated in the near future.

DISPOSABLE

Guide wires

Guide wires are essential for flexible ureterorenoscopy. Two 150-cm-long and 0.035 or 0.038 in. diameter guide wires (one safety, one working wire) should be used. The distal end (straight or curved) must be flexible and atraumatic. Standard floppy-tipped polytetrafluoroethylene (PTFE) could be used, but we strongly recommended to use stiff hydrophilic wires. The Sensor Glidewire from Microvasive Boston Scientific represents a good compromise with a hydrophilic tip and hydrophilic core for the stiffness. This specific wire has shown its superiority over the standard PTFE in gaining access past ureteral stones.(14)

The BiWire (Cook Urological) is also a new hydrophilic guidewire that has an angled tip at one end and a straight tip at the other end making it more versatile and well-adapted to the working channel of F-URS (Figure 13.13).

When two wires are used (safety and working wire), the working guide wire should be hydrophilic, so as to protect the working channel of the scope, the safety guide wire can be a regular PTFE wire. A safety wire should always be employed when the intended procedure involves placing and removing and then replacing the F-URS. The safety wire is fixed to the drape and remains in place for later use to replace the working wire or to place a stent at the end of the procedure.

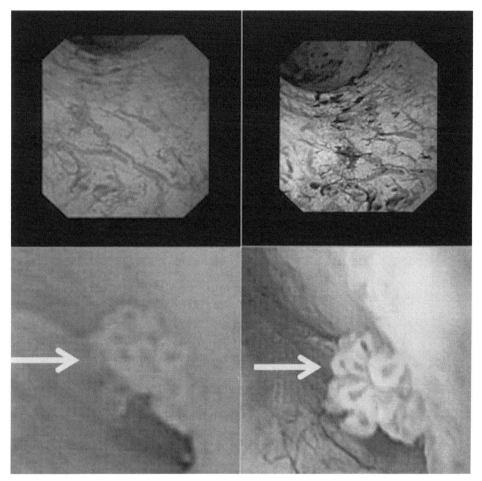

Figure 13.12 Olympus DUR-D with NBI (Narrow band imaging) function. Comparison view of an urothelial tumor (arrow).

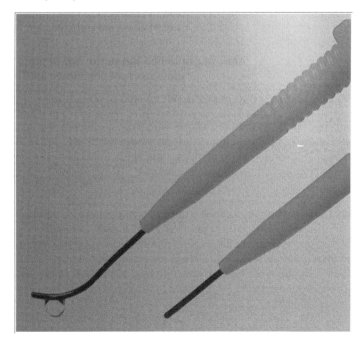

Figure 13.13 BiWire (Cook Medical).

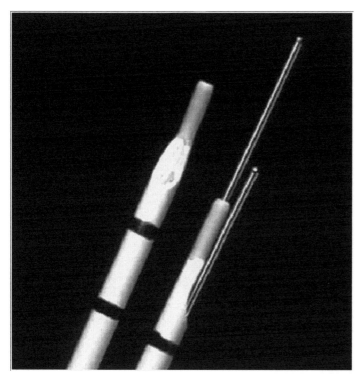

Figure 13.14 Dual lumen catheter (Cook Medical).

Ureteral catheter

At the beginning of the procedure, a 5 or 6 Fr open tip ureteral catheter is used for positioning the guide wire in the ureter. A connector allows contrast agent to be injected for retrograde pyelography (RPG), or to obtain a urine sample for cytology/urine culture.

Dual-lumen catheter

The dual-lumen catheter is a 10Fr ureteral catheter with a flexible, atraumatic 6Fr distal tip. Each lumen accepts a 0.038 in. diameter guide wire (Figure 13.14). It is not always essential, but saves time by eliminating the need for cystoscopy (RPG, insertion of a second guide wire). The dual-lumen catheter allows the operator to insert a second guide wire, with the first wire *in situ*; to inject contrast into the intrarenal collecting system with a guide wire *in situ*; and to dilate the ureter in order to facilitate the passage of the flexible ureterorenoscope. The dual-lumen catheter is placed over a guide wire, under fluoroscopic guidance or under direct visual control during cystoscopy.

Ureteral access sheath (UAS)

UAS were first developed in the 1970s to aid in difficult access to ureters for ureteroscopy. The peel-away sheath was introduced in the 1980s. Over the past few years several new UAS have been made available (Figure 13.15). The Flexor 9,5/11,5 Fr, 12/14 Fr, 14/16 Fr (Cook Medical), The Navigator 11/13 Fr, 13/15 Fr (Boston Scientific) and the UroPass (Gyrus-ACMI) are hydrophilic UAS with a suture hole on the end for securing the UAS in place. The AquaGuide (Bard Urological) and the Flexor DL (Cook Medical) present an additional 3F channel for a safety wire, basket and laser fiber or for another device.

Today, the UAS is routinely used for flexible ureterorenoscopy. It allows the operator to engage the ureter easily and rapidly for multiple reentries and exists; to dilate the ureter; to improve vision by facilitating the return of irrigant; to prevent excessive irrigant pressure rises in the intrarenal collecting system; to encourage stone fragment passage; to protect the F-URS and sometimes to decrease operating time and cost. A theoretical complication of UAS is prolonged pressure on the ureteral wall and ischemia resulting in a ureteral stricture. This has not been demonstrated, and a low rate of stricture 1 to 1.2% or ureteral perforation.

The UAS consists of a two-piece hydrophilic device: the sheath and an internal dilator. The UAS is inserted over a guide wire, under fluoroscopic guidance. The internal dilator has

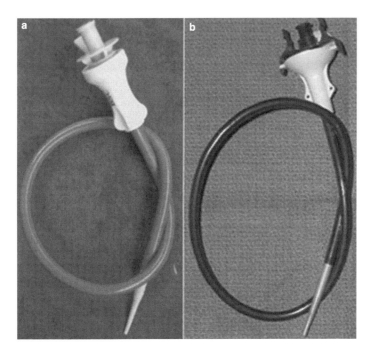

Figure 13.15 Ureteral Access Sheath. A: Navigator (Boston Scientific). B: Flexor (Cook Medical)

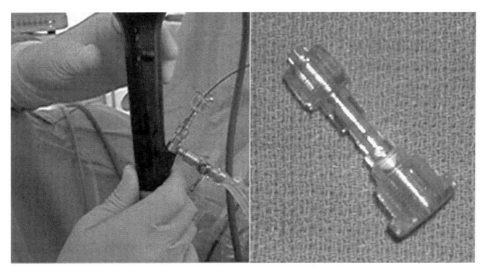

Figure 13.16 Port Seal fitted on the working channel of the flexible URS. The seal allows the operator to conserve irrigant, by preventing leaks; to grip an instrument (such as a laser fiber).

a Luer-Lock fitting for contrast injection, to provide retrograde opacification when the access sheath is *in situ*. When the UAS is in place, the internal dilator can be removed. Depending of the manufacturer, UAS come in various lengths (20–55 cm) and diameter (9.5–14 Fr for internal diameter and 11,5 to 17,5 Fr for the external diameter).

Port Seal

The seal is fitted on the working channel of the flexible URS. The device consists of an O-ring that fits the caliber of all the instruments inserted into the working channel of the scope. The seal allows the operator to conserve irrigant, by preventing leaks and to grip an instrument (such as a laser fiber) with the O-ring (Figure 13.16).

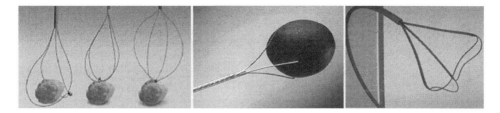

Figure 13.17   Nitinol basket (Bard dimension, N-Circle Cook Medical, Zerotip Boston Scientific), Triceps (Boston Scientific), N-Gage (Cook Medical).

Extraction devices

Baskets : Over the past few years, several new stone retrieval devices have become available. Since its introduction in 1998, Nitinol baskets have become the standard device for stone retrieval and new designs have emerged each year. The Escape from Boston Scientific (Natuck, Mass) was specially designed for use with a small laser fiber (200 µ), trapping the stone which is photo-ablated. The Dimension basket from Bard Urological is an articulating tipless nitinol basket. The new N-Gage 1,7 and 2,2 Fr (Cook Urological) is a compromise between a basket and a grasper. The size of nitinol basket continues top decrease in size : N-Circle 1,5 Fr (Cook Medical), Zerotip 1,9 an 1,3 Fr (Boston Scientific). All these Nitinol baskets are very flexible and designed not to damage the scope and the intrarenal collecting system. The slenderest possible basket should be used. Basket opening and closing are controlled by a proximal handle (15, 16) (Figure 13.17).

Graspers : The recommended device has three or four prongs that allow stone fragments impacted in the renal papillae or in the urothelial mucosa to be extracted. This grasper is also a safe and effective device for removing stones from the kidney. The main advantage of the grasper over nitinol basket is the ability to release the stone at any time.

Biopsy Forceps : The device allows the operator to take biopsy samples from tumors or from the urothelial mucosa.

Irrigation

Achieving adequate irrigation represents an ongoing a major issue for flexible ureterorenoscopy. Saline is the standard irrigant used for flexible ureterorenoscopy. Contrast can be injected through the working channel to opacify the collecting system for fluoroscopic imaging and determination of the position of the F-URS. However, mixing of irrigants causes distorsion of the visual image due to different indices of refraction of the fluid as a result of different densities (i.e: saline and contrast). To avoid this phenomenon, intrarenal cavities should be washed by using saline irrigation during few minutes.

Irrigation is delivered through the same channel used for the working instrument. The flow of irrigant is passed through the side arm so a working instrument can be passed through the channel at the same time. To improve the irrigation flow when an instrument is inserted into the working channel, the irrigant must be pressurized to get an adequate flow at the distal tip of the F-URS. It can be pressurized with a manually powered syringe, pressure irrigation bag, or a mechanical irrigator.

Several irrigation devices have become commercially available over the past few years. Peditrol (EMS medical) is a new irrigation system for flexible and semi-rigid URS.(17) The system is hands-free and activated by foot-pedal. In a recent study, the Peditrol system was superior to gravity irrigation, a handheld 60-cc syringe and a bag irrigation pressurized to 300 cm H_2O.

Gyrus-ACMI offers a system composed of a syringe with a spring and a nonreturn valve. It is connected to the irrigation tubing. It allows brief pulses of raised irrigation pressure to be delivered. Socomed Promepla introduced a new irrigation tube including a manual pressure pomp in conjunction with an automated pressure device (Figure 13.18).

SET-UP AND PATIENT POSITIONING

Endoscopy unit

An endoscopic zoom camera (for optimal image size), with camera programming controls and a focusing ring should be used. A xenon cold-light source will give optimum brightness and

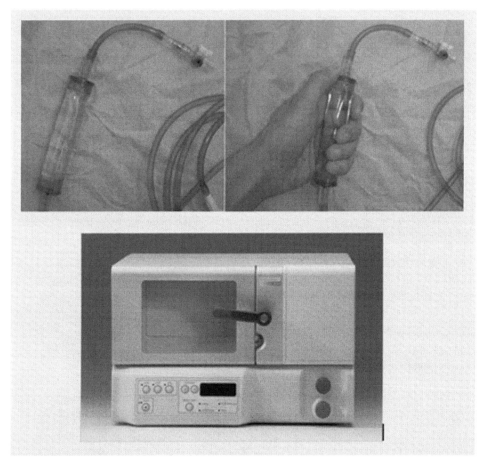

Figure 13.18 Socomed Promepla. Irrigation tube with hand assisted device and automated pressure pomp.

contrast in the intrarenal collecting system. The different components of the endoscopy unit are housed in a mobile endoscopy tower, which also holds the monitor. Significant recent advances include digital imaging, increased resolution of video monitors with high-definition television (HDTV).

Fluoroscopy

Fluoroscopic guidance and monitoring are mandatory in flexible ureteropyeloscopy. Each step in access and placing the F-URS should be followed with real time fluoroscopy. A specialized fluoroscopy technician should be present, and radiation protection regulations (distance, exposure, individual protection) must be stringently observed.(18)

Intracorporeal lithotripsy devices

The introduction of Holmium-YAG laser lithotripsy now allows for the fragmentation of all stones types, converting them to dust-like particles and obviating the need for fragment removal. (19, 20) The Holmium-YAG laser is a solid-state laser made from a rare element (Holmium) and an Yttrium-Aluminium-Garnet crystal (YAG) (Figure 13.19). It delivers pulsatile energy and operates at a wavelength of 2100 nm (in the infrared part of the spectrum, which is invisible to the human eye). The laser allows intracorporeal lithotripsy to be performed, ureteral strictures to be managed, and urothelial tumors to be removed. This is a contact laser: for the system to work, the laser fiber must be placed right against the target (tissue or stone). A flexible ureterorenoscope accommodates two types of laser fibers: a small-diameter (150–200 μm) fiber and a large-diameter (350–400 μm) fiber. The large-diameter fibers will deliver more power, but restrict the deflection of the scope. The reverse is true of the small-diameter fibers: they deliver less energy, but leave the scope free to deflect. A red aiming beam shows where the fiber is in

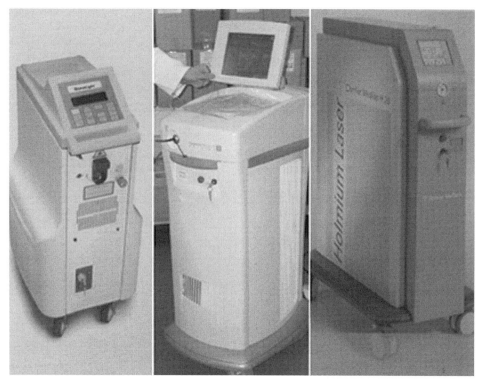

Figure 13.19   Examples of Holmium YAG Lasers.

relation to the target. The Holmium:YAG laser can cut through guide wires and Nitinol instruments. This property may be put to good use when it comes to freeing a stone that has become impacted in a Nitinol extraction basket.(21)

Several new lasers have been evaluated. In an *in vitro* model, the erbium :YAG laser ablate human kidney stones two to five times more efficiently than the Holmium YAG., but the Erbium laser needs improvements in fiber technology before clinical use. Thulium laser is promising but needs to be improved before it becomes clinically useful. Recently, we reported our initial experience with the FREDDY laser in humans, and we found that 72% of stones were completely treated (22–23) (Figure 13.20). However, the FREDDY laser is not very effective in fragmenting hard stones and has no effect oncystine stones. Furthermore, it is not useful for tissue applications (incision, coagulation). (22–24) Today, Holmium YAG laser is still the most versatile laser for upper tract endourologic procedures.(25)

Anesthesia

For diagnostic procedures, I.V. sedation may be sufficient, but for most therapeutic procedures general anesthesia should be used. The urine must be sterile. Urinalysis and culture to rule out a coexisting urinary tract infection is an essential part of the preoperative work-up. Prophylactic antibiotics should be administered.

Patient positioning

As a rule, the patient should be in the dorsal lithotomy position. Pressure points must be protected. It is our practice to place the instrument table under the patient's left leg. In this way, the operator can align all the instruments and the ureterorenoscope level with the patient, without having to involve his or her assistant. The endoscopy tower and the fluoroscopy screens are placed on the patient's right. The screens must be arranged side by side. The foot switches for the fluoroscopy and for the laser are placed under the operator's right foot. The operator stands or sits between the patient's legs. The laser unit is put against the instrument table, to ensure correct positioning and to prevent damage to the laser fiber. The X-ray tube is placed under the operating table, and the image intensifier is placed above the table and as close to the

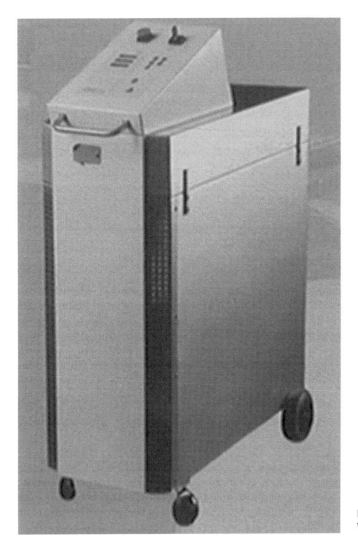

Figure 13.20 FREDDY Nd:YAG laser. World of Medecine.

patient as possible. Sterile drapes with a collecting pocket will allow an assessment, during and after the procedure, of the volume of irrigant used (Figure 13.21).

URETERAL ACCESS

Achievement of ureteral access is necessary for performing retrograde endoscopic procedures such as flexible ureteroscopy. Access into the ureter with a F-URS requires special technique. Technologies such as ureteral access sheaths (UAS), balloon dilators, and coaxial dilators may be useful to facilitate ureteral access especially in difficult cases.

Technique of ureteral dilation and insertion of ureteral access sheath

Systematic dilation of the ureter should be performed only if necessary. If the operator decides to dilate the ureter, it may be achieved in a variety of ways: with a low-pressure ureteral balloon catheter; with a 10Fr dual-lumen catheter or with a hydrophilic UAS (self-dilating).

After standard set-up and patient positioning, cystoscopy is performed and the initial guide wire (working guide wire) is inserted. The bladder is drained and the cystoscope is withdrawn. The ureteral balloon catheter is inserted over the working guide wire, under fluoroscopic guidance. Ureteral dilation is performed (balloon inflated with saline and contrast agent). Under X-ray control, the ureteral balloon catheter is withdrawn.

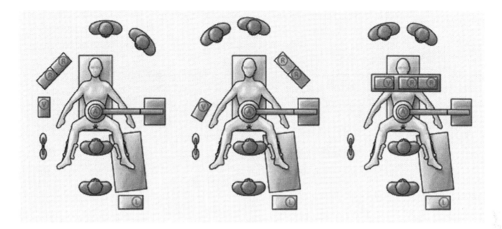

Figure 13.21   Various set-up in operating room. A: C-Arm. R : fluoroscopic control unit. L : Laser unit. V : video unit.

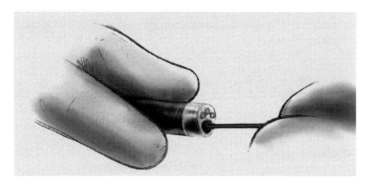

Figure 13.22   placement of the F-URS over the working wire.

The dual-lumen catheter is inserted over the working guide wire, under fluoroscopic guidance. Retrograde pyelogram is performed via the second channel of the dual-lumen catheter, following which the safety guide wire is inserted through the same channel. The dual-lumen catheter is withdrawn and the safety guide wire is secured to the patient's left thigh.

INSERTION OF THE URETERORENOSCOPE INTO THE INTRARENAL COLLECTING SYSTEM

The F-URS may be inserted directly over the working guide wire or through an UAS. If the operator decides not to use UAS (diagnostic procedure), the F-URS should be backloaded over the working wire under fluoroscopic guidance by way of the following steps:

The operator must keep the F-URS straight at all times, using both hands to steady the distal tip of the scope, with the assistant holding the handle of the device. The operator carefully backloads the F-URS over the guide wire, taking care not to damage the working channel, and then slides the F-URS over the guide wire (Figure 13.22). In male patients, the penis is held upwards to straighten the urethra. Fluoroscopy is used to ensure that the scope is advanced to the renal pelvis. At that time, the working guide wire is withdrawn and the cold-light cable, the camera, and the irrigation system are attached.

If the operator decides at the beginning of the procedure to use an UAS, he should take the following steps. The UAS is inserted over the working guide wire, under fluoroscopic guidance. The dilating obturator of the UAS is withdrawn from the ureteral access sheath. At that time, the working guide wire may be or may be not withdrawn. If the operator withdraws the wire, the F-URS is inserted directly into the UAS under endoscopic control after attachment of the cold-light cable, irrigation and camera system. If the working guide wire is saved, the F-URS is inserted over the working guide wire, through the ureteral access sheath. An X-Ray

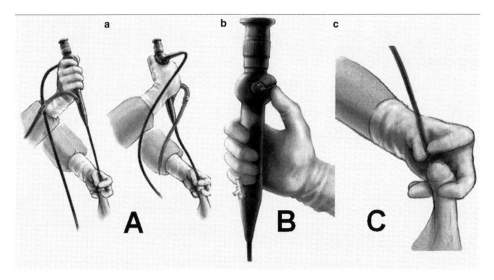

Figure 13.23 The handle of the F-URS is held with the dominant hand (A), the deflection control is worked with the thumb (B). The other hand stabilizes the endoscope sheath at the urethra orifice. In male patients, the non-dominant hand also steadies the penis (C).

control is obtained to ensure that the scope is inside the renal pelvis. At that time, the working guide wire is withdrawn and the cold-light cable, the camera, and the irrigation system are attached.

Recently, Grasso et al. describe a new "wireless and sheathless" technique for the placement of the F-URS.(26)

After the placement of the F-URS into the kidney, with or without the use of an UAS, the intrarenal collecting system is explored, starting with the upper-pole calices, followed by the middle calices and, finally, the lower-pole calices. The exploration is performed under endoscopic vision and fluoroscopic guidance.

The F-URS should always be held with both hands; the hands must work together, to allow the scope to move as a unit. The handle of the F-URS is held with the dominant hand, the deflection control is worked with the thumb (in the ACMI DUR.-8 Elite, with the thumb and the index). The other hand stabilizes the endoscope sheath at the urethra orifice. In male patients, the nondominant hand also steadies the penis (Figure 13.23).

Handling of the ureterorenoscope in the intrarenal collecting system

There are three basic movements for mobilizing the endoscope:

1. Dominant-hand pronation and supination to change the direction of the distal tip of the scope. Supination is essential when the scope is in right renal cavities and pronation is essential when the F-URS is in left renal cavities (Figure 13.24).
2. Thumb (thumb-and-index, in the DUR™-8 Elite) of the dominant-hand controls the deflection to produce downward or upward deflection of the tip of the F-URS.
3. Advancement/withdrawal of the scope is obtained by the non-dominant hand (Figure 13.23).

The F-URS should not be advanced by pushing with the dominant hand that holds the handle. Forward or backward movement is produced by the non-dominant hand that holds the shaft of the endoscope; the dominant hand, which holds the handle, follows the movement of the scope. If, during the procedure, the F-URS is withdrawn (e.g., to allow the removal of a stone), it must be reinserted over a working guide wire if no UAS has been used. In order to do this, the safety guide wire and the dual-lumen catheter must be used to reposition the working guide wire in the intrarenal collecting system.

If an UAS has been used, ureteroscpoe can be reinserted directly or over a reomserted guidewire.

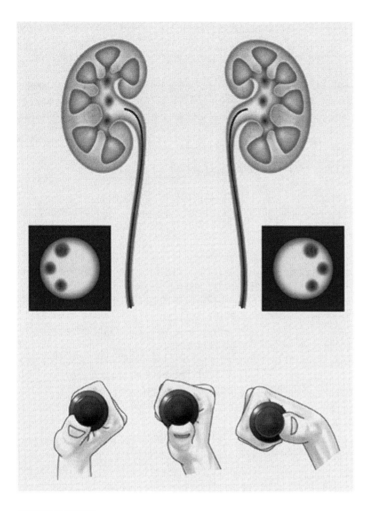

Figure 13.24 Dominant-hand pronation and supination to change the direction of the distal tip of the scope. Supination is essential when the scope is in right renal cavities and pronation is essential when the F-URS is in left renal cavities

INDICATIONS

Flexible ureteroscopy is emerging as a first-line procedure because of miniaturization of F-URS, ancillary devices and introduction of the Holmium Laser. All of these advances have resulted in expanding indications for ureteroscopy.(27, 28)

Flexible ureterorenoscopy represents the ideal technique for the diagnosis of upper tract lesions such as filling defects and other causes of bleeding in unilateral gross hematuria : hemangioma, varicosity, neoplasm, and small vascular lesion. Urinary calculi remain one of the most frequent application for flexible ureterorenoscopy. The F-URS is much more effective than rigid endoscopes to treat urinary stones in the proximal part of the ureter as well as in the kidney.

Although flexible ureterorenoscopy may play a major role in the treatment of proximal ureteral and selected intrarenal calculi smaller than 15 mm (29), the technique seems to play a limited role for renal stones greater than 1.5 cm. However, larger stones are being addressed with retrograde intrarenal surgery. Grasso et al. were the first to report their experience with retrograde ureteroscopic approach for larger renal calculi.(29) Other investigators have similarly treated large stones. Mugiya and colleagues reported a stone free rate of 87% after one single session for stones with a mean stone size of 2.4 cms. Some authors have routinely performed flexible ureterorenoscopy for staghorn calculi, specially for patients with high comorbidities.(30, 31)

For children and prepubertal children, ureteroscopy is becoming more widely accepted as first-line therapy.(32–35) Likewise, ureteroscopy and Holmium laser lithotripsy during pregnancy is becoming more common.(36) Preminger et al. reported that flexible uretroscopy could be considered as a primary option for stone patients with pelvic kidney.(37)

Similarly, ureteroscopy and especially flexible ureteroscopy represents a procedure of choice to treat morbidly obese patients. No significant difference in outcomes has been shown between morbidly obese and normal weight patients undergoing ureteroscopy. (38, 39)

Antegrade or retrograde ureteroscopy in patients who have urinary diversions represents a procedure of choice.(40, 41)

Flexible ureterorenoscopy can be used to treat narrow segments in the ureter and at the ureteropelvic junction (UPJ). Ureteral strictures can be approached with a similar technique as UPJ obstruction. Finally, upper tract neoplasms can also be treated with a F-URS. The Holmium YAG laser can coagulate and ablate tissue.

MANAGEMENT OF KIDNEY STONES (OTHER THAN LOWER-POLE CALCULI)

The intrarenal collecting system is completely explored to identify the exact location of the stone. At that time, a laser fiber (200 or 365 µm) is inserted into the working channel of a straightened F-URS (without any distal tip deflection). The fiber is advanced a few millimetres beyond the end of the working channel; the aiming beam is switched on; and the laser initiated at settings of 5–6 Hz, 1–1.5 J corresponding to 5 to 9 W. When the fragmentation is complete, the laser fiber is withdrawn, and the stone fragments are captured with a Nitinol basket. The F-URS is withdrawn with the fragments, since the fragments cannot pass through the working channel. If a UAS is being used, the F-URS is withdrawn and then repositioned via the UAS. If the fragment will not go through the UAS, it should be grasped against the distal end of the UAS, and the entire unit (scope, grasper holding the stone, and UAS) is removed "in one piece", provided the fragment can be accommodated by the ureter. If the operator has decided not to use a UAS, the F-URS is completely withdrawn, and must be repositioned over a working guide wire. At the end of the procedure, a check is made to ensure that no fragments have been left behind. After this, the surgeon may or may not decide to drain the kidney with a stent. If the kidney is to be drained, a ureteral catheter may be used for 24 hours; alternatively, an internal stent may be left in the ureter for a few days.(42, 43)

MANAGEMENT OF LOWER-POLE CALCULI

When a lower pole calculus is located, a Nitinol basket (1.5–2.4 Fr) is inserted (with the endoscope undeflected) and the stone is captured. The stone is displaced to the upper caliceal system, or into the renal pelvis.(44) The stone is released, and the Nitinol grasper is withdrawn. A laser fiber (200–365 µm-diameter) is introduced into the working channel (Figure 13.25). The fiber is advanced a few millimetres beyond the end of the working channel, and the red aiming beam is switched on. The laser fiber is fixed by using the port seal to avoid back movements of the laser fiber into the working channel. The F-URS with the fiber in place is placed against the stone, and fragmentation is initiated as previously described.(16, 45–47) Displacing a lower pole stone into a more favorable location (upper pole, renal pelvis) before fragmentation has been shown to be more effective with regard to in stone-free rates than treating the stone *in situ*.(48)

If the stone cannot be displaced into the upper pole or the renal pelvis (bulky stone, stricture of the caliceal stem), it may be fragmented *in situ* using a small-diameter (150–200 µm) laser fiber. For the introduction of the laser fiber, the F-URS must always be kept straight (undeflected). Deflection of the scope is not started until the fiber is at the tip of the endoscope. At the end of the procedure, a complete exploration of the intra-renal cavities is obtained to ensure that no fragments have been left behind. If the kidney must to be drained, a ureteral catheter may be used for 24 hours; alternatively, an internal stent may be left in the ureter for a few days.

PREVENTION OF STONE FRAGMENT ACCUMULATION IN LOWER CALYX

If, at the end of the procedure, for any renal calculi regardless of location, many small stone fragments are left in the collecting system, there will be a major risk of fragment re-accumulation in the lower-pole calices. In order to avoid this risk, Fuchs and Patel described a technique to seal the lower pole with an autologous blood clot. For this part of the procedure, the F-URS is placed in the lower pole. Saline is injected into the working channel of the F-URS, to flush the fragments towards the upper calices and the renal pelvis, and to clear any remaining contrast.

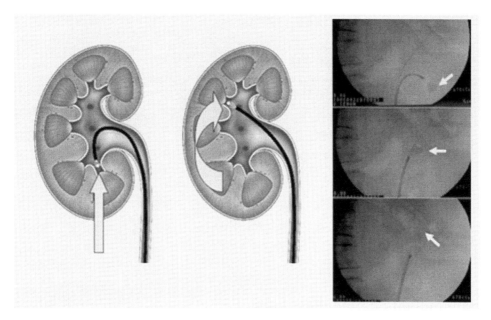

Figure 13.25 Relocation of a lower pole stone. Principle and fluoroscopic control.

Through the working channel of the scope, the operator injects 5 to 10 mL of autologous blood taken from a peripheral venous line. (This will completely obscure endoscopic vision and the position of the F-URS in the lower pole will need to be checked with fluoroscopy). When the injection is complete, the F-URS is withdrawn, and the surgeon waits 5 to 10 minutes for the clot to form. A retrograde pyelogram is performed to check that the lower calyx is no longer visualized, i.e. that the clot are provides a seal.

MANAGEMENT OF CALICEAL DIVERTICULA

A mixture of contrast and methylene blue or indigo carmine is injected through the working channel of the scope. A check is made with fluoroscopy to establish that the diverticulum is properly opacified. Opacification means that the neck of the diverticulum is patent. Saline is injected through the working channel of the scope, to flush the intrarenal collecting system. A detailed inspection of the collecting system is made, to see whether contrast is seen streaming from the diverticular neck. (Delayed emptying of the diverticulum would suggest a narrow neck) (Figure 13.26). Once the diverticulum has been identified, a laser fiber is passed through the working channel of the scope, to incise the neck of the diverticulum. Following incision of the diverticular neck, the F-URS is inserted into the diverticulum. Any stone or stones in the diverticulum may be fragmented *in situ* with the laser or extracted "in one piece" with the Nitinol basket. Following treatment of the stone(s), the neck of the diverticulum is generously incised with the laser, to allow the diverticulum to be marsupialized into the collecting system. At the end of the procedure, a check is made to ensure that no fragments have been left behind. After this, the surgeon may or may not decide to drain the ureter. Ureteral drainage with an internal ureteral stent is strongly recommended. If possible, the renal pigtail of the stent should be placed inside the marsupialized cavity.(49)

MANAGEMENT OF UROTHELIAL TUMORS

A saline wash of the intrarenal collecting system may be obtained and an aspiration sample is collected for cytopathology. If required, retrograde pyelogram may be performed to assist in the localization of the lesion. Retrograde pyelogram must not be performed prior to cytological sampling, since the contrast agent will interfere with the cytolopathological examination. Once

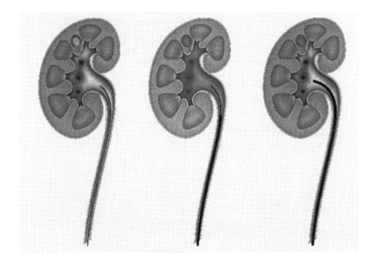

Figure 13.26 Caliceal diverticulum. Methylene blue test.

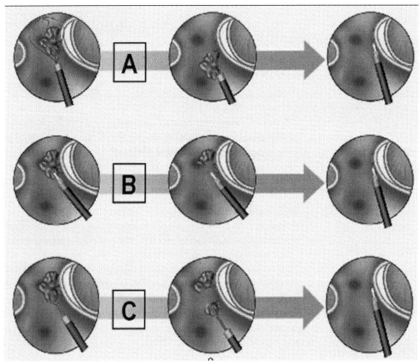

Figure 13.27 Ablation techniques of urothelial tumors. A : nitinol basket cold cutting. B : Laser ablation. C :Biopsy Forceps and laser ablation.

the tumor has been identified, the surgeon must decide which of the three ablation techniques available he prefers (50–52) (Figure 13.27)

A. The first option consists in debulking the tumor by cold-cutting it with a tipless Nitinol basket. This is followed by the collection of tumor stump tissue with biopsy forceps, and the vaporization of the tumor base with the Holmium laser (settings : 10 Hz, 1–1.2 Joules, corresponding to 10 to 12 Watts).

B. The second option consists of taking biopsies and then vaporizing the entire tumor with the holmium:YAG laser, without any prior debulking.

C. The third option consists in completely resecting the tumor with the biopsy forceps, and then vaporizing the tumor base with the Holmium laser.

With all of these techniques, a large-diameter laser fiber is used (generally 365 µm). However, for lesions in the lower pole, a small-diameter fiber (200 µm) is usually used, in order to obtain maximum deflection of the scope. Once the renal urothelial lesion has been treated, the ureter is inspected carefully. To this end, the ureteroscope is gradually withdrawn, and all ureteral surfaces are inspected under endoscopic vision, to the ureteral orifice.

At the end of the procedure, the surgeon may or may not decide to drain the ureter. If the ureter is to be drained, a ureteral catheter may be used for 24 hours; alternatively, an internal stent may be left in the ureter for a few days. Depending on the type of drainage chosen, adjuvant chemotherapy with instillation of a topical therapeutic agent may be started.

RETROGRADE ENDOPYELOTOMY

Retrograde pyelogram is obtained to confirm the UPJ obstruction. A safety guide wire is inserted, through the dual-lumen catheter and the safety guide wire is secured to the patient's left thigh. If required, a UAS is inserted. The F-URS is inserted over the working guide wire. The position of the F-URS is checked with the fluoroscopoic control : the F-URS could be in the renal pelvis, if the ureteropyelic junction (UPJ) is passable or the F-URS is distal to the UPJ if the junction is not passable. The working guide wire is withdrawn. The cold-light cable, the camera, and the irrigation system are attached. If possible, the intrarenal collecting system and the UPJ are explored. With the F-URS kept straight (distal tip undeflected), a 365 µm diameter laser fiber is introduced into the working channel of the scope. The fiber is advanced a few millimetres beyond the end of the working channel; the red aiming beam is switched on; and the laser is set at Ready. Power setting: 12 to 15 Hz, 1 to 1,5 J corresponding to 15 to 22 W. If the F-URS is in the intrarenal collecting system, the UPJ is incised as the scope is being withdrawn towards the ureter. If the ureterorenoscope is below the UPJ, the incision is made as the scope is being advanced towards the renal pelvis. Repeated passes with the laser fiber are made, until the periureteral fat appears. The F-URS is withdrawn. A high-pressure ureteral balloon catheter is inserted over the safety guide wire and under fluoroscopic guidance, the high-pressure balloon is inflated with contrast agent, to dilate the incised area. The high-pressure ureteral balloon catheter is withdrawn. The dual-lumen catheter is inserted over the safety guide wire, and retrograde pyelogram is performed. If the endopyelotomy has been correctly performed, there will be an extravasation of contrast from the ureter. At the end of the procedure, an internal ureteral stent (8Fr, or 12/8Fr) should be inserted and left in place for 4 to 6 weeks; a urinary catheter should be left in place for 24 hours.(53)

ANTEGRADE FLEXIBLE URETEROSCOPY

Flexible ureteroscopy may be performed using an antegrade approach; however, the procedure is rarely indicated. It is considered in cases where a retrograde route is not feasible, such as with external and, particularly, with internal urinary diversion. The technique is well established; however, the antegrade approach places great mechanical stress on the scope, and weakens the equipment.

The patient is positioned prone. The intrarenal collecting system is identified and punctured, under ultrasound or fluoroscopic guidance. Preferentially, the middle or upper caliceal system should be punctured, to ensure that the scope is aligned with the ureter. Contrast is injected through the puncture needle to opacify the intrarenal collecting system and the ureter, and the working guide wire is inserted into the ureter, under fluoroscopic guidance. The puncture needle is withdrawn. A dual-lumen catheter is inserted over the working guide wire and the safety guide wire is inserted through the second channel of the dual-lumen catheter. The dual-lumen catheter is then withdrawn and the safety guide wire is secured to the patient's body. The high-pressure ureteral balloon catheter is inserted over the working guide wire. Under fluoroscopic guidance, the high-pressure balloon catheter is inflated with contrast agent, to dilate the puncture needle tract. The high-pressure ureteral balloon catheter is withdrawn. The ureteral access sheath is inserted over the working guide wire, under fluoroscopic guidance. The dilating obturator is withdrawn from the ureteral access sheath.

Table 13.1 Characteristics of new generation flexible URS.

	Length (cm)	Distal tip diameter (Fr)	Midshaft diameter (Fr)	Proximal Diameter (Fr)	Field of view (Degrees)	Angle of visualization (Degrees)	Working channel (F)	Deflection Ventral/ Dorsal (Degrees)
Olympus URFP5	67	5.9	8	8.9	85	0	3.6	275/180
Karl Storz FLEX-X2	67	6.5	7.5	8.4	88	0	3.6	270/270
WOLF Viper	68	6	7.5	8.8	85	0	3.6	270/270
Gyrus-ACMI DUR8 Elite	64	6.75	8.7–9.4	10.1	80	9	3.6	270/180
Gyrus-ACMI DUR-D	65	8.7	9.3	10.9	80	0	3.6	250/250
Olympus URF-V	67	9	9.5	10.9	85	0	3,6	275/180

Through the ureteral access sheath, the F-URS is inserted over the working guide wire, under fluoroscopic guidance. The working guide wire is withdrawn and the cold-light cable, the camera, and the irrigation system are attached. Antegrade exploration of the ureter is performed. Any calculi, tumors, or ureteral strictures are addressed in customary fashion.

At the end of the procedure, the ureterorenoscope is withdrawn. The ureteral access sheath is removed. Over the safety guide wire, a percutaneous nephrostomy tube is inserted, under fluoroscopic guidance. The safety guide wire is withdrawn, and the nephrostomy tube is secured to the skin.(40, 41)

CONCLUSIONS

Flexible URS combined with Holmium-YAG laser is an effective, reproducible and minimally traumatic diagnostic and therapeutic technique perfectly adapted to diseases of the upper urinary tract, and especially for the management of lower pole stone less than 15mm. This technology must be part of the therapeutic armamentarium of any centre involved in the management of urinary stones.

The equipment has improved dramatically over the past two decades in several areas: ureteroscope design, intracorporeal lithotripter, accessory devices and especially video and imaging. Advances in electro-optics continue to improve the urologist's ability to perform minimally invasive procedures. While the development of flexible fiberoptic ureteroscopes (URS) has greatly facilitated upper tract procedures, distal sensor/ digital technology may represent the next step in the evolution of endoscopy. Better image quality could translate into greater precision for diagnostic and therapeutic procedures and could potentially shorten procedures. Collectively, all these improvements allow excellent results in the management of upper tract diseases, with high stone free rate particularly for the lower pole stone with lower morbidity.

There are no reasons to think that such improvements will stop in the future and due to the past improvements of the equipment and ancillary accessories, we can easily imagine that manufacturers will produce in the near future new flexible endoscopes with improved characteristics for an optimal ability to access virtually any area of the intrarenal collecting system including patients with anomalous or reconstructed urinary tract anatomy.

REFERENCES

1. Grasso M, Bagleyd. Small diameter, actively defectable flexible ureteropyeloscopy. J. Urol 1998; 160: 1648–53.
2. Beiko DT, Denstedt JD. Advances in ureterorenoscopy. Urol Clin N Am 2007; 34: 397–408.
3. Michel M, Knoll T, Ptaschnyk T, Kohrmann KU, Alken P. Flexible ureterorenopyeloscopy for the treatment of lower pole calyx stones: influence of different lithotripsy probes and stone extraction tools on scope deflection and irrigation flow. Eur Urol 2002; 41: 312.

4. Pasqui F, Dubosq F, Tchala K et al. Impact on active scope deflection and irrigation flow of all endoscopic working tools during flexible ureteroscopy. Eur Urol 2004; 45: 58–64.

5. White MD, Moran ME. Fatigability on the latest generation ureteropyeloscopes: Richrad Wolf vs Karl Storz. J Endourol 1998; supp 12: 182.

6. Afane JS, Olweny EO, Bercowsky E et al. Flexible ureteroscopes: a single center evaluation of the durability and function of the new endoscopes smaller than 9Fr. J. Urol 2001; 164: 1164–8.

7. Traxer O, Pasqui F, Dubosq F et al. Etude comparative de deux urétérorénoscopes souples de dernière génération. Prog Urol 2005; 15: 656–61.

8. Lobik L, Lopez Pujals A, Leveillee RJ. Variables affecting deflection of a new third-generation flexible ureteropyeloscope (DUR-8 Elite). J Endourol 2003; 17: 733–6.

9. Chiu KY, Cai Y, Marcovich R, Smith AD, Lee BR. Are new-generation flexible ureteroscopes better than their predecessors? BJU Int 2004; 93: 115–9.

10. Ankem MK, Lowry PS, Slovick RW, Munoz Del Rio A, Nakada SY. Clinical utility of dual active deflection flexible ureteroscope during upper tract ureteropyeloscopy. Urology 2004; 64: 430–4.

11. Traxer O, Pasqui F, Dubosq F et al. Urétérorénoscope souple à double déflexion active. Expérience initiale. Prog Urol 2003; 13: 592–7.

12. Traxer O, Dubosq F, Jamali K, Gattegno B, Thibault P. New-generation flexible ureterorenoscopes are more durable than previous ones. Urology 2006; 68: 276–9.

13. Bultitude M.F, Dasgupta P, Tiptaft RC, Glass JM. Prolonging the life of the flexible ureterorenoscope. Int J Clin Pract 2004; 8: 756–7.

14. Mostafavi MR. Clinical evaluation of differents wires in gaining access during ureteroscopy for ureteral stones disease. J Endourol 2006; 20(1): Abst A117.

15. Landman J, Monga M, El-gabry EA et al. Bare naked baskets: ureteroscope deflection and flow characteristics with intact and disassembled ureteroscopic nitinol stone baskets. J Urol 2002; 167: 2377.

16. Kourambas J, Delvecchio FC. Munver R, Preminger GM. Nitinol stone retrieval-assisted ureteroscopic management of lower pole renal calculi. Urology 2000; 20: 56: 935–9.

17. Blew BD, Dagnone AJ, Pace KT et al. Comparison of Peditrol irrigation device and common methods of irrigation. J Endourol 2005; 19: 562–5.

18. Bagley DH, Fabrizio M, EL Gabry E. Ureteroscopic and radiographic imaging of the upper urinary tract. J Endourol 1998; 12: 313–24.

19. Saïdi A, Combes F, Delaporte V et al. Urétéroscopie souple-Laser Holmium :YAG. Matériel et technique. Prog Urol 2006; 16: 19–24.

20. Denstedt JD. Preliminary experience with Holmium YAG laser lithotripsy. J Endourol. 1995; 9: 255–8.

21. Grasso M, Chalik Y. Principles and applications of laser lithotripsy: experience with the Holmium laser lithotrite. J Clin Laser Med Surg 1998; 16: 3–7.

22. Dubosq F, Pasqui F, Girard F et al. Endoscopic lithotripsy and the FREDDY laser: initial experience. J Endourol 2006; 20: 296–9.

23. Dubosq F, Pasqui F, Girard F et al. Intérêt et place de la lithotritie endocorporelle Nd:YAG en urétéroscopie souple et semi-rigide : une alternative au laser Holmium:YAG ? Prog Urol 2005; 15: 662–6.

24. Del Vecchio F, Auge BK, Brizuela RM et al. In vitro analysis of stone fragmentation ability of the Freddy Laser. J Endourol 2003; 17: 177.

25. GOULD DL. Retrograde flexible ureterorenoscopic Holmium-Yag laser lithotripsy: the new gold standard. Tech Urol 1998; 1: 22–4.

26. Johnson GB, Portela D, Grasso M. Advanced ureteroscopy: wireless and sheathless. J Endourol 2006; 20: 552–5.

27. Elashry OM, Elbahnasy AM, Rao GS, Nakada SY, Clayman RV. Flexible ureteroscopy: Washingtown University experience with the 9,3F and 7,5F flexible ureteroscopes. J Urol 1997; 157: 2074–80.

28. Parkin J, Keeley FX Jr, Timoney AG. Flexible ureteroscopes: a user's guide. BJU Intern 2002; 90: 640.

29. Grasso M, Conlin M, Bagley DH. Retrograde ureteropyeloscopic treatment of large upper urinary tract (2 cm) and minor staghorn calculi. J Urol 1998; 160: 346–51.

30. Mugiya S, Ozono S, Nagata M et al. Retrograde endoscopic management of ureteral stones more than 2 cm in size. Urology 2006; 67: 1164–8.

31. Diner EK, Rosenblum M, Patel SV et al. Primary ureterorenoscopy and holmium laser lithotripsy for large renal stone and staghorn calculi. J Urol 2005; 173(suppl 4): 457.

32. Raza A, Smith G, Moussa S et al. Ureteroscopy in the management of pediatric urinary tract calculi. J Endourol 2005; 19: 151–8.

33. Minevich E, Sheldon CA. The role of ureteroscopy in pediatric urology. Curr Opin Urol 2006; 16: 295–8.

34. Minevitch E, Defoor W, Reddy P et al. Ureteroscopy is safe and effective in prepubertal kids. J Urol 2005; 174: 276–9.

35. Tan AH, Al-Omar M, Denstedt JD et al. Ureteroscopy for pediatric urolithiasis : an evolving first line therapy. Urology 2005; 65: 153–6.

36. Akpinar H, Tufek I, Alici B et al. Ureteroscopy and Holmium laser lithotripsy in pregnancy: stents must be used postoperatively. J Endourol 2006; 20: 107–10.
37. Weizer AZ, Springhart WP, Ekeruo WO et al. Ureteroscopic management of renal calculi in anomalous kidneys. Urology 2006; 67: 1164–8.
38. Bultitude MF, Tiptaft RC, Dasgupta P et al. Treatment of urolithiasis in the morbidly obese. Obes Surg 2004; 14: 300–4.
39. Dash A, Schuster TG, Hollenbeck BK et al. Ureteroscopic treatment of renal calculi in morbidly obese patients: a stone matched comparison. Urology 2002; 60: 393–7.
40. L'Esperance JO, Sung J, Marguet C et al. The surgical management of stones in patients with urinary diversions. Curr Opin Urol 2004; 14: 129–34.
41. Kieran K, Nelson CP, Wolf S Jr et al. Retrograde ureterosopy in patients with orthotopic ileal neobladder urinary diversion : an update. J Urol 2006; 175(Suppl 4): 349.
42. Fabrizio MD, Behari A, Bagley DH. Ureteroscopic management of intrarenal calculi. J Urol 1998; 159: 1139–43.
43. Tawfiek ER, Bagley DH. Management of upper urinary calculi with ureteroscopic techniques. Urology 1999; 53: 25.
44. Grasso M, Ficazzola M. Retrograde ureteropyeloscopy for lower pole caliceal calculi. J Urol 1999; 162: 1904–8.
45. Auge BK, Dahm P, Wu NZ et al. Ureteroscopic management of lower pole renal calculi : technique of calculus displacement. J Endourol 2001; 15: 835–8.
46. Traxer O, Thibault F, Niang L et al. Inferior calyx stone and flexible ureterorenoscopy to mobilize the stone before fragmentation. Prog Urol 2006; 16: 198–200.
47. Preminger GM. Management of lower pole renal calculi : shock wave lithotripsy vs. percutaneous nephrolithotomy vs. flexible ureteroscopy. Urol Res 2006; 34: 108–11.
48. Schuster TG, Hollenbeck BK, Faerber GJ et al. Ureteroscopic treatment of lower pole calculi: comparison of lithotripsy in situ and after displacement. J Urol 2002; 168: 43–5.
49. Traxer O, Sebe P, Chambade D et al. Comment repérer le collet d'un diverticule caliciel en urétérorénoscopie souple. Prog Urol 2005; 15: 100–2.
50. Grasso M, Fraiman M, Levine M. Ureteropyeloscopic diagnostis and treatment of upper urinary tract urothelial malignancies. Urology 1999; 54: 240–6.
51. Lam JS, et Gupta M. ureteroscopic management of upper tract transitional cell carcinoma. Urol Clin N Am: JS LAM 2004; 31: 115–28.
52. Chen GL, EL-Gabry EA, Bagley DH. Surveillance of upper urinary tract transitional cell carcinoma: the role of ureteroscopy, retrograde pyelography, cytology and urinalysis. J Urol 2000; 164: 1901–4.
53. Conlin MJ, Bagley DH. Ureteroscopic endopyelotomy in a single setting. J Urol 1998; 159: 727–31.

14 | Renal calculi: Treatment outcomes

Benjamin K Canales and Manoj Monga

INTRODUCTION

Since the first reported successful shock wave lithotripsy (SWL) of a patient with a renal stone in 1980 (1), minimally invasive surgery has supplanted open surgery in the management of renal calculi. The renal anatomy, the mineral composition of the stone, and the patient's body habitus all play major roles in determining the type of operative approach and the expected results. This chapter will attempt to better define renal "stone-free" and "success" rates by reviewing the outcomes of patients with residual stone fragments following renal procedures and by stratifying surgical outcomes based on traditional predictive factors (stone size, location, and composition). In addition, we will briefly review some of the more recent risk-stratification techniques based on imaging modalities as well as the use of adjuvant therapies to better define both their roles in kidney stone surgical outcomes.

DEFINITION OF OUTCOMES

The definition of success in the management of kidney stone treatment has undergone a series of metamorphosis over the last 25 years. As early as 1988 (2), residual fragments between 1 and 4 mm following SWL, once thought to be evidence of failure in open or percutaneous therapies, were termed "clinically insignificant" as long as they were asymptomatic and non-infected. Despite the widespread acceptance of this term, there was no consensus within the urologic community as to what constituted a "clinically insignificant" fragment. Furthermore, re-growth rates and symptomatic/interventional episodes for these fragments in long-term studies have been reported to range up to 78% and 43% respectively (Table 14.1). Therefore, most urologists agree that attempts should be made to render a patient stone-free at the time of the first procedure, as any residual stone fragment may require continued radiological monitoring and has the potential for growth or symptoms.

Noncontrast, spiral computed tomography (CT) has become the imaging modality of choice in the assessment of urinary stone disease, offering highly specific information such as stone location, size, number, density, and renal anatomy.(3) This increase in diagnostic accuracy has lead to the detection of smaller residual fragments following renal stone procedures than what has previously been seen on KUB (kidneys-ureters-bladder) films, tomography, or renal ultrasound, and as such has raised the bar for the definition of stone-free outcomes for renal calculi.

For example, "stone-free" rates for SWL in the 2005 Lower Pole II study (4), based on CT criteria, were almost 30% less than the reported success rates by KUB/tomography for similar-sized stones in the 2001 Lower Pole I study.(5) CT scan imaging was similarly

Table 14.1 Reported stone-free rates and outcomes of clinically insignificant fragments (< 5 mm, seen @ 1–3 months by KUB) for any stone type following SWL; ≥one year follow-up.

Author	Number of Patients	Stone-Free Rate (KUB)	Stone Growth	Symptomatic Stones
Newman et al. 1988(2)	227	N/A	22–43%	N/A
Zanetti et al. 1997(113)	129	47%	10%	15–23%
Yu et al. 1993(114)	44	16%	64%	7%
Beck et al.1991(115)	18	11%	78%	6%
Fine et al. 1995(77)	39	55%	41%	N/A
Streem et al. 1996(116)	160	24%	18%	43%
Buchholz et al. 1997(117)	44	88%	2%	0%
Candau et al. 2000(118)	86	33%	37%	20%

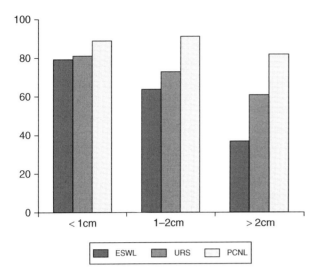

Figure 14.1 Renal KUB stone-free success rates stratified by procedure type and stone size. Means calculated by the weighted average of multiple SWL (9, 37, 79–91), URS (6, 26, 92–102), and PCNL(37, 48, 102–109) studies.

demonstrated to impact the definition of stone-free outcomes by Portis et al. (6), who reported only 54% stone-free results following ureteroscopy for intrarenal calculi when post-operative imaging was performed using CT. This discrepancy is not trivial when comparing old and new outcomes and highlights the need to apply strict criteria for the design and implementation of future studies in urologic stone disease.

The challenge therefore in summarizing 25 years of outcomes for renal calculi using minimally invasive procedures is that not only has technology evolved over time, but so has our definition and means of detecting outcomes. In the proceeding sections, we will attempt to report KUB stone free (no residual seen), KUB "success" (stone fragments 1–4 mm in size), and CT stone-free (no residual by CT) when at all possible. As the use of CT as an outcome measure in clinical trials expands, one might anticipate that lower reported success rates for many of our surgical procedures may not be due to technique or a regression in technology but perhaps due to an artifact of more accurate and sensitive results reporting.

TRADITIONAL OUTCOMES

Stone Size

A wealth of clinical series has been published on shock wave lithotripsy using a variety of device types, and it would be impractical to attempt to compare all of these studies. In general, the best indication for SWL is a solitary renal stone < 2 cm in diameter located in a nonlower pole, unobstructed part of the collecting system. KUB-determined success rates for patients with solitary, nonstaghorn stones based on size are shown in Figure 14.1. These figures, in particular ureteroscopy, were calculated by a "weighted average" approach, with the reported mean representing the additive total reported success rates based on stone size divided by total number of patients included from all studies. Overall, stone-free rates are proportional to degree of surgical invasiveness (higher morbidity usually accompanies higher success rates) and inversely proportional to stone burden.

When examining the efficacy of SWL for renal stone disease, complete stone clearance has replaced "fragmentation" as the primary outcome of treatment. For stone fragments that do not pass spontaneously after 2–3 months, some authors have proposed early re-treatment with the goal of complete residual fragment clearance. Table 14.2 summarizes the results from three such studies. While it appears that an additional SWL treatment following primary SWL may promote the passage of residual debris and calyceal stone fragments, the advantage of this higher stone-free rate is thought to be limited to one additional SWL session or a total of two SWL sessions.

Stone Composition

Several stone types have been identified as resistant to SWL. Brushite (composed of calcium phosphate dihydrate), cystine (a genetic disorder caused by the inability to process certain

Table 14.2   Reported SWL re-treatment success rates for residual stone fragments after shock wave lithotripsy.

Author	Number of Patients	Stone-Free Rates (KUB)	Reduction in Size	Stable Fragments or Growth
Krings et al. 1992(119)	24	42%	42%	16%
Parr et al. 1991(120)	22	14%	18%	68%
Moon et al. 1993(121)	16	75%	N/A	25%

urinary amino acids), and calcium oxalate monohydrate (COM) stones account for almost all SWL treatment failures. In addition, cystine and COM stones are notorious for fragmenting into relatively large pieces that do not spontaneously pass from the collecting system (7), eventually requiring URS extraction to clear remaining fragments. For patients with these stone types, if SWL is considered, it should be reserved for stone burdens less than 1.0 cm with a low threshold to advance to more invasive modalities (URS, PCNL) for larger stones or should SWL fail with one session.

Lower Pole Location: Shock wave Lithotripsy

Despite success in SWL treatment of ureteral and renal stones, lower pole renal calculi remain one of the more challenging technical aspects of endourology. First noticed only as an increased incidence of lower pole SWL treatments (8), it readily became apparent that small, lower pole, KUB stone-free rates were about 25% less than the expected 70–90% stone-free rates for middle calyceal and upper pole stones.(9) Single treatment outcomes (Figure 14.2) have traditionally been much more favorable for patients with stones less than 1 cm (35%–74%) compared to patients with stones 1–2 cm (23%–57%) or greater than 2 cm (14–33%). These findings questioned the role of SWL in the management of larger, lower pole stones and opened the door for numerous retrospective and prospective studies concerning the management of these calculi. (10–15) A summary of the most recent lower pole stone-free success rates stratified by procedure type and stone size are listed in Figure 14.2. Where at all possible, stone-free rates are provided for single treatments with the longest recorded follow-up based on strict CT criteria. Occasionally, mean stone size was used due to lack of individual stone size reporting.

   Although a number of explanations have been offered for the poor stone-free rates in lower-pole stones following SWL, the cause is likely multi-factorial, including the anatomical characteristics of the lower pole infundibulum and gravity dependent clearance of calculi in this area. The four most commonly reported infundibular anatomical factors that are believed to play a role in fragment clearance include: 1) lower pole infundibulo-pelvic (I-P) angle (four studies have shown no effect (5, 16–18), six studies have shown a negative effect on clearance rates (19–24)); 2) infundibular width (three studies no effect (5, 17, 23), six studies negative effect (16, 18, 20, 21, 24, 25); 3) infundibular length (five studies no effect (5, 17, 18, 23, 24), two studies negative effect (16, 21); and 4) infundibular height (three studies negative effect (18, 23, 25)). Despite multiple cadaveric, retrospective, and randomized prospective studies in this area, no single clear LP anatomic factor has been identified that best predicts LP SWL success. In general, urologists consider "favorable" lower pole anatomy to be infundibulo-pelvic (I-P) angles >70 degrees (also known as an "obtuse" angle), infundibular width ≥ 5 mm, and infundibular length ≤ 3 cm. Reproducibility throughout all the above studies is one of the largest confounders as no standard exists for lower pole measurements and as technical and stone factors may have impacted the published study results. Overall, it is likely that each of these factors play some role in SWL success rates, but their role in prediction of fragment clearance remains to be determined. In addition, as CT scan imaging has replaced intravenous pyelograms as the primary diagnostic test for stones, the preoperative availability of information on lower pole anatomy is at times limited.

   In 2001, the Lower Pole Study Group published a prospective, randomized trial comparing SWL and PCNL for the treatment of lower pole stones.(5) A total of 128 patients with symptomatic lower pole calculi were randomized to receive either PCNL or SWL. Overall, KUB stone-free rates at 3 months were 95% for PCNL as opposed to only 37% for the SWL group (p<0.001). When stratified by size, SWL success rates declined as stone size increased. The KUB stone-free rates following SWL for stones 11 – 20 mm and 21 – 30 mm were 23% and 14% respectively as compared with 93% and 86% for PCNL. Re-treatment and the need for

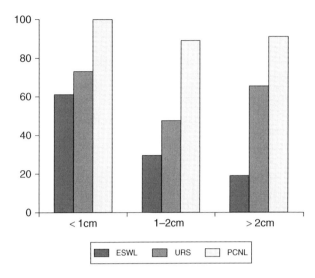

Figure 14.2 Lower pole stone-free success rates stratified by procedure type and stone size. Means calculated by the weighted average of multiple studies. SWL: <1 cm (4, 5, 8, 16, 24, 61, 110), 1–2 cm (5, 8, 17, 18, 24, 82, 110), >2 cm (5, 8)); URS: <1 cm (4, 16, 26–28, 111, 112), 1–2 cm (26, 28, 29, 95, 112), >2 cm (95, 96); and PCNL: <1 cm (5, 8), 1–2 cm (5, 8, 29), >2 cm (5, 8)

auxiliary procedures were more common in the SWL group, while hospital stay was significantly longer in the PCNL group. Overall morbidity was not significantly different between the two groups. The authors concluded that stones greater than 10 mm in diameter are better managed initially with PCNL due to the higher stone-free rates and acceptable rate of morbidity.

Lower Pole Location: Ureteroscopy

As with SWL, ureteroscopic management of lower pole stones is frequently more challenging than ureteroscopy for stones located elsewhere in the ureter or kidney. Grasso and Ficazzola reported overall stone-free rates of 82%, 71%, and 65% in patients with lower pole stones measuring 10 mm or less, 11–20 mm, and greater than 20 mm respectively managed with retrograde ureteropyeloscopy.(26) Several factors contribute to these success rates including difficulty accessing the stone due to acute infundibular angles and reduction in active ureteroscope deflection with the passage of stiff laser fibers. With the advent of newer, smaller flexible endoscopes as well as tipless nitinol stone baskets, many urologists have taken to relocating lower pole stones into a more favorable location prior to fragmentation. Kourambas and colleagues describe the use of either a 3.2F nitinol basket or 2.6F nitinol grasper in 10 cases where access to the lower pole was inhibited by decreased ureteroscopic deflection.(27) Fragmentation was achieved in all 10 cases after stones were manipulated into a more favorable location. Schuster and associates reviewed their experience in 78 patients undergoing ureteroscopy for lower pole stones.(28) Success rates were significantly better in cases where stones were displaced into a more favorable location than in those where lithotripsy was performed in situ. This was statistically significant for stones measuring 1–2 cm, as only 29% of cases in the in situ, lower pole group were successful compared to 100% success in the displacement group.

Recognizing the potential application of URS for mid-sized lower pole stones, the Lower Pole Stone Study Group compared URS to PCNL for stones 11–25 mm.(29) Based on strict CT criteria, significant differences were seen in CT stone-free rates for URS (31% at 4 months) vs. PCNL (76% at 4 months). (29) When "clinically insignificant" fragments are considered, success rates improve to 80% for URS and 100% for PCNL. In perhaps one of the most important papers to date in the management of upper tract stones, Pearle and her associates in the Lower Pole Stone Study Group reported their results of a 19-center trial comparing SWL and flexible ureteroscopy (URS) for the treatment of lower pole calculi less than or equal to 1 cm in diameter (the Lower Pole II study group). (4)

In this randomized, prospective trial, 78 patients were enrolled, and 67 remained on protocol. Despite the study's early termination due to poor enrolment and lack of difference between the groups, several outcomes are notable. First, although a trend in higher success for URS cohort was seen, there was no significant difference in stone-free rates for SWL (35% at 4 months by CT) vs. URS (50% at 4 months by CT, p = 0.92). SWL took significantly less time to complete than URS (66 vs. 90 minutes) and had fewer intra-operative complications (one nonvisualized stone) compared to URS (14% failed lower pole access, 2% ureteral perforation rate). Post-operative complication rates were similar between the groups (23% SWL, 21% URS), and no differences were seen in the number of patients requiring retreatment or ancillary treatments. SWL was associated with greater patient acceptance (more rapid return to driving, return to work) and shorter convalescence (8.1 vs. 15.6 days) than URS. In total, 90% of patients who underwent SWL would choose the procedure again as opposed to 63% in the URS group (p<0.05). The results of this study would seem to support SWL treatment over URS for lower pole stones 1 cm or less in diameter due to superior patient acceptance and low morbidity although the required numbers calculated to show such a significant difference in stone-free outcomes were not reached. The authors do point out, however, that many of the symptoms encountered by the URS group could be attributed to the presence of a ureteral stent. The design of future studies in this particular area of ureteroscopy will continue to focus on the implementation of validated urinary questionnaires that better address the irritative voiding symptoms that accompany ureteral stents.

Lower pole conclusion

While lower pole calculi continue to present challenges for the urologist, new technologies and improved techniques offer the promise of better success rates in these cases. As a general rule, lower pole calculi 1 cm or less are best managed initially with SWL when feasible while most stones between 1 – 2 cm may be well managed with either URS or PCNL as primary therapy. Large calculi, especially those greater than 2 cm, have profoundly lower success rates in the lower pole and are best managed with PCNL when possible as this modality is the least influenced by a lower calyceal anatomy. As always, patient and stone factors including comorbidities, anatomic factors, and stone composition should be taken into account when choosing the treatment with the best chance of success.

COMPLICATIONS

SWL

In general, the noninvasive nature of shock wave lithotripsy translates into low morbidity and high tolerability for many patients. It is well established that shock wave lithotripsy causes tissue damage (primarily injury to small vessels) that ranges from mild parenchymal bruising to severe subcapsular hematomas.(30) Very large hematomas causing acute renal failure or requiring blood transfusion are rare (31), and most agree that asymptomatic hematomas occur about in about 1–12% of SWL cases and usually resolve without lasting sequelae.(32) Steinstrasse occurs in 1–4% of patients who undergo SWL (33), increasing to 5–10% for stones >2 cm in size (34) and up to 40% in patients with partial or full staghorn calculi.(35) Although the rates of asymptomatic bacteremia are thought to be fairly high following SWL (14%)(36), true infectious-related sepsis occurs in 2.7% of cases with struvite stones and in <1% of nonstruvite stones.(37)

New onset hypertension, primarily diastolic, is a potential consequence of SWL, with the development likely being dose dependent(38). Despite multiple retrospective reports, three prospective randomized trials in this area failed to demonstrate SWL-mediated changes in blood pressure.(39) In a recent retrospective, case-control study, development of diabetes and hypertension was found to be higher in patients who underwent SWL in 1985 (odds ratio of 3.23 and 1.47 respectively) than in control patients who were treated conservatively.(40) Despite the study limitations and potential biases, the results of this analysis must be viewed as significant potential long-term complications of SWL, and patients should be counseled appropriately.

Ureteroscopy

Urologists cause 84% of iatrogenic ureteral injuries, the most common being mucosal perforations, and the bulk of these occur during ureteroscopic interventions for stones.(41) The reported risk of perforation ranges greatly, depending on whether it is defined as a complete perforation (0.1–0.7%) (42, 43), partial perforation (1.6%) (44), or mucosal tear (4.7%).(45) The risk of avulsion or stricture is rare, around 0–0.2%.(42–45) Similarly, the risk of bleeding (2%) or infection (1–2%) is low.(42, 45) In a multivariate analysis of ureteroscopic procedures, the only predictive variable of a complication was operative time. However, one might argue that the complication may have contributed to the increase in operative time.(45) Ureteral injuries can occur at any time during a ureteroscopic procedure, and as such a high vigilance must be maintained.

PCNL

Due to its more invasive nature, PCNL has the highest rate complication rate and most morbid profile of all minimally invasive approaches. Percutaneous surgeries result in a variety of vascular complications, ranging from minor hemodynamically stable bleeding to major hemorrhage requiring blood transfusion (7.5%) (46) or embolization (1.4% (47)). In the most recent and largest retrospective series to date, Duvdevani et al. report only a 0.8% transfusion rate in over 1,500 percutaneous procedures (48) compared to the traditional 5% blood transfusion rate that is commonly quoted to patients.(49) Though likely a reflection of the high-volume experience of the investigators, the lower incidence of transfusion could also be due to balloon dilation of the tract by this group, as Amplatz serial dilation has been reported to have more than twice the blood transfusion rate than balloon dilation.(50) Incidence of pleural injury during PCNL is directly related to the level of access (5% when below the 12th rib, and 10–25% with supracostal tracts (49, 51)), and rare reports of splenic or colonic injury as well as reno-cutaneous fistulas have been reported.

OBESITY AND IMAGE-BASED OUTCOMES

Obesity

As the waistlines of those in both underdeveloped and developed countries continue to expand, urologists will increasingly be presented with the therapeutic challenge of stone disease in obese and morbidly obese patients.(52, 53) From a technical standpoint, ureteroscopic, SWL, and percutaneous approaches to the obese patient with stone disease bring about its own unique set of nuances. . In general, special attention to thromboembolic prophylaxis and prevention of pressure-induced iatrogenic injuries during prolonged dorsal lithotomy or prone positioning may be warranted in the morbidly obese. Specific limits for SWL include: patient's weight that exceeds gantry or table limits; size that exceeds the focal length of the lithotripter; or inadequate visualization of stone due to poor penetration or body habitus.(54, 55) PCNL has been shown to be safe and effective in both nonobese and obese populations. Modifications in technique for the obese include specialized long equipment sets and the ability of the obese patient to tolerate the prone position.(56) Although the anatomy is similar and standard equipment will suffice for the ureteroscopic approach, the obese patient who requires ureteroscopy must be able to tolerate general anesthesia and must be able to fit on the operating table without interfering with fluoroscopy. (57) In an attempt to maximize therapy and avoid unnecessary anesthetics and surgery, more urologists are using image-based surrogate measures of obesity (skin to stone distance) and stone composition (noncontrast spiral CT stone Hounsfield units) not only in the morbidly obese but also in normal patients. The hope is that these surrogate measures will aid in selection of surgical approach as well as aid in the prediction of successful SWL surgical outcomes.

Skin to Stone Distance

Excluding positioning and technical concerns, obese patients may still receive a suboptimal outcome after SWL due to inadequate shockwave focusing or penetration. In 1994, Ackermann et al. performed SWL using a Dornier HM-3 lithotriptor and first described body mass index (BMI) as an independent predictor of SWL failure.(58) Their data suggested that patients with BMI >28 had less chance at successful SWL and implied that SWL failure in obese patients may be due to hampered stone targeting or dampened shock wave blast path. In two more recent studies using second generation electrohydraulic lithotriptors, Portis and associates and Pareek et al. both reported a causal relationship between SWL failures and BMI.(59, 60) Both groups hypothesized that fat may be distributed differently in two patients with the same BMI. In order to quantitatively measure the distance from the shockhead to the kidney, the term "skin to stone distance" (or SSD) was coined. SSD is calculated using radiographic calipers or computational measuring device by measuring three distances (0 degree, 45 degrees, and 90 degrees) from the stone to the skin.(61) The averaged value of these three represents the SSD for a given stone. In a series of 64 lower pole stone patients undergoing SWL, Pareek and colleagues found that SSD > 10 cm was a better predictor of SWL failure than BMI or HU measurements.(60) Conversely, El-Nahas et al. published their series of 120 patients who underwent SWL for solitary renal stones 5–25 mm in size.(62) SSD was shown to be predictive of SWL stone disintegration failure by univariate analysis (p=0.033) but did not reach significance on their multivariate analysis. Interestingly, BMI was a more reliable predictor of stone fragmentation failure and need for more than three SWL sessions than any other surrogate marker that they studied. Overall, obesity itself appears to be a risk factor for SWL failure, and prospective randomized studies in this area are needed to clarify the role that SSD should play when counseling patients on outcomes.

Hounsfield units –in vitro studies

Because larger cystine, brushite, and calcium oxalate monohydrate stones are known to be more resistant to SWL fragmentation (10–12), some success has been achieved by attempting to differentiate stone composition by evaluating CT attenuation values of urinary calculi in Hounsfield units (HU), a quantitative scale used to describe radiodensity. In vitro studies have demonstrated that calcium oxalate and phosphate stones HU usually exceed 1,000 (13–15), while uric acid stones have attenuation levels below 1,000 HU. Many urate stones are less than 500 HU. The first criticism in using HU to predict stone composition are the overlap/mixed nature of many stones. Two separate studies have demonstrated that the range of HU for struvite and COM overlap, suggesting that these two stone types cannot be reliably predicted by CT.(13, 63) Second, HU may be unreliable for small stones as several studies have shown that small size may falsely lower HU density calculations. In the early 1980s, Parienty et al. (64) found that stones of the same composition <5 mm in diameter had lower attenuation value than sized at 5–9 mm. The group also proposed that the routine use of low-resolution beam (5 mm) collimation, or CT cuts, can yield artificially low attenuation values due to volume averaging of dark spaces around the stone. More recently, Saw et al. developed a model based on helical CT physics. Their group scanned 127 human calculi (ex vivo) and predicted the effect of scan collimation width on HU density based on stone size.(65) As stone size decreased, HU for the same stone types also decreased, implying that smaller stones may falsely decrease attenuation readings and produce misleading results.

Hounsfield units: in vivo studies

In 2002, Joseph et al. introduced the concept of correlating SWL success rates with stone HU attenuation levels. Their group studied 30 patients with renal calculi undergoing SWL therapy using an electromagnetic lithotripter.(66) Patients with calculi <500 HU (n=12) required fewer shocks (median of 2,500) and were found to have 100% stone clearance rates. Patients with stone HU ranging from 500 to 1,000 (n=7) required a median of 3,390 shocks and had an overall success rate of 86%. Patients with calculi HU > 1,000 (n=11) had a clearance rate of 56% and required a median of 7,300 shocks. Along the same lines, Gupta et al. used high-resolution CT protocols to report a linear relationship between calculus density and number of SWL sessions in patients with renal and proximal ureteral stones.(67) For stones less than 1.1 cm with HU <750, they reported that 34 patients had three or fewer SWL sessions and a stone-free rate of 90%. In patients with HU > 750 and stone size > 1.1 cm, almost 80% required three or more SWL treatments with stone-free rates of only 60%.(67)

One of the first prospective trials in this area was published in 2005 by Wang et al.(68) Their group followed the outcomes of 80 patients who underwent SWL and described three important predictive factors of failure based on multivariate analysis: stone burden >700 mm3, stone density >900 HU, and presence of nonoval (branched, irregular) stones.(68) As a follow-up, El-Nahas and colleagues looked at very similar factors and found that stone density > 1,000 HU and body mass index (BMI) were the only variables that predicted stone disintegration failure by multivariate analysis.(62) They went on to attempt to link stone morphology to stone fragility with the use of high-resolution bone windows (for accurate stone size measurements) and narrow slide width protocols (with 3 different stone HU calculations) to predict a high risk SWL failure group.(62) In contrast, Pareek and colleagues analyzed 64 patients with lower pole renal calculi sized 5 – 15 mm undergoing SWL and did not find HU to be an independent risk factor for stone clearance.(61) Since their stone-free group had significantly smaller lower pole stone sizes prior to SWL (p<0.01), it is likely that stone size, stone density, and stone location along with other patient factors are linked in the context of lower pole clearance rates. Further studies in the clinical area of HU and stone density (in particular lower pole stones) will undoubtedly aid in stratifying SWL outcomes.

ADJUVANTS TO SURGICAL THERAPY TO IMPROVE OUTCOMES

Mechanical adjuvants
Complementary and pharmacological adjuncts have been utilized to try to improve stone-free outcomes after extracorporeal shock wave lithotripsy. Pace et al. utilized inversion, mechanical percussion, and forced diuresis (MPI) to improve stone clearance afters SWL for lower pole calculi.(69) Sixty-nine patients with residual lower pole fragments 3 months following SWL were randomized to receive either MPI or observation for 1 month. The group receiving MPI had a significantly better KUB stone-free rates than the observed group (40% vs. 3%) as well as a greater reduction in total stone area (-63.3% vs. +2.7%) in patients who were not free of stones.

Phyllanthus niruri
Micali et al. evaluated the impact of *Phyllanthus niruri*, an herbal remedy that grows in India and China, on KUB and renal ultrasound stone-free rates after SWL in a prospective randomized trial of 150 patients with renal stones.(70) Patients received a minimum 3 months therapy with 2 grams of *P. niruri*, and KUB stone-free rates were defined as residual fragments <3mm in size. For the group that received the adjuvant therapy, the KUB stone-free rate was 94% at 6 month follow-up, compared to 83% for those patients treated with ESWL alone. The improvement in stone-free rates reached statistical significance specifically for lower caliceal stones (94% vs. 71%, p = 0.01).(70)

Citrates
Cicerello et al. evaluated the impact of sodium potassium citrate (6–8 gm/d in 3 divided doses) compared to forced oral diuresis (to achieve a urine output of 2–3L/d) in 70 patients with 2–5 residual fragments less than 5mm in diameter on plain radiography 6–8 weeks after SWL.(71) Citrate supplementation improved stone clearance rates (74% vs. 32%) and decreased the risk of stone regrowth (5% vs. 47%) at one-year follow-up. Soygur et al. evaluated the impact of potassium citrate supplementation (60 mEq/day) in 110 patients with lower caliceal calcium oxalate stones who underwent SWL monotherapy.(72) Patients with residual fragments who were treated with potassium citrate had a higher rate of stone remission (44% vs. 12%) and a lower rate of stone growth (0% vs. 63%) than patients treated with diet alone.

Spasmolytics
Though calcium channel antagonists and alpha antagonists have improved stone clearance and decreased renal colic after SWL for ureteral calculi (73, 74), there have been few studies on their impact on outcomes after SWL for renal calculi. Sarica et al. evaluated the impact of verapamil (250 mg TID) compared to forced diuresis or no intervention on spontaneous stone passage after SWL.(75) In this small nonblinded study of 70 patients, they reported that stone clearance was similar whether Verapamil (46%) or forced diuresis (46%) was initiated, and both approaches were superior to no intervention (18%). Similarly, Gravina and colleagues reported that at 3-month follow-up, KUB stone clearance was higher in patients treated with tamsulosin (79% vs. 60%).(76) Interestingly, this effect was most pronounced for patients with calculi larger than 1 cm.(76)

Medical therapy for stone growth
While the above studies have focused on the impact of adjuvant therapy on stone clearance, others have evaluated the impact of directed medical therapy on the clinical significance and stone growth of residual fragments after SWL. Fine et al. reported a reduction in growth of residual fragments (81% vs. 17%) in patients treated with medical therapy after SWL.(77) More

recently Kang and colleagues reported similar results in patients with residual fragments after undergoing percutaneous nephrolithotomy, with stone remission rates of 77% in patients with who were treated with medical therapy compared to only 21% in controls.(78)

Overall, it is clear that adjuvant therapies have a potential role to improve stone-free outcomes after SWL and possibly after endoscopic procedures. As such, complementary and medical approaches should be considered for further investigation in larger scale clinical trials. Indeed, multi-agent therapy initiated immediately after SWL may prove more beneficial than waiting until an adjuvant setting of 4–8 weeks.

CONCLUSION

Improvements in instrumentation and surgeon experience have driven improvements in outcomes for renal calculi over the past 25 years. In some areas, such as SWL, outcomes seem to have regressed, perhaps due to more reliable imaging measurements of success. Despite this apparent dichotomy, the uniform reliability of CT imaging has identified predictive factors for success that have lead to improvements in both patient selection and outcomes. Further stratification of "scope vs. shock" will be driven by the development of high-level evidence from randomized clinical trials. Standardization of the radiographic definition of success and development of adjuvant approaches to facilitate stone clearance and minimize surgical morbidity will undoubtedly be critical as urologists strive to continually improve kidney stone surgical outcomes.

REFERENCES

1. Chaussy C, Brendel W, Schmiedt E. Extracorporeally induced destruction of kidney stones by shock waves. Lancet 1980; 2: 1265–68.
2. Newman D, Scott J, Lingeman J. Two-year follow-up of patients treated with extracorporeal shock wave lithotripsy. J Endourol 1988; 2: 163–71.
3. Smith RC, Rosenfield AT, Choe KA et al. Acute flank pain: comparison of non-contrast-enhanced CT and intravenous urography. Radiology 1995; 194: 789–94.
4. Pearle MS, Lingeman JE, Leveillee R et al. Prospective, randomized trial comparing shock wave lithotripsy and ureteroscopy for lower pole caliceal calculi 1 cm or less. J Urol 2005; 173: 2005–09.
5. Albala DM, Assimos DG, Clayman RV et al. Lower pole I: a prospective randomized trial of extracorporeal shock wave lithotripsy and percutaneous nephrostolithotomy for lower pole nephrolithiasis-initial results. J Urol 2001; 166: 2072–80.
6. Portis AJ, Rygwall R, Holtz C, Pshon N, Laliberte M. Ureteroscopic laser lithotripsy for upper urinary tract calculi with active fragment extraction and computerized tomography followup. J Urol 2006; 175: 2129–33.
7. Pittomvils G, Vandeursen H, Wevers M et al. The influence of internal stone structure upon the fracture behaviour of urinary calculi. Ultrasound Med Biol 1994; 20: 803–10.
8. Lingeman JE, Siegel YI, Steele B, Nyhuis AW, Woods JR. Management of lower pole nephrolithiasis: a critical analysis. J Urol 1994; 151: 663–67.
9. Renner C, Rassweiler J. Treatment of renal stones by extracorporeal shock wave lithotripsy. Nephron 1999; 81(Suppl 1): 71–81.
10. Dretler SP. Stone fragility--a new therapeutic distinction. J Urol 1988; 139: 1124–27.
11. Klee LW, Brito CG, Lingeman JE. The clinical implications of brushite calculi. J Urol 1991; 145: 715–18.
12. Zhong P, Preminger GM. Mechanisms of differing stone fragility in extracorporeal shockwave lithotripsy. J Endourol 1994; 8: 263–68.
13. Mostafavi MR, Ernst RD, Saltzman B. Accurate determination of chemical composition of urinary calculi by spiral computerized tomography. J Urol 1998; 159: 673–75.
14. Nakada SY, Hoff DG, Attai S et al. Determination of stone composition by noncontrast spiral computed tomography in the clinical setting. Urology 2000; 55: 816–19.
15. Zarse CA, McAteer JA, Tann M et al. Helical computed tomography accurately reports urinary stone composition using attenuation values: in vitro verification using high-resolution micro-computed tomography calibrated to fourier transform infrared microspectroscopy. Urology 2004; 63: 828–33.
16. Elbahnasy AM, Shalhav AL, Hoenig DM et al. Lower caliceal stone clearance after shock wave lithotripsy or ureteroscopy: the impact of lower pole radiographic anatomy. J Urol 1998; 159: 67682.
17. Madbouly K, Sheir KZ, Elsobky E. Impact of lower pole renal anatomy on stone clearance after shock wave lithotripsy: fact or fiction? J Urol 2001; 165: 1415–18.

18. Sumino Y, Mimata H, Tasaki Y et al. Predictors of lower pole renal stone clearance after extracorporeal shock wave lithotripsy. J Urol 2002; 168: 1344–47.

19. Sampaio FJ, D'Anunciacao AL, Silva EC. Comparative follow-up of patients with acute and obtuse infundibulum-pelvic angle submitted to extracorporeal shockwave lithotripsy for lower caliceal stones: preliminary report and proposed study design. J Endourol 1997; 11: 157–61.

20. Sabnis RB, Naik K, Patel SH, Desai MR, Bapat SD. Extracorporeal shock wave lithotripsy for lower calyceal stones: can clearance be predicted? Br J Urol 1997; 80: 853–57.

21. Elbahnasy AM, Clayman RV, Shalhav AL et al. Lower-pole caliceal stone clearance after shockwave lithotripsy, percutaneous nephrolithotomy, and flexible ureteroscopy: impact of radiographic spatial anatomy. J Endourol 1998; 12: 113–19.

22. Lojanapiwat B, Soonthornpun S, Wudhikarn S. Lower pole caliceal stone clearance after ESWL: the effect of infundibulopelvic angle. J Med Assoc Thai 1999; 82: 891–94.

23. Keeley FX Jr, Moussa SA, Smith G, Tolley DA. Clearance of lower-pole stones following shock wave lithotripsy: effect of the infundibulopelvic angle. Eur Urol 1999; 36: 371–75.

24. Gupta NP, Singh DV, Hemal AK, Mandal S. Infundibulopelvic anatomy and clearance of inferior caliceal calculi with shock wave lithotripsy. J Urol 2000; 163: 24–7.

25. Tuckey J, Devasia A, Murthy L, Ramsden P, Thomas D. Is there a simpler method for predicting lower pole stone clearance after shockwave lithotripsy than measuring infundibulopelvic angle? J Endourol 2000; 14: 475–78.

26. Grasso M, Ficazzola M. Retrograde ureteropyeloscopy for lower pole caliceal calculi. J Urol 1999; 162: 1904–08.

27. Kourambas J, Delvecchio FC, Munver R, Preminger GM. Nitinol stone retrieval-assisted ureteroscopic management of lower pole renal calculi. Urology 2000; 56: 935–39.

28. Schuster TG, Hollenbeck BK, Faerber GJ, Wolf JS Jr. Ureteroscopic treatment of lower pole calculi: comparison of lithotripsy in situ and after displacement. J Urol 2002; 168: 43–5.

29. Kuo R, Lingeman J, Leveillee R et al. A randomized clinical trial of ureteroscopy and percutaneous nephrolithotomy for lower pole stones between 11 and 25 mm. J Endourol 2003; 17: A31.

30. Kaude JV, Williams CM, Millner MR, Scott KN, Finlayson B. Renal morphology and function immediately after extracorporeal shock-wave lithotripsy. AJR Am J Roentgenol 1985; 145: 305–13.

31. Tuteja AK, Pulliam JP, Lehman TH, Elzinga LW. Anuric renal failure from massive bilateral renal hematoma following extracorporeal shock wave lithotripsy. Urology 1997; 50: 606–08.

32. Krishnamurthi V, Streem SB. Long-term radiographic and functional outcome of extracorporeal shock wave lithotripsy induced perirenal hematomas. J Urol 1995; 154: 1673–75.

33. Madbouly K, Sheir KZ, Elsobky E, Eraky I, Kenawy M. Risk factors for the formation of a steinstrasse after extracorporeal shock wave lithotripsy: a statistical model. J Urol 2002; 167: 1239–42.

34. Bierkens AF, Hendrikx AJ, Lemmens WA, Debruyne FM. Extracorporeal shock wave lithotripsy for large renal calculi: the role of ureteral stents. A randomized trial. J Urol 1991; 145: 699–702.

35. Wirth MP, Theiss M, Frohmuller HG. Primary extracorporeal shock wave lithotripsy of staghorn renal calculi. Urol Int 1992; 48: 71–5.

36. Muller-Mattheis VG, Schmale D, Seewald M, Rosin H, Ackermann R. Bacteremia during extracorporeal shock wave lithotripsy of renal calculi. J Urol 1991; 146: 733–36.

37. Lingeman JE, Coury TA, Newman DM et al. Comparison of results and morbidity of percutaneous nephrostolithotomy and extracorporeal shock wave lithotripsy. J Urol 1987; 138: 485–90.

38. Lingeman JE, Woods JR, Toth PD. Blood pressure changes following extracorporeal shock wave lithotripsy and other forms of treatment for nephrolithiasis. JAMA 1990; 263: 1789–94.

39. Skolarikos A, Alivizatos G, de la Rosette J. Extracorporeal shock wave lithotripsy 25 years later: complications and their prevention. Eur Urol 2006; 50: 981–90.

40. Krambeck AE, Gettman MT, Rohlinger AL et al. Diabetes mellitus and hypertension associated with shock wave lithotripsy of renal and proximal ureteral stones at 19 years of followup. J Urol 2006; 175: 1742–47.

41. Al-Awadi K, Kehinde EO, Al-Hunayan A, Al-Khayat A. Iatrogenic ureteric injuries: incidence, aetiological factors and the effect of early management on subsequent outcome. Int Urol Nephrol 2005; 37: 235–41.

42. Geavlete P, Georgescu D, Nita G, Mirciulescu V, Cauni V. Complications of 2735 retrograde semirigid ureteroscopy procedures: a single-center experience. J Endourol 2006; 20: 179–85.

43. Butler MR, Power RE, Thornhill JA et al. An audit of 2273 ureteroscopies--a focus on intra-operative complications to justify proactive management of ureteric calculi. Surgeon 2004; 2: 42–6.

44. Krambeck AE, Murat FJ, Gettman MT et al. The evolution of ureteroscopy: a modern single-institution series. Mayo Clin Proc 2006; 81: 468–73.

45. Schuster TG, Hollenbeck BK, Faerber GJ, Wolf JS Jr. Complications of ureteroscopy: analysis of predictive factors. J Urol 2001; 166: 538–40.

46. Osman M, Wendt-Nordahl G, Heger K et al. Percutaneous nephrolithotomy with ultrasonography-guided renal access: experience from over 300 cases. BJU Int 2005; 96: 875–78.

47. Srivastava A, Singh KJ, Suri A et al. Vascular complications after percutaneous nephrolithotomy: are there any predictive factors? Urology 2005; 66: 38–40.

48. Duvdevani M, Razvi H, Sofer M et al. Third prize: contemporary percutaneous nephrolithotripsy: 1585 procedures in 1338 consecutive patients. J Endourol 2007; 21: 824–29.

49. Kim SC, Kuo RL, Lingeman JE. Percutaneous nephrolithotomy: an update. Curr Opin Urol 2003; 13: 235–41.

50. Davidoff R, Bellman GC. Influence of technique of percutaneous tract creation on incidence of renal hemorrhage. J Urol 1997; 157: 1229–31.

51. Lallas CD, Delvecchio FC, Evans BR et al. Management of nephropleural fistula after supracostal percutaneous nephrolithotomy. Urology 2004; 64: 241–45.

52. Koo BC, Burtt G, Burgess NA. Percutaneous stone surgery in the obese: outcome stratified according to body mass index. BJU Int 2004; 93: 1296–99.

53. Rigby N, Baillie K. Challenging the future: the Global Prevention Alliance. Lancet 2006; 368: 1629–31.

54. Cass AS. Equivalence of mobile and fixed lithotriptors for upper tract stones. J Urol 1991; 146: 290–93.

55. Busby JE, Low RK. Ureteroscopic treatment of renal calculi. Urol Clin North Am 2004; 31: 89–98.

56. Pearle MS, Nakada SY, Womack JS, Kryger JV. Outcomes of contemporary percutaneous nephrostolithotomy in morbidly obese patients. J Urol 1998; 160: 669–73.

57. Dash A, Schuster TG, Hollenbeck BK, Faerber GJ, Wolf JS Jr. Ureteroscopic treatment of renal calculi in morbidly obese patients: a stone-matched comparison. Urology 2002; 60: 393–97.

58. Ackermann DK, Fuhrimann R, Pfluger D, Studer UE, Zingg EJ. Prognosis after extracorporeal shock wave lithotripsy of radiopaque renal calculi: a multivariate analysis. Eur Urol 1994; 25: 105–09.

59. Portis AJ, Yan Y, Pattaras JG et al. Matched pair analysis of shock wave lithotripsy effectiveness for comparison of lithotriptors. J Urol 2003; 169: 58–62.

60. Pareek G, Armenakas NA, Panagopoulos G, Bruno JJ, Fracchia JA. Extracorporeal shock wave lithotripsy success based on body mass index and Hounsfield units. Urology 2005; 65: 33–6.

61. Pareek G, Hedican SP, Lee FT Jr, Nakada SY. Shock wave lithotripsy success determined by skin-to-stone distance on computed tomography. Urology 2005; 66: 941–44.

62. El-Nahas AR, El-Assmy AM, Mansour O, Sheir KZ. A prospective multivariate analysis of factors predicting stone disintegration by extracorporeal shock wave lithotripsy: the value of high-resolution noncontrast computed tomography. Eur Urol 2007; 51: 1688–93.

63. Motley G, Dalrymple N, Keesling C, Fischer J, Harmon W. Hounsfield unit density in the determination of urinary stone composition. Urology 2001; 58: 170–73.

64. Parienty RA, Ducellier R, Pradel J et al. Diagnostic value of CT numbers in pelvocalyceal filling defects. Radiology 1982; 145: 743–47.

65. Saw KC, McAteer JA, Monga AG et al. Helical CT of urinary calculi: effect of stone composition, stone size, and scan collimation. AJR Am J Roentgenol 2000; 175: 329–32.

66. Joseph P, Mandal AK, Singh SK et al. Computerized tomography attenuation value of renal calculus: can it predict successful fragmentation of the calculus by extracorporeal shock wave lithotripsy? A preliminary study. J Urol 2002; 167: 1968–71.

67. Gupta NP, Ansari MS, Kesarvani P, Kapoor A, Mukhopadhyay S. Role of computed tomography with no contrast medium enhancement in predicting the outcome of extracorporeal shock wave lithotripsy for urinary calculi. BJU Int 2005; 95: 1285–88.

68. Wang LJ, Wong YC, Chuang CK et al. Predictions of outcomes of renal stones after extracorporeal shock wave lithotripsy from stone characteristics determined by unenhanced helical computed tomography: a multivariate analysis. Eur Radiol 2005; 15: 2238–43.

69. Pace KT, Tariq N, Dyer SJ, Weir MJ, Dah RJ. Mechanical percussion, inversion and diuresis for residual lower pole fragments after shock wave lithotripsy: a prospective, single blind, randomized controlled trial. J Urol 2001; 166: 2065–71.

70. Micali S, Sighinolfi MC, Celia A et al. Can Phyllanthus niruri affect the efficacy of extracorporeal shock wave lithotripsy for renal stones? A randomized, prospective, long-term study. J Urol 2006; 176: 1020–22.

71. Cicerello E, Merlo F, Gambaro G et al. Effect of alkaline citrate therapy on clearance of residual renal stone fragments after extracorporeal shock wave lithotripsy in sterile calcium and infection nephrolithiasis patients. J Urol 1994; 151: 5–9.

72. Soygur T, Akbay A, Kupeli S. Effect of potassium citrate therapy on stone recurrence and residual fragments after shockwave lithotripsy in lower caliceal calcium oxalate urolithiasis: a randomized controlled trial. J Endourol 2002; 16: 149–52.

73. Micali S, Grande M, Sighinolfi MC, De Stefani S, Bianchi G. Efficacy of expulsive therapy using nifedipine or tamsulosin, both associated with ketoprofene, after shock wave lithotripsy of ureteral stones. Urol Res 2007; 35: 133–37.

74. Kupeli B, Irkilata L, Gurocak S et al. Does tamsulosin enhance lower ureteral stone clearance with or without shock wave lithotripsy? Urology 2004; 64: 1111–15.

75. Sarica K, Inal Y, Erturhan S, Yagci F. The effect of calcium channel blockers on stone regrowth and recurrence after shock wave lithotripsy. Urol Res 2006; 34: 184–89.

76. Gravina GL, Costa AM, Ronchi P et al. Tamsulosin treatment increases clinical success rate of single extracorporeal shock wave lithotripsy of renal stones. Urology 2005; 66: 24–8.
77. Fine JK, Pak CY, Preminger GM. Effect of medical management and residual fragments on recurrent stone formation following shock wave lithotripsy. J Urol 1995; 153: 27–32.
78. Kang DE, Maloney MM, Haleblian GE et al. Effect of medical management on recurrent stone formation following percutaneous nephrolithotomy. J Urol 2007; 177: 1785–88.
79. Psihramis KE, Jewett MA, Bombardier C, Caron D, Ryan M. Lithostar extracorporeal shock wave lithotripsy: the first 1,000 patients. Toronto Lithotripsy Associates. J Urol 1992; 147: 1006–09.
80. Cass AS. Comparison of first generation (Dornier HM3) and second generation (Medstone STS) lithotriptors: treatment results with 13,864 renal and ureteral calculi. J Urol 1995; 153: 588–92.
81. Logarakis NF, Jewett MA, Luymes J, Honey RJ. Variation in clinical outcome following shock wave lithotripsy. J Urol 2000; 163: 721–25.
82. Saw KC, Lingeman JE. Management of calyceal stones. AUA Update Series 1999; 20: 154–59.
83. Ng CF, Thompson TJ, McLornan L, Tolley DA. Single-center experience using three shockwave lithotripters with different generator designs in management of urinary calculi. J Endourol 2006;20: 1–8.
84. Lingeman JE, Newman D, Mertz JH et al. Extracorporeal shock wave lithotripsy: the Methodist Hospital of Indiana experience. J Urol 1986; 135: 1134–37.
85. Kanao K, Nakashima J, Nakagawa K et al. Preoperative nomograms for predicting stone-free rate after extracorporeal shock wave lithotripsy. J Urol 2006; 176: 1453–56.
86. Clayman RV, McClennan BL, Garvin TJ et al. An electromagnetic acoustic shock wave unit for extracorporeal lithotripsy. J Endourol 1989; 3: 307–13.
87. Al-Ansari A, As-Sadiq K, Al-Said S et al. Prognostic factors of success of extracorporeal shock wave lithotripsy (ESWL) in the treatment of renal stones. Int Urol Nephrol 2006; 38: 63–7.
88. Nomikos MS, Sowter SJ, Tolley DA. Outcomes using a fourth-generation lithotripter: a new benchmark for comparison? BJU Int 2007; 100: 1356–60.
89. Hoag CC, Taylor WN, Rowley VA. The efficacy of the Dornier Doli S lithotripter for renal stones. Can J Urol 2006; 13: 3358–63.
90. Lalak NJ, Moussa SA, Smith G, Tolley DA. The Dornier Compact Delta lithotripter: the first 500 renal calculi. J Endourol 2002; 16: 3–7.
91. Abe T, Akakura K, Kawaguchi M et al. Outcomes of shockwave lithotripsy for upper urinary-tract stones: a large-scale study at a single institution. J Endourol 2005; 19: 768–73.
92. Johnson GB, Portela D, Grasso M. Advanced ureteroscopy: wireless and sheathless. J Endourol 2006; 20: 552–55.
93. Holland R, Margel D, Livne PM, Lask DM, Lifshitz DA. Retrograde intrarenal surgery as second-line therapy yields a lower success rate. J Endourol 2006; 20: 556–59.
94. Stav K, Cooper A, Zisman A et al. Retrograde intrarenal lithotripsy outcome after failure of shock wave lithotripsy. J Urol 2003; 170: 2198–201.
95. Grasso M, Conlin M, Bagley D. Retrograde ureteropyeloscopic treatment of 2 cm. or greater upper urinary tract and minor Staghorn calculi. J Urol 1998; 160: 346–51.
96. El-Anany FG, Hammouda HM, Maghraby HA, Elakkad MA. Retrograde ureteropyeloscopic holmium laser lithotripsy for large renal calculi. BJU Int 2001; 88: 850–53.
97. Sofer M, Watterson JD, Wollin TA et al. Holmium:YAG laser lithotripsy for upper urinary tract calculi in 598 patients. J Urol 2002; 167: 31–4.
98. Fabrizio MD, Behari A, Bagley DH. Ureteroscopic management of intrarenal calculi. J Urol 1998; 159: 1139–43.
99. Dasgupta P, Cynk MS, Bultitude MF, Tiptaft RC, Glass JM. Flexible ureterorenoscopy: prospective analysis of the Guy's experience. Ann R Coll Surg Engl 2004; 86: 367–70.
100. Tawfiek ER, Bagley DH. Management of upper urinary tract calculi with ureteroscopic techniques. Urology 1999; 53: 25–31.
101. Menezes P, Dickinson A, Timoney AG. Flexible ureterorenoscopy for the treatment of refractory upper urinary tract stones. BJU Int 1999; 84: 257–60.
102. Chung BI, Aron M, Hegarty NJ, Desai MM. Ureteroscopic vs. percutaneous treatment for medium-size (1–2 cm) renal calculi. J Endourol 2008; 22: 343–46.
103. Brown MW, Carson CC 3rd, Dunnick NR, Weinerth JL. Comparison of the costs and morbidity of percutaneous and open flank procedures. J Urol 1986; 135: 1150–52.
104. Davol PE, Wood C, Fulmer B. Success in treating renal calculi with single-access, single-event percutaneous nephrolithotomy: is a routine „second look" necessary? J Endourol 2006; 20: 289–92.
105. Al-Kohlany KM, Shokeir AA, Mosbah A et al. Treatment of complete staghorn stones: a prospective randomized comparison of open surgery vs. percutaneous nephrolithotomy. J Urol 2005; 173: 469–73.
106. Pearle MS, Watamull LM, Mullican MA. Sensitivity of noncontrast helical computerized tomography and plain film radiography compared to flexible nephroscopy for detecting residual fragments after percutaneous nephrostolithotomy. J Urol 1999; 162: 23–6.

107. Olbert PJ, Hegele A, Schrader AJ, Scherag A, Hofmann R. Pre- and perioperative predictors of short-term clinical outcomes in patients undergoing percutaneous nephrolitholapaxy. Urol Res 2007; 35: 225–30.
108. Lam HS, Lingeman JE, Barron M et al. Staghorn calculi: analysis of treatment results between initial percutaneous nephrostolithotomy and extracorporeal shock wave lithotripsy monotherapy with reference to surface area. J Urol 1992; 147: 1219–25.
109. Meretyk S, Gofrit ON, Gafni O et al. Complete staghorn calculi: random prospective comparison between extracorporeal shock wave lithotripsy monotherapy and combined with percutaneous nephrostolithotomy. J Urol 1997; 157: 780–86.
110. Sorensen CM, Chandhoke PS. Is lower pole caliceal anatomy predictive of extracorporeal shock wave lithotripsy success for primary lower pole kidney stones? J Urol 2002; 168: 2377–82.
111. Elashry OM, Nakada SY, Pearle MS, Clayman RV. Endourologic management of stone-bearing excluded calices: contrasting case reports. J Endourol 1996; 10: 21–6.
112. Hollenbeck BK, Schuster TG, Faerber GJ, Wolf JS. Flexible ureteroscopy in conjunction with in situ lithotripsy for lower pole calculi. Urology 2001; 58: 859–63.
113. Zanetti G, Seveso M, Montanari E et al. Renal stone fragments following shock wave lithotripsy. J Urol 1997; 158: 352–55.
114. Yu CC, Lee YH, Huang JK et al. Long-term stone regrowth and recurrence rates after extracorporeal shock wave lithotripsy. Br J Urol 1993; 72: 688–91.
115. Beck EM, Riehle RA Jr. The fate of residual fragments after extracorporeal shock wave lithotripsy monotherapy of infection stones. J Urol 1991; 145: 6–9.
116. Streem SB, Yost A, Mascha E. Clinical implications of clinically insignificant store fragments after extracorporeal shock wave lithotripsy. J Urol 1996; 155: 1186–90.
117. Buchholz NP, Meier-Padel S, Rutishauser G. Minor residual fragments after extracorporeal shockwave lithotripsy: spontaneous clearance or risk factor for recurrent stone formation? J Endourol 1997; 11: 227–32.
118. Candau C, Saussine C, Lang H et al. Natural history of residual renal stone fragments after ESWL. Eur Urol 2000; 37: 18–22.
119. Krings F, Tuerk C, Steinkogler I, Marberger M. Extracorporeal shock wave lithotripsy retreatment ("stir-up") promotes discharge of persistent caliceal stone fragments after primary extracorporeal shock wave lithotripsy. J Urol 1992; 148: 1040-1.
120. Parr NJ, Ritchie AW, Moussa SA, Tolley DA. The impact of extracorporeal piezoelectric lithotripsy on the management of ureteric calculi: an audit. Br J Urol 1991; 67: 18–23.
121. Moon YT, Kim SC. Fate of clinically insignificant residual fragments after extracorporeal shock wave lithotripsy with EDAP LT-01 lithotripter. J Endourol 1993; 7: 453–56.

15 | Ureteral calculi: Treatment outcomes

Michael K Louie and Ralph V Clayman

INTRODUCTION

The treatment of ureteral calculi has undergone major changes in the past three decades. Driven by the advancement of shock wave lithotripsy, flexible ureteroscopes, laser lithotripsy, percutaneous access, laparoscopy, and medical therapy, the open surgical approach to ureteral calculi has all but been laid to rest. The development of nephrolithiasis guidelines by the American Urological Association (AUA) in 1991 and the subsequent ureteral stone treatment guidelines and outcomes analysis updates in 1997 and 2007 have outlined the standard of care recommendations.(1, 2) The latest update in 2007 is the first international set of ureteral stone treatment guidelines made possible by a cooperative effort between the European Association of Urology (EAU) and the AUA.

As in the recently published guidelines, examination of ureteral calculi treatment outcomes in this chapter have been separated by location, size, treatment type, and any special conditions of the patient such as pregnancy. Of note, the guidelines did not find enough evidence to stratify treatment outcomes according to stone composition. When stating the location of a stone within the ureter, the proximal ureter has been classified most commonly as above the superior border of the iliac crest to the renal pelvis on a plain abdominal pelvic radiograph, the mid-ureter refers to the region of the ureter overlying the bony pelvis, and the distal ureter is the ureter below the inferior border of the sacro-iliac joint. For convenience, treatment outcomes stratified by stone size are usually divided into <10mm or ≥10mm for surgical intervention data and <5mm or ≥5mm for observation or medical expulsive therapy data. The main treatment types for ureteral calculi are observation, medical expulsive therapy, ureteroscopy, and extracorporeal shock wave lithotripsy; less commonly used approaches include percutaneous antegrade ureteroscopy, laparoscopic ureterolithotomy, and rarely, open ureterolithotomy. Additionally, new perspectives on the role of ureteral stents and the use of access sheaths to facilitate ureteroscopy have garnered renewed interest in the literature. While percutaneous antegrade ureteroscopy is reserved for the unique situation of a large impacted ureteral stone or a stone associated with a distal ureteral stricture, some experts believe this endourological procedure has supplanted laparoscopic and open ureterolithotomy as the most invasive treatment necessary for ureteral stones. The use of open or laparoscopic ureterolithotomy is commonly employed in underdeveloped nations where access to the latest endourological tools is rare. Finally, the special condition of pregnancy warrants review of the current treatment paradigm and of the treatment outcomes. The advancement of technology to treat ureteral stones results inevitably with an increase in the cost of delivering the technology to the patient and health-care system. Despite the initial cost, the benefit of this technology in decreasing patient morbidity and increasing urologic surgical efficiency is being proven with time. To this end, a review of some of the recent, albeit small number of cost analyses regarding the treatment of ureteral calculi will also be presented.

OBSERVATION AND MEDICAL EXPULSIVE THERAPY

Observation therapy

Conservative treatment of ureteral stones encompasses observation and observation with medical expulsion therapy. The decision to use conservative treatment for ureteral stones is based on the size of the stone, its location, and patient factors such as pain, infection, hydronephrosis, and renal reserve. Based on the 2007 AUA guidelines, for stones in any location that are ≤ 5 mm a period of observation is recommended if there is little pain or co-morbidity; this recommendation is based on a documented spontaneous passage rate of 68% (46–85%) in a meta-analysis of 224 patients.(1) For calculi 5–10 mm, the rate decreases to 47% (36–59%) in 104 patients. For

Table 15.1   Spontaneous stone passage rates from selected series.

| Size | Location | | | Notes |
	Proximal Ureter	Mid-Ureter	Distal Ureter	
< 5 mm	68% (46–85%)			Meta-analysis (1)
	29–98%		71–98%	Range only (2)
	47%	80%	77%	(3)
	86%	67%	94%	(4)
5–10 mm	47% (36–59%)			Meta-analysis (1)
	10–53%		25–53%	Range only (2)
	63%	0%	71%	Stones 5–7 mm; Only 3 patients in mid-ureter group (3)
	50%	50%	50%	Stones 4–6 mm (4)
> 10 mm	59% (45–72%)			Meta-analysis (1)
	25%	100%	67%	Stones > 7mm (3)

ureteral calculi ≥10 mm, observation or medical expulsive therapy is not recommended due to the unlikely event of spontaneous stone passage and the risk of further morbidity. The wide range of passage rates was culled mostly from retrospective case series with varying imaging and treatment modalities. Complicating analysis further were nonstandardized patient control groups.

Noncontrast or unenhanced CT scan of the upper abdomen and pelvis has become the standard imaging procedure when a patient is suspected of having a kidney stone. Coll et al. reviewed the spontaneous passage rates of stones in one of the few studies strictly utilizing unenhanced CT imaging to determine initial stone size and stone passage.(3) In their study, the stone passage rate for stones of all sizes were 48% for proximal stones, 60% for mid-ureteral stones, 75% for distal stones, and 79% for stones located at the ureterovesical junction. When stone passage rates were stratified according to size, they found that for proximal stones (n = 62) 1–4 mm it was 47%, for 5–7 mm stones it was 63%, and for stones >7 mm it was 25%. Similarly, stone free rates for mid-ureteral stones (n = 10) 1–4 mm was 80%, 5–7 mm was 0%, >7 mm was 100%. In the distal ureter and ureterovesical junction (n = 90), the stone free rates for stones 1–4 mm was 83%, for 5–7 mm stones was 65%, and for stones >7 mm was 50%. Overall stone passage rates were significantly correlated with location, but not with stone size at each location. These results are a more accurate representation of stone passage rates as most patients are currently diagnosed with ureteral calculi using unenhanced CT imaging. Table 15.1 shows selected stone passage rates for observation therapy.

The duration of observation after which spontaneous stone passage is unlikely remains undefined as there are no randomized clinical trials in this regard. Miller et al. analyzed the natural history of ureterolithiasis by observing the time to spontaneous stone passage for stones 2– 6 mm.(4) Seventy-five patients were followed every 2 weeks using clinical symptoms, stone recovery, and plain radiography. The mean number of days for stone passage according to stone size was 8 days for stones 2 mm or smaller, 12 days for stones 2–4 mm, and 22 days for stones 4–6 mm. The mean number of days for 95% of stones to pass was 31 days (0–36 days) for stones 2 mm or smaller, 40 days (0–40 days) for stones 2–4 mm, and 39 days (0–105 days) for stones 4–6 mm. Intervention was required due to pain or failure to progress in 4.8% (2 of 41 patients) in the 2 mm or smaller group, while 50% (8 of 16 patients) of those with stones 4–6 mm required intervention. The authors concluded that spontaneous stone passage was a highly variable event with 95% of stones 4 mm or smaller passing by 40 days, and that stones 5 mm or larger had a 50% chance of requiring intervention. Roberts et al. examined the rate of ureteral stricture after stone impaction in 21 patients.(5) Stone impaction was defined as nonprogression of a ureteral stone for two months. Despite their small series, of the 21 patients who were treated for stone impaction, 5 (24%) developed ureteral strictures at a mean of 2.6 months (1–5 months). As such, it would appear that if a stone has not passed by 4–6 weeks, intervention is reasonable.

Medical expulsive therapy

The use of medical expulsive therapy for ureteral stones is not a new idea. The use of hormones, nonsteroidal anti-inflammatories, calcium channel blockers, corticosteroids, and alpha adrenergic antagonists have all been used to try to expedite stone passage.(6) Hormones such as prostaglandins and glucagon are now of historical interest only. The 2007 AUA guidelines summary on medical expulsive therapy shows that only the calcium channel blocker, nifedipine, and alpha-1-adrenergic blockers had sufficient data for meta-analysis.(1) There was no subgroup analysis regarding the use of medical expulsive therapy in relation to the location of the stone. There were 4 studies with 160 patients analyzed from the nifedipine group with a 75% passage rate. For alpha blockers, 6 studies with 280 patients yielded a passage rate of 81%. When compared to control groups, nifedipine realized an absolute increase of 8% in the stone passage rate which was not significant, and alpha blockers showed an absolute increase of 29% in stone passage rates which was significant. Two randomized-controlled trials compared tamsulosin and nifedipine.(7, 8) Porpiglia et al. found the stone passage rates to be similar in both the nifedipine and tamsulosin groups while the Dellabella et al. study found tamsulosin to be superior. Both studies found either medical therapy to be superior to control. Yilmaz et al. randomized 114 patients with distal ureteral calculi to either control, tamsulosin, doxazosin, or terazosin.(9) Use of any alpha blocker resulted in a passage rate of >75% compared with the control group passage rate of 54%. However, the expulsion rate was highest in the tamsulosin group with 79.3%. All other outcomes such as number of pain episodes, expulsion time, and analgesic dose were also found to be lower than the control group. Although not reported consistently in all trials, a pooled analysis of adverse effects by Singh et al. showed that alpha blockers had an overall 4% incidence of adverse effects while the overall incidence for calcium channel blockers was 15.2%.(10) The addition in particular of an alpha blocker to observational therapy improves the passage rate of stones and confers little excess morbidity to the patient. The use of corticosteroids to decrease ureteral inflammation in conjunction with nifedipine or an alpha blocker or by itself has garnered mixed results, and recent literature indicates that although likely to be synergistic with either drug in the expulsion of ureteral stones, the use of corticosteroids is not a requirement for medical expulsive therapy and may lead to adverse side effects.(11) Borghi et al. in 1994 conducted a small randomized-controlled trial comparing methylprednisolone with nifedipine vs. methylprednisolone given with a placebo. Their results showed that the nifedipine and methylprednisolone group was significantly better than the methylprednisolone and placebo group in terms of stone passage without surgical manipulation, 87% success vs. 65% success rate, respectively.(12) A recent prospective randomized placebo controlled trial by Porpiglia et al. studied the use of corticosteroids in medical expulsive therapy of symptomatic distal ureteral stones by comparing deflazacort alone, in conjunction with the alpha blocker tamsulosin, tamsulosin alone, and a control group receiving only analgesics.(13) They enrolled 114 patients with stones ≥5 mm into these four groups. They evaluated the success of the therapies after 10 days, which was previously determined by Dellabella et al. to be a sufficient duration of treatment. (8) The expulsion rate was 60% in the tamsulosin alone group, 37.5% in the deflazacort alone group, 84.8% in the tamsulosin and deflazacort group, and 33.3% in the analgesics only group. The difference in analgesic use was only significant between the combined therapy group and the analgesics only group. Interestingly, of those who failed medical therapy and were waiting for ureteroscopic treatment, the combined therapy group eventually expelled all stones without any further treatment while the tamsulosin alone and deflazacort alone groups did not expel any more stones and in fact did worse in this regard when compared with the analgesics alone group. The authors concluded that for distal stones, corticosteroids alone were only as effective as analgesics, but corticosteroids in conjunction with tamsulosin improved the success of stone passage over a shorter period of time. Dellabella et al. in their own randomized-controlled trial looked at tamsulosin vs. tamsulosin with deflazacort.(14) They treated for 28 days or until stone expulsion, whichever came first. Their results did not show a significant difference in stone expulsion rates, but the combined therapy group expelled the stones in a shorter time period.

Paralleling the popularization of medical expulsive therapy for ureteral stones has been the use of medical expulsive therapy as an adjunct to shock wave lithotripsy. A prospective randomized double blind placebo controlled trial by Bhagat et al. evaluated 60 patients with a single renal (6 mm–24 mm) or ureteral calculus (6 mm–15 mm).(15) These patients underwent shock wave lithotripsy and were randomized to placebo or tamsulosin treatment. The tamsulosin success rate of 96.6% was significantly better than the placebo success rate of 79.3%. Besides the expulsion rate, the tamsulosin group used less analgesia. In other recent trials, most have shown an increased stone expulsion rate with the use of tamsulosin after shock

Table 15.2   Ureteroscopy vs. shock-wave lithotripsy as primary/first treatment.

Size	Location		
	Proximal Ureter	**Mid-Ureteral**	**Distal Ureter**
<10 mm	90% - SWL	84% - SWL	86% - SWL
	80% - URS	91% - URS	97% - URS
>10 mm	68% - SWL	76% - SWL	74% - SWL
	79% - URS	78% - URS	93% - URS

Adapted from the 2007 AUA/EUA Management of Ureteral Calculi Guide.

wave lithotripsy, and a decreased need for additional analgesia with tamsulosin treatment. (16–21) The optimal duration of treatment with medical therapy has not been standardized, but in most studies the median follow-up period was 4 weeks with alpha blockers expediting the expulsion of most ureteral stones within 14 days, while calcium channel blockers required up to 28 days.(10)

Bensalah et al. assessed the cost-effectiveness of medical expulsive therapy for distal ureteral calculi using cost data from the United States and four European countries.(22) Based on assumptions from prior studies that the base rate of spontaneous distal ureteral stone passage was 45%, that the use of alpha blocker medical expulsive therapy increased the passage of the stone by 54%, that after medical expulsive therapy failure URS would be used ($4,773) to treat the stone, and that the cost of alpha blocker therapy was $2.08 per tablet of tamsulosin, the authors created a decision analysis model. Medical expulsive therapy was associated with a $1,132 cost advantage over initial observation. This was mainly due to the high cost of URS in the United States. Compared to Germany, where the cost of URS was $160, medical expulsive therapy was only marginally superior from a fiscal standpoint; however this did not include the postprocedure costs of stent removal.

EXTRACORPOREAL SHOCK WAVE LITHOTRIPSY AND URETEROSCOPY

If initial treatment of a ureteral stone fails with observation alone or with medical expulsive therapy then definitive treatment with extracorporeal shock wave lithotripsy (SWL) or ureteroscopy (URS) should be the next step. Overall stone-free rates for SWL and URS for stones in the proximal ureter show no significant difference according to the most recent 2007 AUA guidelines. However, when stratified according to stone size, SWL stone-free rates of proximal ureteral stones <10 mm was significantly higher than URS. Conversely, URS of proximal ureteral stones >10 mm had superior stone-free rates compared to SWL. The panel noted that the stone-free rate did not vary with URS in regard to stone size, but did vary inversely with SWL. Overall mid-ureteral stone-free rates were higher with URS, but did not reach statistical significance due to the small number of patients. Distal stone-free rates showed URS as superior to SWL for all stone sizes. (Table 15.2)

Outcomes for SWL

Since the introduction of SWL, there has been a great debate regarding the optimal primary method of ureteral calculi treatment. Adding to the controversy, is the ongoing introduction of new technologies for ureteroscopy, such as nitinol guidewires and baskets, the holmium laser, ureteral access sheaths, and ever smaller and more deflectable, flexible ureteroscopes. As such, ureteroscopy is ever improving as an efficient single procedure for the treatment of ureteral stones. The caveat is that although more efficient as a single procedure, ureteroscopy with intracorporeal lithotripsy requires general or spinal anesthesia and carries an infrequent, but higher risk of complications such as ureteral perforation, ureteral stricture, or ureteral avulsion.

Shock wave lithotripsy on the other hand has become stagnant in its ability to improve stone free rates or decrease secondary procedures.(23) The Dornier HM3 lithotripter is the original SWL machine, and the standard by which all other SWL machines are judged. The HM3 stone-free rates are among the highest for SWL despite being introduced over two decades ago. Newer SWL machines appear to be unable to equal or exceed the stone-free rates of the HM3 in the ureter perhaps due to decreasing focal areas and shock head coupling problems. Tiselius et al. recently reported on the efficacy of two modern lithotripters, the Modulith SLX Classic and the Modulith SLX-F2.(24) The F2 allowed extension of the focal area from the default of 6 x 28 mm to 10 x 50 mm, while the Classic did not have this feature. They treated 580 patients and after a single treatment with either the Classic or F2, the success rates were almost identical: for proximal ureteral stones 80% and 66%, for mid-ureteral stones 69% and 64%, and for distal stones 82% and 86%, respectively. In order to achieve stone-free rates >95%, the average number of SWL sessions per patient was 1.37 for proximal stones, 1.47 for mid-ureteral stones, and 1.22 for distal stones. These results highlight some of the best results in the literature for SWL of ureteral stones. The stone-free rates based on the AUA guidelines meta-analysis were 82% for the proximal ureter (6,428 patients), 73% in the mid-ureter (1,607 patients), and 74% in the distal ureter (6,981 patients). The distal ureter showed a significant worsening in the results and it was unclear why this occurred. In terms of the number of SWL sessions per patient, for proximal stones it was 1.31, for mid-ureteral stones it was 1.11, and for distal stones it was 1.22. These results were similar to the data compiled by the AUA guidelines panel despite large differences in lithotripters.

Pre-SWL stenting

In their conclusion, the 2007 AUA guidelines did not find sufficient or significant evidence to suggest that pre-SWL stent placement made a difference in treatment outcomes, nor enough data to make meaningful interpretations regarding procedure counts. The guidelines also did not find any significant differences between stent bypass, pushback, or *in situ* SWL, and therefore did not recommend routine pre-operative ureteral stent placement for ureteral stones. This was further substantiated by Nakada et al.(25) for mid-ureteral stones treated with SWL. More recently, El-Assmy et al.(26) performed a randomized prospective study comparing pre-SWL stenting to no stenting in patients with stones up to 2 cm associated with moderate or severe hydronephrosis. They found that pre-SWL stenting did not increase the stone free rate or decrease the number of additional procedures, but instead significantly increased morbidity directly related to the stent.

Long-term complications of SWL

Shock wave lithotripsy carries relatively little acute morbidity, but a controversial 19 year follow-up study by Krambeck et al. shows an association of SWL with the development of diabetes mellitus and hypertension.(27) A total of 578 patients received a questionnaire regarding possible adverse effects related to SWL, and 59% responded. The patients had been treated with the HM3 lithotripter for renal or proximal ureteral stones, and were matched by age, sex, and year of presentation to patients with stones not undergoing surgical therapy. Overall, 93.8% received only one SWL treatment with a median of 20kV and 1,100 shocks. Hypertension was found in 36% of the SWL group compared to 27.9% in the control group (O.R. = 1.47, p=0.034). Diabetes mellitus was found in 16.8% of the SWL group compared to 6.7% of the control group (O.R. = 3.23, p=0.001). They concluded that SWL caused renal and pancreatic damage that was related to the number and frequency of shocks. In contrast to Krambeck et al., a long-term (10–22 years of follow up) retrospective study was published by Sato et al., with 1,277 HM-3 patients responding (30% response rate).(28) The patients were stratified according to renal and ureteral treatment groups because the authors believed that ureteral treatment would not affect either the kidney or the pancreas in the blast zone. They found no statistical difference between the two groups with regard to hypertension and diabetes. With a low rate of response and a possible bias in the control group, further studies need to be performed to determine the nature of long-term SWL complications. Also, it needs to be realized that these results only apply to the HM3 which at this point in time is present at very few stone centers.

Outcomes of URS

While the revolution of SWL has now become a standard of care for many ureteral stones, its efficacy has been challenged by the evolution of URS. Smaller and more flexible ureteroscopes have supplanted rigid ureteroscopes for all but the distal ureter, and the use of Holmium laser lithotripsy allows disintegration of even the hardest stones. The development of nitinol baskets and guidewires in <2 French sizes allows for the direct vision manipulation and removal of stone fragments from even the most difficult areas with relative safety.(29) The overall complication rate for URS has decreased with flexible ureteroscopes; in particular ureteral perforation (<5%) and long-term complications such as stricture formation (<2%) are much less common than in the 1990's.(30) Additionally, the rebirth of the ureteral access sheath, in a safer and more functional form, has been shown to allow for more rapid and more complete stone clearance; however, the concerns related to ureteral trauma and post-operative stricture formation are unanswered as the data remain sparse and to date, no postureteroscopy stricture has been directly attributed to use of an access sheath.

The presented data in the recent AUA guidelines highlights the changes in technology that have made an impact on first treatment stone-free rates when stratified by location and size, and when compared to SWL. For proximal stones <10 mm and >10 mm, URS has a stone-free rate of about 80% for both, compared to SWL which has a stone-free rate of 90% and 68%, respectively. SWL is dependent on stone size and location for clearance while the stone size effect on URS efficacy appears to be much less. For mid-ureteral and distal stones of either <10 mm or >10 mm treated with URS, the stone-free rates are 91% and 78% for the mid-ureter, and for the distal ureter 97% and 93%. SWL comparatively has lower stone-free rates for middle and distal ureteral calculi. For middle ureteral calculi, this difference is not significant as the number of patients is too small, while for distal ureteral calculi, SWL has stone-free rates significantly lower than URS with 86% for stones <10 mm and 74% for stones >10 mm.

Flexible vs. rigid URS

The introduction of flexible ureteroscopy allowed proximal stones of almost any size to be endoscopically treated. The stone-free rates were superior for flexible ureteroscopy (87%) compared to rigid ureteroscopy (77%).(1) However, these differences were negligible in the mid-ureter. In the distal ureter, the opposite was true with rigid ureteroscopy (94%) performing better than flexible ureteroscopy (79%) for stones >10 mm. This is attributed to the difficulty maintaining vision and access in the distal ureter with flexible URS. As such it is understandable why only a few studies in the literature used strictly flexible ureteroscopy and most used semi-rigid ureteroscopy for distal ureteral stones, saving flexible ureteroscopy for middle and proximal stones.(31–34)

Intracorporeal lithotripters

The holmium:YAG (Ho: YAG) laser is now ubiquitous as the intracorporeal lithotripter of choice. It is a laser whose active medium is a crystal of yttrium, aluminum, and garnet (YAG) doped with holmium, and whose beam falls in the near infrared portion of the electromagnetic spectrum (2,150 nm). The laser energy is absorbed in <0.5 mm of fluid making it an ideal surgical laser for endourologic applications such as laser lithotripsy. The nominal hazard zone if the laser is discharged in air is approximately 1 meter. The Ho:YAG laser is a robust tool that is able to destroy all types of stones and delivers its energy through the smallest fibers (i.e. 200 microns).(35) Ho:YAG fragments stones by a photothermal chemical decomposition of the stone (i.e. vaporization). The complication rates are very low (0–4%) with no major complications and the Ho: YAG can even be used in patients with uncorrected coagulopathies.(36, 37)

Due to the efficiency and safety profile of the Ho:YAG laser in the ureter, the other intracorporeal lithotripters are mainly only of historical interest. These lithotripters include the electrohydraulic, ultrasonic, pneumatic, and the pulsed dye laser.(37) The ultrasonic lithotripter can only be used through a rigid ureteroscope with larger working channels and is now not used at the majority of medical centers. The pulsed dye laser is a nonthermal laser employing a coumarin dye system operating at a wavelength of 504 nm. Laser light is absorbed by the stone, leading to gaseous plasma formation on the surface, which expands to create a shockwave. The pulsed dye laser has excellent stone-free rates, but is unable to fragment some types of stones (e.g., cystine); it also has a much larger footprint in the operating room and has higher maintenance requirements than the holmium laser. . Electrohydraulic (EHL) probes, like laser fibers, are smaller in diameter and flexible. With EHL, although effective for stone fragmentation; it is not as successful as the holmium laser; in addition, a 10–15% rate of ureteral damage that is proportional to the number of shocks and energy applied can occur.(37) Pneumatic probes like the Swiss Lithoclast also have high stone fragmentation and clearance rates, but due to and the need for a rigid or semi-rigid ureteroscope and increased retropulsion of stone fragments it has become less popular than the holmium laser. Complication rates for pneumatic lithotripsy are slightly higher for ureteral perforation (5–7.7%) than holmium laser.(38, 39) All ureteral perforations were due to the direct transmission of force from the pneumatic lithotrite on impacted stones. In terms of cost, EHL ($12,000 generator, $200 disposable probe) and pneumatic lithotripsy ($25,000 generator cost, $150 re-usable probe) are the least expensive to use, but the Ho: YAG laser ($50,000 generator cost, $150–300 disposable fibers of varying size) by increasing stone-free rates, decreasing morbidity, decreasing operative times, allowing access to difficult to reach areas in the collecting system, and providing multi-disciplinary usage may compensate for its steep initial purchase price.(37, 40–42)

Ureteral access sheath

The use of access sheaths for use with flexible URS remains controversial. While there is ample evidence that the sheath allows for improved and more rapid stone clearance and decreased intra-renal pressure during ureteroscopy, concerns regarding potential morbidity remain.(43–45) Stone-free rates for intra-renal calculi have been reported by L'Esperance et al. in 173 patients using a ureteral access sheath compared to 83 patient who did not have a ureteral access sheath used. There was a significant improvement in the stone free rate using an access sheath vs. not using an access sheath (79% vs. 67%, p<0.05). Besides stone clearance, the benefits of using an access sheath are the ability to access the ureter multiple times and actively basket stone fragments without continual trauma to the ureter, improved flow of irrigation thereby improving vision, decreasing the intrarenal pressure during URS to decrease the risk of pyelovenous and pyelosinus backflow, and hypothetically increasing the durability of flexible ureteroscopes by decreasing endoscope buckling. However, when using a ureteral access sheath, the post-ureteroscopy placement of an indwelling stent is indicated. Landman et al. studied the intrarenal pressure in fresh *ex-vivo* cadaveric urinary tracts, and found that an access sheath significantly reduces the intrarenal pressure.(46) Auge et al. reported on a series of five patients with percutaneous nephrostomies who underwent URS without and then with an access sheath and noted that at all locations in the ureter, URS with a sheath produced lower pressures than without one.(47) A randomized prospective trial by Kourambas et al. showed that usage of an access sheath compared to no access sheath decreased operative time by a mean of 10.5 min with a cost savings benefit at their institution of $350 per ureteroscopic procedure.(48) Additionally, compared to balloon dilatation, the access sheath saved a mean of 10 min from the operative time and $700 when the cost of the balloon dilator is considered.

There have been no direct reports of a stricture associated with access sheath placement. An assessment by Delvecchio et al. (49) of 71 procedures performed with a ureteral access sheath found a single asymptomatic ureteropelvic junction stricture. The stricture was found after a second ureteroscopy for a distal ureteral stone in a T6 paraplegic patient with recurrent struvite stones who had two prior percutaneous and one shock wave lithotripsy procedures. The first ureteroscopy was for a proximal ureteral stone. For the second ureteroscopy, a 12/14F sheath was placed only to the level of the iliac vessels and not passed above the UPJ. As such the authors note that this finding of a stricture at the UPJ was likely due to his long history of stone disease and subsequent treatments and not due to the use of a ureteral access sheath. A ureteral perforation has been noted during placement of the access sheath, but again is a rare event.(43) In the animal laboratory, placement of an access sheath has been shown to cause transient ischemia of the ureter as Lallas et al. (50) showed in the *in vivo* pig model, but after 70 min there is a trend toward the return of blood flow. At 72 hours the ureters were harvested, and did not show ischemic damage in the mucosa or muscularis. To date, while concern has been expressed and hypothesized, there has in fact, been little evidence regarding any complications from using the current models of ureteral access sheaths.

Of note, while the access sheath was specifically designed for use with the flexible ureteroscope; it has also been combined with semi-rigid ureteroscopy. Kourambas et al. noted no difference in stone-free rates between 6.5F semi-rigid (17% of patients) and 7.5F flexible ureteroscopes (83% of patients) when used with a ureteral access sheath in treating proximal ureteral and renal calculi.(48) However, De Sio et al. reported on 12 patients with difficult distal ureteral calculi (8 patients with stones >1 cm, and 4 patients with large prostates). The authors noted that in 5 of the 12 patients they were unable to complete lithotripsy with a semi rigid ureteroscope unless they removed the access sheath.(51) Rapoport et al. found that 7 of 19 (37%) patients who were not stented after having a ureteral access sheath returned to the emergency room, and recommended placing a stent after using a ureteral access sheath as it precludes uncomplicated ureteroscopy.(52) In sum, the ureteral access sheath is most beneficial for use with the flexible ureteroscope in the cost effective treatment of proximal and middle ureteral stones, especially larger stones (>10 mm) that require multiple passes with the flexible ureteroscope to clear stone fragments.

Routine stenting after URS

Routine stenting of the ureter after ureteroscopy is commonplace. The stated concept is that a stent would decrease the risk of obstruction from ureteral edema or residual fragments, and prevent ureteral strictures from forming.(53) However, a stent is not without its own morbidity and cost. A majority of patients complain of irritative voiding symptoms and may have stent colic. The additional cost is not only related to the stent and its initial placement, but also with the need to remove the stent cystoscopically unless a suture is left on the bladder portion of the stent. Haleblian et al. (54) reviewed the randomized prospective trials of stented and nonstented patients after ureteroscopy for peri-operative morbidity.(52, 55–66) One of these studies by Borboroglu et al., was a multi-institutional randomized controlled prospective study of stented vs. nonstented patients with a distal ureteral stone (mean size 6.6 ± 1.7 mm).(55) Only semi-rigid ureteroscopes (6F–9.5F) were used with 55% of the stented group undergoing ureteral dilation, and 57% of the non-stented group undergoing dilation. Mean scores for flank pain, bladder pain, urinary symptoms, and overall pain were assessed preoperatively, at 48 hours post-procedure, and then at 1 and 4 weeks. Patients with stents all had significantly worse scores than in those without stents. Readmission due to unremitting flank pain was necessary in four patients in the non-stented group. No patients in the stented group required readmission, but this was not statistically significant. This study and the others similar to it demonstrate that routine stenting is not required after uncomplicated ureteroscopy. However, the definition of uncomplicated ureteroscopy has not been established and includes any of the following: minimal or no trauma to the ureter, no excess dilation, no use of an access sheath, lithotripsy of smaller stones, and shorter operative times.

Bleeding diatheses

One of the distinct advantages of SWL over URS has been that the procedure is more easily performed with intravenous sedation or other minimal anesthetic techniques. However, only with URS can one operate on a patient who is pregnant or has a bleeding diathesis. Watterson et al. reviewed the safety and efficacy of URS and holmium laser lithotripsy in 25 patients with bleeding diatheses at two tertiary care stone centers.(67) The stone-free rate was 96% overall (89% for intra-renal and proximal stones, and 100% for mid-ureteral and distal stones). The authors reported only one bleeding complication due to electrohydraulic lithotripsy use resulting in a retroperitoneal hemorrhage which required blood transfusion and no bleeding complications if the patient was treated only with holmium laser.

PERCUTANEOUS ANTEGRADE URS

Percutaneous antegrade URS is particularly suited for large impacted proximal ureteral calculi where retrograde URS cannot be performed due to the inability to place a guidewire past the stone or due to anatomic constraints, ureteral tortuosity, or previous lower urinary tract surgery.(68) Percutaneous access allows larger instruments to be passed into the proximal ureter such as a cystoscope or nephroscope with their attendant larger working ports and larger instruments. Goel et al. performed antegrade rigid ureteroscopy using a nephroscope in 66 patients for impacted proximal ureteral calculi with a mean size of 21 mm (16–29 mm), and were able to achieve complete stone clearance in 65 patients through a single tract and single session based on post-operative KUB. (69) Antegrade URS is relatively safe and very effective, and fills the less invasive niche when an impacted proximal ureteral stone cannot be approached successfully in a retrograde manner.

OPEN AND LAPAROSCOPIC URETEROLITHOTOMY

The 1997 AUA guidelines stated that open surgery for ureteral calculi should not be a primary procedure. This holds true today especially with the advancements that have been made in ureteroscopic and percutaneous renal procedures. Many underdeveloped nations continue to use open stone surgery as primary therapy for difficult ureteral calculi, because of this, they are at the forefront of laparoscopic treatment of ureteral calculi.(70–74) From 1997 to 2005, 15 case series of laparoscopic ureterolithotomy published in the English language literature detailed the results in 458 patients; most procedures were for large or impacted calculi.(75) The overall success rate is 96%. Stone size does not appear to be associated with outcome, but distal ureterolithotomy was less successful than in the middle or proximal ureter. Both transperitoneal and retroperitoneoscopic ureterolithotomy techniques have shown similar stone free rates as open surgery in small case series. However, the retroperitoneoscopic approach lends itself well to proximal and middle ureteral calculi while the transperitoneal approach allows better access to the distal ureter.(74) Again, this is largely being done outside of the United States; in locales without full access to flexible ureteroscopes and holmium lasers.

PREGNANCY

For pregnant women with ureteral calculi, ionizing radiation should be limited due to its teratogenic effects on the embryo during the first trimester (>1 Gy).(76) However, there are to date no evidence in animals or humans of diagnostic radiation (<0.5 Gy) causing congenital malformations.(76) Nevertheless, the recommended initial exam should be an ultrasound of the kidneys.(1) If this is indeterminate of the size and location of the stone, then a limited intravenous pyelogram may be used. Noncontrast CT scan is not routinely used in this scenario due to the increased radiation dose. Low-dose noncontrast CT scans have been used as a compromise between decreasing radiation exposure and increasing the sensitivity to find ureteral calculi. White et al. reviewed their own institution's use of low dose noncontrast CT scanning in 20 pregnant women (average gestational age 26.45 weeks, range 18–40 weeks) presenting with acute flank pain.(77) Prior to 2004, if a CT scan was warranted in a pregnant woman, their institution used a standard scan (2.3 cGy). After 2004, a low-dose (0.7cGy, range 0.2–1.3 cGy) protocol was used in pregnant women. All women received a renal ultrasound prior to urologic consultation and subsequent CT scan. The authors found that the low-dose CT scan diagnosed stones in 65% of the patients, while the renal ultrasound could only detect hydronephrosis and did not diagnose any stones. While promising, the authors conclude that low-dose noncontrast CT scans should be reserved for pregnant women with refractory flank pain or indeterminate ultrasound findings given the small numbers of patients in their study and the need for more evidence regarding the clinical impact of even low-dose CT scans on fetal health. In addition, MRI imaging may be used to define the anatomic level of hydronephrosis, but is poor for localizing the stone.

While 70–80% of stones in pregnant patients pass spontaneously, temporizing measures help alleviate the pregnant patient's renal colic with either a ureteral stent or a percutaneous nephrostomy tube depending on the clinical situation.(78) However, this involves multiple stent changes or nephrostomy tube changes until the delivery of the baby, and carries the added morbidity of having a stent or tube. Watterson et al. reviewed their results using ureteroscopy and holmium laser lithotripsy to treat symptomatic pregnant women with ureteral calculi.(79) A total of 8 patients with 10 calculi were treated with URS and holmium laser lithotripsy, and achieved a stone-free rate of 89% without any complications. Additionally, there was no need to dilate any of the ureters. The safety of holmium laser lithotripsy for both mother and baby makes this technique feasible as a definitive treatment for ureteral stones in the pregnant patient.

COST ANALYSIS OF THE TREATMENT OF URETERAL CALCULI

The overall cost of URS for the treatment of ureteral calculi is less than the cost of SWL. Grasso et al. compared SWL to URS to establish the most efficacious and cost-effective treatment for ureteral calculi.(80) Stone-free rates at 3 months were 97% for URS and 62% for SWL with 3% of URS patients undergoing a second procedure and 31% of SWL patients undergoing auxiliary procedures. A cost comparison between the two procedures surprisingly shows that they were similar. However, the auxiliary procedures, multiple office visits, and repeat imaging increase the cost of SWL to a level far greater than URS. Parker et al. studied the cost of treating proximal ureteral stones with either URS or SWL. A total of 220 patients underwent treatment for their proximal ureteral stones. In the URS group, 91% were stone free after a single treatment, while for SWL it was 55%. Lotan et al. used a decision tree model to determine the cost of treating ureteral calculi. (81, 82) Observation was the least costly pathway if no cost was incurred by failure of observation. URS was less costly than SWL for stones at all ureteral locations. The difference between the two modalities was $1,440, $1,670, and $1,750 for proximal, middle, and distal ureteral calculi. Only if the cost of SWL decreased by $1,489 would it reach equivalence with URS.

CONCLUSION

The recent 2007 AUA guidelines for the management of ureteral calculi highlight the difficulty in recommending treatments for ureteral calculi due to the lack of randomized-controlled trials. However, the evidence gleaned from meta-analyses of the many retrospective studies and from the smaller randomized mostly uncontrolled trials allows some conclusions to be made. First, medical expulsive therapy increases the spontaneous passage rate of stones in the ureter at all locations, but distal stones have a high rate of passage regardless; the drug of choice in this regard appears to be tamsulosin for upwards of 2 weeks. For stones failing to pass within a 5–6 week period, definitive therapy is indicated. Ureteroscopy and shock wave lithotripsy are both considered first-line therapy. Ureteroscopy is more cost effective and efficient particularly, for larger (i.e. $\geq$ 10 mm) stones in the proximal or mid-ureter especially when combined with use of a ureteral access sheath. Shock wave lithotripsy is at least as effective as ureteroscopy for small < 10 mm stones in the proximal ureter. Percutaneous antegrade ureteroscopy is an option if the patient fails retrograde ureteroscopy or the anatomy of the patient precludes retrograde access. Open ureterolithotomy is rarely indicated and even when indicated it has been supplanted at many places, by laparoscopic ureterolithotomy, especially in developing nations; we believe that open ureterolithotomy will continue to wane and indeed, at some major medical centers is an operation that has not been performed by specialists in urolothiasis therapy in decades. Pregnant patients who do not have active urinary tract infections may be definitively treated safely with holmium laser lithotripsy and ureteroscopy. The introduction of new technologies for the treatment of ureteral calculi gives the urologist a wealth of tools by which to improve the outcomes of the patients he treats. Conversely, each patient's clinical characteristics will guide the clinician in reaching for the tools he needs. At the end of the day, however, for the patient with a ureteral calculus in 2008, the need for incisional therapy is indeed, exceedingly rare.

REFERENCES

1. Preminger GM, Tiselius HG, Assimos DG et al. 2007 guideline for the management of ureteral calculi. J Urol 2007; 178(6): 2418–34.
2. Segura JW, Preminger GM, Assimos DG et al. Ureteral Stones Clinical Guidelines Panel summary report on the management of ureteral calculi. The American Urological Association. J Urol 1997; 158(5): 1915–21.
3. Coll DM, Varanelli MJ, Smith RC. Relationship of spontaneous passage of ureteral calculi to stone size and location as revealed by unenhanced helical CT. AJR Am J Roentgenol. 2002; 178(1): 101–3.
4. Miller OF, Kane CJ. Time to stone passage for observed ureteral calculi: a guide for patient education. J Urol 1999; 162: 688–90.
5. Roberts WW, Cadeddu JA, Micali S, Kavoussi LR, Moore RG. Ureteral stricture formation after removal of impacted calculi. J Urol 1998; 159(3): 723–6.
6. Sterrett SP, Nakada SY. Medical expulsive therapy. Curr Opin Urol 2008; 18(2): 210–3.
7. Porpiglia F, Ghignone G, Fiori C, Fontana D, Scarpa RM. Nifedipine vs. tamsulosin for the management of lower ureteral stones. J Urol 2004; 172(2): 568–71.
8. Dellabella M, Milanese G, Muzzonigro G. Randomized trial of the efficacy of tamsulosin, nifedipine and phloroglucinol in medical expulsive therapy for distal ureteral calculi. J Urol 2005; 174(1): 167–72.
9. Yilmaz E, Batislam E, Basar MM et al. The comparison and efficacy of 3 different alpha1-adrenergic blockers for distal ureteral stones. J Urol 2005; 173(6): 2010–2.
10. Singh A, Alter HJ, Littlepage A. A systematic review of medical therapy to facilitate passage of ureteral calculi. Ann Emerg Med 2007; 50(5): 552–63.
11. Hollingsworth JM, Rogers MA, Kaufman SR et al. Medical therapy to facilitate urinary stone passage: a meta-analysis. Lancet 2006; 368(9542): 1171–9.

12. Borghi L, Meschi T, Amato F et al. Nifedipine and methylprednisolone in facilitating ureteral stone passage: a randomized, double-blind, placebo-controlled study. J Urol 1994; 152(4): 1095–8.

13. Porpiglia F, Vaccino D, Billia M et al. Corticosteroids and tamsulosin in the medical expulsive therapy for symptomatic distal ureter stones: single drug or association? Eur Urol 2006; 50(2): 339–44.

14. Dellabella M, Milanese G, Muzzonigro G. Medical-expulsive therapy for distal ureterolithiasis: randomized prospective study on role of corticosteroids used in combination with tamsulosin-simplified treatment regimen and health-related quality of life. Urology 2005; 66(4): 712–5.

15. Bhagat SK, Chacko NK, Kekre NS et al. Is there a role for tamsulosin in shock wave lithotripsy for renal and ureteral calculi? J Urol 2007; 177(6): 2185–8.

16. Porpiglia F, Destefanis P, Fiori C, Scarpa RM, Fontana D. Role of adjunctive medical therapy with nifedipine and deflazacort after extracorporeal shock wave lithotripsy of ureteral stones. Urology 2002; 59(6): 835–8.

17. Kupeli B, Irkilata L, Gurocak S et al. Does tamsulosin enhance lower ureteral stone clearance with or without shock wave lithotripsy? Urology 2004; 64(6): 1111–5.

18. Gravina GL, Costa AM, Ronchi P et al. Tamsulosin treatment increases clinical success rate of single extracorporeal shock wave lithotripsy of renal stones. Urology 2005; 66(1): 24–8.

19. Resim S, Ekerbicer HC, Ciftci A. Role of tamsulosin in treatment of patients with steinstrasse developing after extracorporeal shock wave lithotripsy. Urology 2005; 66(5): 945–8.

20. Gravas S, Tzortzis V, Karatzas A, Oeconomou A, Melekos MD. The use of tamsulozin as adjunctive treatment after ESWL in patients with distal ureteral stone: do we really need it? Results from a randomised study. Urol Res 2007; 35(5): 231–5.

21. Kekre NS, Kumar S. Optimizing the fragmentation and clearance after shock wave lithotripsy. Curr Opin Urol 2008; 18(2): 205–9.

22. Bensalah K, Pearle M, Lotan Y. Cost-effectiveness of medical expulsive therapy using alpha-blockers for the treatment of distal ureteral stones. Eur Urol 2008; 53(2): 411–8.

23. Miller NL, Lingeman JE. Treatment of kidney stones: current lithotripsy devices are proving less effective in some cases. Nat Clin Pract Urol 2006; 3(5): 236–7.

24. Tiselius HG. How efficient is extracorporeal shockwave lithotripsy with modern lithotripters for removal of ureteral stones? J Endourol 2008; 22(2): 249–56.

25. Nakada SY, Pearle MS, Soble JJ et al. Extracorporeal shock-wave lithotripsy of middle ureteral stones: are ureteral stents necessary? Urology 1995; 46(5): 649–52.

26. El-Assmy A, El-Nahas AR, Sheir KZ. Is pre-shock wave lithotripsy stenting necessary for ureteral stones with moderate or severe hydronephrosis? J Urol 2006; 176(5): 2059–62.

27. Krambeck AE, Gettman MT, Rohlinger AL et al. Diabetes mellitus and hypertension associated with shock wave lithotripsy of renal and proximal ureteral stones at 19 years of followup. J Urol 2006; 175(5): 1742–7.

28. Sato Y, Tanda H, Kato S et al. Shock wave lithotripsy for renal stones is not associated with hypertension and diabetes mellitus. Urology 2008; 71(4): 586–91.

29. Honey RJ. Assessment of a new tipless nitinol stone basket and comparison with an existing flat-wire basket. J Endourol 1998; 12(6): 529–31.

30. Johnson DB, Pearle MS. Complications of ureteroscopy. Urol Clin North Am 2004; 31(1): 157–71.

31. Turna B, Stein RJ, Smaldone MC et al. Safety and efficacy of flexible ureterorenoscopy and holmium:YAG lithotripsy for intrarenal stones in anticoagulated cases. J Urol 2008; 179(4): 1415–9.

32. Gur U, Holland R, Lask DM, Livne PM, Lifshitz DA. Expanding use of ureteral access sheath for stones larger than access sheath's internal diameter. Urology 2007; 69(1): 170–2.

33. Krambeck AE, Murat FJ, Gettman MT et al. The evolution of ureteroscopy: a modern single-institution series. Mayo Clin Proc 2006; 81(4): 468–73.

34. Dasgupta P, Cynk MS, Bultitude MF, Tiptaft RC, Glass JM. Flexible ureterorenoscopy: prospective analysis of the Guy's experience. Ann R Coll Surg Engl 2004; 86(5): 367–70.

35. Gupta PK. Is the holmium:YAG laser the best intracorporeal lithotripter for the ureter? A 3-year retrospective study. J Endourol 2007; 21(3): 305–9.

36. Leveillee RJ, Lobik L. Intracorporeal lithotripsy: which modality is best? Curr Opin Urol 2003; 13(3): 249–53.

37. Noor Buchholz NP. Intracorporeal lithotripters: selecting the optimum machine. BJU Int 2002; 89(2): 157–61.

38. Sun Y, Wang L, Liao G et al. Pneumatic lithotripsy vs. laser lithotripsy in the endoscopic treatment of ureteral calculi. J Endourol 2001; 15(6): 587–90.

39. Jeon SS, Hyun JH, Lee KS. A comparison of holmium:YAG laser with Lithoclast lithotripsy in ureteral calculi fragmentation. Int J Urol 2005; 12(6): 544–7.

40. Malik HA, Tipu SA, Mohayuddin N et al. Comparison of holmium: Yag laser and pneumatic lithoclast in percutaneous nephrolithotomy. J Pak Med Assoc 2007; 57(8): 385–7.

41. Huang S, Patel H, Bellman GC. Cost effectiveness of electrohydraulic lithotripsy v Candela pulsed-dye laser in management of the distal ureteral stone. J Endourol 1998; 12(3): 237–40.

42. Zheng W, Denstedt JD. Intracorporeal lithotripsy. Update on technology. Urol Clin North Am 2000; 27(2): 301–13.

43. Portis AJ, Rygwall R, Holtz C, Pshon N, Laliberte M. Ureteroscopic laser lithotripsy for upper urinary tract calculi with active fragment extraction and computerized tomography followup. J Urol 2006; 175(6): 2129–33.

44. L'Esperance JO, Ekeruo WO, Scales CD Jr et al. Effect of ureteral access sheath on stone-free rates in patients undergoing ureteroscopic management of renal calculi. Urology 2005; 66(2): 252–5.

45. Stern JM, Yiee J, Park S. Safety and efficacy of ureteral access sheaths. J Endourol 2007; 21(2): 119–23.

46. Landman J, Venkatesh R, Ragab M et al. Comparison of intrarenal pressure and irrigant flow during percutaneous nephroscopy with an indwelling ureteral catheter, ureteral occlusion balloon, and ureteral access sheath. Urology 2002; 60(4): 584–7.

47. Auge BK, Pietrow PK, Lallas CD et al. Ureteral access sheath provides protection against elevated renal pressures during routine flexible ureteroscopic stone manipulation. J Endourol 2004; 18(1): 33–6.

48. Kourambas J, Byrne RR, Preminger GM. Does a ureteral access sheath facilitate ureteroscopy? J Urol 2001; 165(3): 789–93.

49. Delvecchio FC, Auge BK, Brizuela RM et al. Assessment of stricture formation with the ureteral access sheath. Urology 2003; 61(3): 518–22.

50. Lallas CD, Auge BK, Raj GV et al. Laser Doppler flowmetric determination of ureteral blood flow after ureteral access sheath placement. J Endourol 2002; 16(8): 583–90.

51. De Sio M, Autorino R, Damiano R et al. Expanding applications of the access sheath to ureterolithotripsy of distal ureteral stones. A frustrating experience. Urol Int 2004; 72(Suppl 1): 55–7.

52. Rapoport D, Perks AE, Teichman JM. Ureteral access sheath use and stenting in ureteroscopy: effect on unplanned emergency room visits and cost. J Endourol 2007; 21(9): 993–7.

53. Auge BK, Sarvis JA, L'Esperance JO, Preminger GM. Practice patterns of ureteral stenting after routine ureteroscopic stone surgery: a survey of practicing urologists. J Endourol 2007; 21(11): 1287–91.

54. Haleblian G, Kijvikai K, de la Rosette J, Preminger G. Ureteral stenting and urinary stone management: a systematic review. J Urol 2008; 179(2): 424–30.

55. Borboroglu PG, Amling CL, Schenkman NS et al. Ureteral stenting after ureteroscopy for distal ureteral calculi: a multi-institutional prospective randomized controlled study assessing pain, outcomes and complications. J Urol 2001; 166(5): 1651–7.

56. Byrne RR, Auge BK, Kourambas J et al. Routine ureteral stenting is not necessary after ureteroscopy and ureteropyeloscopy: a randomized trial. J Endourol 2002; 16(1): 9–13.

57. Chen YT, Chen J, Wong WY et al. Is ureteral stenting necessary after uncomplicated ureteroscopic lithotripsy? A prospective, randomized controlled trial. J Urol 2002; 167(5): 1977–80.

58. Cheung MC, Lee F, Leung YL, Wong BB, Tam PC. A prospective randomized controlled trial on ureteral stenting after ureteroscopic holmium laser lithotripsy. J Urol 2003; 169(4): 1257–60.

59. Damiano R, Autorino R, Esposito C et al. Stent positioning after ureteroscopy for urinary calculi: the question is still open. Eur Urol 2004; 46(3): 381–7.

60. Denstedt JD, Wollin TA, Sofer M et al. A prospective randomized controlled trial comparing nonstented vs. stented ureteroscopic lithotripsy. J Urol 2001; 165(5): 1419–22.

61. Harmon WJ, Sershon PD, Blute ML, Patterson DE, Segura JW. Ureteroscopy: current practice and long-term complications. J Urol 1997; 157(1): 28–32.

62. Hollenbeck BK, Schuster TG, Seifman BD, Faerber GJ, Wolf JS Jr. Identifying patients who are suitable for stentless ureteroscopy following treatment of urolithiasis. J Urol 2003; 170(1): 103–6.

63. Jeong H, Kwak C, Lee SE. Ureteric stenting after ureteroscopy for ureteric stones: a prospective randomized study assessing symptoms and complications. BJU Int 2004; 93(7): 1032–4.

64. Knudsen BE, Beiko DT, Denstedt JD. Stenting after ureteroscopy: pros and cons. Urol Clin North Am 2004; 31(1): 173–80.

65. Nabi G, Cook J, N'Dow J, McClinton S. Outcomes of stenting after uncomplicated ureteroscopy: systematic review and meta-analysis. BMJ 2007; 334(7593): 572.

66. Netto NR Jr, Ikonomidis J, Zillo C. Routine ureteral stenting after ureteroscopy for ureteral lithiasis: is it really necessary? J Urol 2001; 166(4): 1252–4.

67. Watterson JD, Girvan AR, Cook AJ et al. Safety and efficacy of holmium: YAG laser lithotripsy in patients with bleeding diatheses. J Urol 2002; 168(2): 442–5.

68. Maheshwari PN, Oswal AT, Andankar M, Nanjappa KM, Bansal M. Is antegrade ureteroscopy better than retrograde ureteroscopy for impacted large upper ureteral calculi? J Endourol 1999; 13(6):441–4.

69. Goel R, Aron M, Kesarwani PK et al. Percutaneous antegrade removal of impacted upper-ureteral calculi: still the treatment of choice in developing countries. J Endourol 2005; 19(1): 54–7.

70. Kijvikai K, Patcharatrakul S. Laparoscopic ureterolithotomy: its role and some controversial technical considerations. Int J Urol 2006; 13(3): 206–10.

71. Hemal AK, Goel A, Goel R. Minimally invasive retroperitoneoscopic ureterolithotomy. J Urol 2003; 169(2): 480–2.

72. Goel A, Hemal AK. Upper and mid-ureteric stones: a prospective unrandomized comparison of retroperitoneoscopic and open ureterolithotomy. BJU Int 2001; 88(7): 679–82.

73. El-Feel A, Abouel-Fettouh H, Abdel-Hakim AM. Laparoscopic transperitoneal ureterolithotomy. J Endourol 2007; 21(1): 50–4.

74. Gaur DD, Trivedi S, Prabhudesai MR, Madhusudhana HR, Gopichand M. Laparoscopic ureterolithotomy: technical considerations and long-term follow-up. BJU Int 2002; 89(4): 339–43.

75. Wolf JS Jr. Treatment selection and outcomes: ureteral calculi. Urol Clin North Am 2007; 34(3): 421–30.

76. De Santis M, Di Gianantonio E, Straface G et al. Ionizing radiations in pregnancy and teratogenesis: a review of literature. Reprod Toxicol 2005; 20(3): 323–9.

77. White WM, Zite NB, Gash J et al. Low-dose computed tomography for the evaluation of flank pain in the pregnant population. J Endourol 2007; 21(11): 1255–60.

78. Evans HJ, Wollin TA. The management of urinary calculi in pregnancy. Curr Opin Urol 2001; 11(4): 379–84.

79. Watterson JD, Girvan AR, Beiko DT et al. Ureteroscopy and holmium:YAG laser lithotripsy: an emerging definitive management strategy for symptomatic ureteral calculi in pregnancy Urology 2002; 60(3): 383–7.

80. Grasso M, Beaghler M, Loisides P. The case for primary endoscopic management of upper urinary tract calculi: II. Cost and outcome assessment of 112 primary ureteral calculi. Urology 1995; 45(3): 372–6.

81. Lotan Y, Gettman MT, Roehrborn CG, Cadeddu JA, Pearle MS. Management of ureteral calculi: a cost comparison and decision making analysis. J Urol 2002; 167(4): 1621–9.

82. Lotan Y, Pearle MS. Economics of stone management. Urol Clin North Am 2007; 34(3): 443–53.

16 | Stones in patients with renal anomalies: Techniques and outcomes

Alana Desai and Ramakrishna Venkatesh

INTRODUCTION

Management of stones in patients with renal anomalies can pose unique technical challenges for the treating urologist. Anatomic anomalies resulting in obstruction, stasis or both may predispose patients to stone formation in addition to metabolic stone risk factors seen in urolithiasis patients with normal renal units. Stone composition is not known to be different compared to patients with normal renal anatomy, with calcium oxalate being the prevalent stone type. Horseshoe kidney is the most common congenital renal anomaly and the rate of stone formation in these patients is up to 20%. The other renal anomalies associated with increased risk of stone formation include calyceal diverticulum and other fusion anomalies such as crossed fused ectopia. Some authors categorize congenital ureteropelvic junction obstruction as a renal anomaly due to anomalous orientation of the ureteral smooth muscle leading to obstruction and stone formation. Hydronephrosis is the most common finding in an ectopic kidney, but its relation to stone formation when there is no renal obstruction is unclear. In a retrospective study of 82 ectopic kidneys, hydronephrosis was associated in 56% of ectopic kidneys, obstruction in 25% and nonrenal conditions such as sacral agenesis, undescended testis, ventricular septal defects, etc. in 52% of patients.(1) However, the above study did not include horseshoe kidneys.

Although the general principles remain the same, approach to treat stones in anomalous kidneys must be tailored to the individual patient due to altered renal anatomy or ectopic position compared to the treatment strategies used in an anatomically normal kidney. It is essential to treat associated obstruction in addition to stones in an anomalous kidney (e.g., calyceal diverticulum, ureteropelvic junction obstruction in a horseshoe kidney). Therefore, it is not surprising that the reported stone-free rates after Extracorporeal Shock Wave Lithotripsy (ESWL) for patients with stones in a calyceal diverticulum or other anomalous kidneys with hydronephrosis are poor.(2, 3) A thorough metabolic evaluation including stone analysis, serum and 24-hour urine stone risk profile is mandatory in the work up to minimize stone recurrence and growth of small residual stone fragments into clinically significant ones in the above anatomically and technically challenging group of patients. For uric acid stones medical management to dissolve the stones should be the first line of treatment. This chapter describes the various treatment techniques and reported outcomes in the management of patients with stones in an anomalous kidney including stones in a transplant kidney.

FUSION ANOMALIES

Horseshoe Kidney

It is the most common of the renal fusion anomalies with a prevalence of 0.25%.(4)On evaluation, up to 2/3rds of patients with horseshoe kidney (HSK) have hydronephrosis, infection, or urolithiasis.(5) The fused lower pole crosses the ventral aorta and, during ascent, is halted by the inferior mesenteric artery; hence the fused kidney lies more caudad in position compared to normal kidneys. Fusion occurs prior to rotation on their long axis resulting in anteriorly placed renal pelvis and ureters that cross the isthmus and posteriorly placed calyces. The calyces are directed posterior and the lower-pole calyces point caudally and medially (Figure 16.1). In contrast, the normal kidneys have calyces positioned lateral to the renal pelvis. The ureters may also have a high insertion into the renal pelves, and this combined with the abnormal anterior course, may contribute to obstruction and secondary stone formation. Apart from the renal ectopia and anomalous pelvicalyceal system, aberrant renal vasculature and relation of

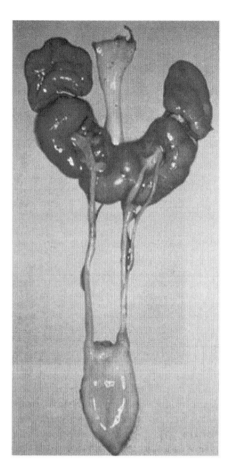

Figure 16.1 Horseshoe kidney in neonate with multiple anomalies. Note thick parenchymatous tissue of isthmus, anterior location and course of ureters.

adjacent bowel should be taken into careful consideration while planning surgical intervention for stones in a horseshoe kidney.

The etiology of stone formation in a HSK is attributed to impaired urinary drainage, stasis, and metabolic stone risk factors. The most common stone type is calcium oxalate and the most common location is the medial posterior lower calyx, followed by the renal pelvis. Raj and co-authors in 2004 evaluated a metabolic etiology for stone formation in 37 patients with horseshoe kidneys.(6) Metabolic derangements were found in all of them, the most common being hypovolemia, hypercalcuria, and hypocitraturia suggesting that increased stone formation in these patients may not solely be due to anatomical causes. Thus, metabolic evaluation is warranted with the goal of initiating medical therapy to reduce the risk of stone formation in this difficult to treat population.

ESWL

The challenge in treating horseshoe kidneys with ESWL lies in stone localization in a medially positioned HSK, because of obscured vision by bowel and skeletal structures including spine and pelvic bone. Positioning of the lithotripter head for coupling in the usual supine patient position can be challenging in the low-lying kidney because of the iliac bone. Also, the shock wave path is longer for these kidneys with difficult stone localization over F2 focal point. Lithotripsy in the prone position has been studied without adverse effect on bowel; however the potential for injury remains a possibility.(7) If ESWL is performed in the traditional prone position, this creates a longer shock wave path. Gupta and co-authors in their experience have found a wedge placed beneath the contralateral side in the supine position separating the medially located stones from the spine for fluoroscopic vision.(8) Also, a shorter path is created, the iliac crest is avoided, allowing placement of the stone within the F2 focal zone. Alternatively, if the stone cannot be positioned over F2, the "blast path" technique may be employed, wherein stone fragmentation is possible with sufficient acoustic pressure beyond F2 along the axis of the shock wave.(9)

Table 16.1 ESWL in anomalous kidneys.

Author	No. Patient anomaly	Stone size	Stone free rate One session	Ancillaly procedures	Overall Stone free rate
Smith *et al*, 1989	14 horseshoe kidneys	na	57%	4 ESWL, 2 URS, 1 PCNL	79%
Lock *et al*, 1990	10 horseshoe kidneys	13.4 mm	55%	3 ESWL,2 PCNL, 1 pyelolithotomy	73%
Serrate *et al*, 1991	11 horseshoe kidneys	na	80%	5 ESWL	na
Vandeursen and Baert, 1992	10 horseshoe kidneys	8.9 mm	na	31 ESWL	83%
Bhatia *et al*, 1994	27 horseshoe kidneys	28 mm			70%
Kirkali *et al*, 1996	18 horseshoe kidneys	24 mm	28%	57%	
Lampel *et al*, 1996	37 horseshoe kidneys	14 mm	na	7 ESWL, 2URS	76%
Sheir *et al*, 2003	49 horseshoe kidneys	13.5 mm	na	35 ESWL	71%
Tunc *et al*, 2004	150 57 duplex systems 45 horseshoe kidneys 30 malrotated kidneys 14 pelvic kidneys 4 crossed fused ectopia	16.9 mm 22.4 mm 19.2 mm 23.5 mm 30 mm	na	159 ESWL, 8 open, 5 URS	80.7% duplex 66.7% horseshoe 56.7% malrotated 57.2% pelvic 25% crossed fused
Jenkins and Gilllenwater, 1988	4 2 horseshoe kidneys 1 pelvic 2 crossed-fused ectopia	Na	50% horseshoe 100% pelvic 100% crossed fused	none	
Theiss *et al*, 1993	24 21 horseshoe kidneys 1 pelvic 2 crossed-fused ectopia	14 mm	na	6 ESWL	62.7% horseshoe 100% pelvic 100% crossed fused
Semerci *et al*, 1997	53 27 duplex 18 horseshoe kidneys 2 pelvic kidneys 1 sigmoid kidney 1 L shaped kidney	26.4 mm 39.3 mm 31 mm 23 mm 22 mm 10 mm		2.9 ESWL 2.5 ESWL 3.3 ESWL 1.5 ESWL 1 ESWL 1 ESWL	60.7% duplex 50% horseshoe 75% renal agenesis 100% pelvic kidney 100% sigmoid kidney 100% L shaphed Kidney

URS=Ureteroscopy, PCNL= percutaneous nephrolithotomy
Na= not available
*Average number of sessions per patient

Extracorporeal shock wave lithotripsy has been used in the treatment of renal anomalies with variable success with stone-free rates ranging from 28 to 80% in one session (Table 16.1) and even higher rates with retreatment.(10–22) Though ESWL is the least invasive treatment method, despite adequate fragmentation, stone passage may be impeded by the ureteral course, collecting system dilatation, and urinary stasis. Patients with HSK with stones have higher re-treatment rates (30%) compared to similar stone size and location in orthotopic kidneys (10%), and hence patients should be counseled accordingly.(23, 24) In a carefully selected patient with a stone of < 1.5 cm in size, located in the renal pelvis or nondependent calyces, in a nonobstructed system satisfactory results can be obtained by ESWL therapy.(2) In a series of 28 patients with calculi in horseshoe kidneys over a period of three years, fragmentation rate was 82.7%, and stone-free rate was 55.2% due to retained fragments, especially for stones in lower pole calyces.(8) The degree of dilation and stone size were found to be the main contributors to failure, and ESWL is not recommended as the treatment of choice for stones larger than 2 cm or those in hydronephrotic kidneys.

Ureteroscopy

Although the mainstay of management of calculi in anomalous kidneys has been PCNL and ESWL, there are occasions when these treatment modalities are contraindicated. These include bleeding dyscrasias, patients on anticoagulation, and obese patients. In addition, ESWL failures, impacted stones, and stones in systems with distal ureteral obstruction may be better served by an endoscopic approach.(25) Refinements in endoscopic technology have allowed access, fragmentation, and stone retrieval in difficult anatomic situations. Smaller caliber semi-rigid ureteroscopes allow treatment of distal and mid-ureteral stones and do not always require ureteral dilation.(26) Flexible ureteroscopes as small as 7.5 French with active deflection and adequate working channels allow access to the entire collecting system.(27) The development of small caliber flexible ureteroscopies with active deflection up to 270 degrees and accessory tools such as the 200 μ holmium laser fiber and ureteral access sheaths has allowed wider use of endoscopic treatment of stone disease in patients with renal anomalies.(28–30)

There are few studies, however, reporting on the outcomes of renal calculi in anomalous kidneys treated endoscopically. Weizer and co-authors treated eight patients, 4 each with horseshoe and pelvic kidneys with flexible ureteroscopy and holmium laser lithotripsy to achieve stone-free rates of 75% in both groups of patients.(31) Lakmichi et al. also reported on the endoscopic laser lithotripsy of calculi in patients with fusion anomalies who were previously treated with ESWL or PCNL. Six patients with HSK and one with L-shaped kidney with stone-free rate of 85.7% considering over 5 patients required 2 treatments. Ureteroscopy with the use of laser lithotripsy and nitinol basket is a reasonable approach in select patients with stones < 2 cm in fusion anomalies, however more than one session may be necessary for optimal results.(32) Semi-rigid ureteroscopy for proximal ureteral stones in horseshoe kidneys is difficult and potentially dangerous due to the aberrant anatomical course, but mid and distal ureteral stones can be managed similar to those within normal kidneys. Due to impaired drainage, complete extraction of stone fragments is recommended with the aid of the ureteral access sheath and use of nitinol basket.(28)

Percutaneous nephrolithotomy (PCNL)

PCNL should be employed in those patients with large (> 2 cm) stone burden with inadequate drainage.(33) The percutaneous approach in patients with renal anomalies requires a thorough knowledge of the anatomy and vascularity, and a preoperative CT scan delineating the above is useful. A defect in the normal development of the laterocoronal fascia and the absence of the kidney in its normal anatomic position may result in a retrorenal colon in patients with horseshoe kidney, increasing the risk of a colonic injury.(34, 35) Treatment for colonic perforation has been described and consists of withdrawal of the nephrostomy tube into the colon, ureteral stent placement, and intravenous antibiotics. The ureteral stent may be removed after nephrostogram demonstrates no fistula.(36) Janetschek and Kunzel studied the arterial supply of the horseshoe kidney in 6 cadaveric specimens and examined 8 patients who underwent percutaneous stone removal. The orientation of the collecting system offered good access and they in fact found this almost easier than in normally oriented kidneys. They found three groups of arteries: (1) the normal renal arteries (2) accessory arteries originating from different levels of the aorta including the bifurcation, the internal and common iliac arteries and entering the renal hilum, and (3) aberrant arteries entering the poles or the isthmus originating from the renal artery, aorta, bifurcation, middle sacral and common iliac artery. There was found to be no dorsally located vessels except for some of the arteries to the isthmus. Thus a dorsal or dorsolateral approach would avoid these blood vessels. There is no increased risk of bleeding in horseshoe kidneys compared to the normal population.(37) The most favorable approach is through the most superior posterior calyx which allows access to the pelvis

Table 2   PCNL in anomalous kidneys.

Author	No. patients	Anomaly	Stone free rate	Ancillary procedures	Complications
Janetschek and Kuknzel (1988)	8	Horseshoe	100%	1 pcnl	None
Jones et al. (1991	15	Horseshoe	77.8%	2 ESWL	Tx (2), fever
Salas et al. (1992)	6	Horseshoe	80%	None	UTI
Al-Otaibi and Hosking (1999)	12	Horseshoe	75%	1 ESWL (83%)	Prolonged urine leak
Desai et al. (2000)	9	Pelvic ectopic	100%	32nd stage	Ileus, nephrostomy site leak
Shokeir et al. (2004)	34	Horseshoe	73.5%	8 ESWL, 1 URS	Tx(3), sepsis, obs, colonic injury
Matlaga et al. (2006)	8	Pelvic ectopic*	100%	None	None
Gupta et al. (2006)	16	Pelvic	100%	52nd stage	Bowel injury, perinephric hematoma, ileus

*Laproscopic assisted in six cases.

and other calyces. Often the lower calyces face antero-medially and are inaccessible for a safe percutaneous puncture. The site of access is located more medial than in normal kidneys due to the posteriorly directed calyces. Once access is achieved, the distance to stones within the renal pelvis or lower pole may be found to be too long for rigid nephroscopy and flexible nephroscopy may be required.(38) Percutaneous access should be guided by fluoroscopy or ultrasound. Alternatively, a 3D CT-guided puncture in patients with anatomical abnormalities has been described and this allows visualization of stone size as well as calyceal anatomy.(39, 40) Multiple tracts and nephrostomies may be required to achieve a stone-free status.(34)

The results of PCNL are superior to those of ESWL with an average stone-free rate of 84% (range 73%–100%) (Table 16.2) (34, 35, 41–46). Shokeir et al. reported on 34 patients with stones in HSK with a stone-free rate of 82% upon discharge and 89% at three months. However, on follow-up 56% demonstrated recurrence.(35) Complications occurred in six cases and included hematuria, sepsis, ureteral obstruction, and colonic injury. Despite the risk of colonic injury described, this is the only incidence of this in three recent series consisting of a total of 50 patients.(34, 35, 38) Thoracic injury is minimized with the inferior location of the horseshoe kidney, even with upper pole access.(8, 28)

Laparoscopy

There have been case reports of laparoscopic pyelolithotomy in horseshoe kidneys with a large stone burden.(47–49) This approach is especially suitable for patients with renal pelvic stone or small caliceal stone with associated uretero pelvic junction obstruction. Care should be taken not to compromise the renal vascularity in view of possible aberrant vascular anatomy and crossing vessels.(50) Typically the camera and the working trocars are positioned in the midline or close to midline to facilitate stone extraction and pyeloplasty in a more medially located UPJ in a low lying HSK. The renal pelvic stone can be removed through a pyelotomy and caliceal stone(s) with the aid of a flexible cystoscope and a grasper or a nitinol basket through a laparoscopic trocar. Laparoscopy has also been used to assist in PCNL allowing percutaneous access under direct vision to avoid bowel or vessel injury. Results of laparoscopic techniques for stone disease in horseshoe kidneys are limited, but encouraging (Table 16.3). (48, 51–58) Most studies consist of one to two patients, but stone-free rates are close to 100% and none have required additional procedures. In addition, the number of reported complications was negligible.

OTHER FUSION ANOMALIES

Crossed renal ectopia is a condition in which the kidney is located contralateral to its ureteral insertion into the bladder and 90% of the ectopic kidneys are fused to the ipsilateral kidney.

Table 3 Laparascopic approaches in anomalous kidneys.

Author	No. patients	Anomaly	Technique	Stone free rate	Ancillary procedures	Complications
Eshghi et al. (1985)	1	Pelvic kidney	Laparoscopic assisted PCNL	100%	None	None
Valdivia-Uria et al. (1994)	2	Horseshoe kidney	Laparoscopic pyelolithotomy	100%	None	Urine leak
Hoenig et al. (1997)	1	Pelvic kidney	Laparoscopic pyelolithotomy	100%	None	None
Holman and Toth (1998)	15	Pelvic kidney	Laparoscopic assisted PCNL	100%	None	Urine leak
Ramakumar et al. (2002)	19	UPJ obstruction	Laparoscopic* pyelolithotomy and pyeloplasty	90%	None	None
Maheshwari et al. (2004)	3	Pelvic kidney	Laparoscopic assisted PCNL	100%	None	None
Maheshwari et al. (2004)	1	Horseshoe kidney	Laparoscopic assisted PCNL	100%	None	None
Obek et al. (2004)	1	Horseshoe kidney	Laparoscopic pyelolithotomy	100%	None	None
Goel et al. (2006)	2	Pelvic kidney	Laparoscopic assisted PCNL	100%	None	None

Depending on the position relative to the ipsilateral kidney, the anomalies are termed sigmoid, lump, L-shaped, disc, unilateral fused kidney with superior ectopia, and unilateral fused kidney with inferior ectopia. The abnormal position of the kidney may predispose to calculus formation.(8) Much of the literature regarding ESWL for the management of stones in patients with other renal anomalies such as malrotation and crossed renal ectopia is based upon case reports or in series with limited numbers (Table 16.1). Limited reports of ESWL for stones in crossed renal ectopia and pelvic ectopia has excellent success rates similar to results in normal kidneys; however, dismal rates are to be expected for larger stone burden.

Pelvic Kidney

Renal ectopia occurs when, during its ascent, the kidney does not reach its normal anatomic location. Pelvic ectopia is the most common and has an estimated occurrence of 1in 2,200 to 3,000 in autopsy series, the left side occurring slightly more commonly than the right.(33) The kidney does not rotate completely resulting in an anterior renal pelvis and hydronephrosis from obstruction at the uretero-pelvic or ureterovesical junction, vesicoureteral reflux, and from the malrotation itself.(1) Thus, it is important to evaluate for concomitant obstruction with imaging prior to surgical treatment.

ESWL

Due to its location, intervening bowel and bony structures may make treatment of stones within pelvic kidneys with ESWL difficult. However, with accurate localization and position, ESWL should be considered the primary treatment option if these two goals are achieved. Similar to treatment of stones in HSK, due to its ectopic position, technique may be modified to account for overlying structures. Patients may be treated in the prone position. The use of ureteral catheters to assist in stone localization has been described as well.(64) Indications for placement of a ureteral stent do not differ from that in normal kidneys, although a shorter stent is required due to the shorter ureteral length.

Talic and co-workers reported on 14 patients with stones in renal pelvic ectopia. Twelve with stones over the sacroiliac joint were treated in the prone position and ureteral catheters were placed to aid in fluoroscopic localization. Most required a single session (64%), 2 required 2 sessions and 2 required multiple sessions. Steinstrasse occurred in 2 patients requiring repeat ESWL for both patients and one required ureteroscopy. Overall, 82% were stone free at 3 months.(59) Kupeli et al. reported on seven patients with stones in pelvic kidneys with a stone-free rate of 54% at 3 months.(60) Others have reported rates ranging from 57.2% to 100% (Table

16.1).(28, 61–63) It is important to recognize that in many of these series, additional ESWL sessions were required. In a large series of 150 patients, Tunc and co-workers reported on the results of ESWL in renal anomalies and found that the type of anomaly, stone burden and stone location all affected treatment success.(18) By location stone-free rates for upper pole, middle pole, lower pole, pelvic, and ureteral stones was found to be 100%, 60%, 50%, 90%, and 92%, respectively. In summary, ESWL should be considered for small stones in the pelvic kidney in a nonobstructed collecting system.

Ureteroscopy

In those situations where ESWL or PCNL are contraindicated, ureteroscopy may be used to treat stones in pelvic kidneys. Weizer et al. reported on 4 patients with pelvic kidneys undergoing ureteroscopy, holmium laser lithotripsy, and stone extraction with a nitinol basket or graspers with a 75% stone-free rate and no ancillary procedures were required. The authors challenged the "noninvasiveness" of ESWL in this population due to the need for multiple sessions and ancillary procedures. In this series, no patient had a contraindication to ESWL, but stone composition, size (1.5 cm or greater), or location in the lower pole limited ESWL efficacy. They found that the ureteral access sheath helped to "straighten" the ureter, allowing ease of access to the renal pelvis and kept the ureteroscope in line, improving deflectability.(24) Ureteroscopy should thus be considered for managing renal calculi in select patients with renal stones in pelvic kidneys prior to more invasive procedures.

PCNL

Calculi in ectopic kidneys have traditionally been treated with open stone surgery. Due to potential injury to abdominal viscera and vessels, PCNL has not been traditionally performed in pelvic ectopic kidneys. Percutaneous access in pelvic kidneys is obtained with the patient in the supine position as the pelvic bones preclude access in the prone position. Desai and co-workers described treatment of stones in pelvic ectopic kidneys with the use of ultrasound guided puncture. The calyx of entry was located with the ultrasound and pressure on the probe was used to displace bowel loops from the puncture site. Under ultrasound guidance, the calyx was punctured and dilated. Pre-operative bowel preparation with an enema was performed although gas in the sigmoid colon was found to be helpful for its identification. One tract was used in seven patients and 2 required 2 tracts.(44, 46) They performed PCNL in 16 patients with stones in pelvic ectopic kidneys with the use of ultrasound guided puncture. There was one bowel injury and a perinephric hematoma. Another patient showed intraperitoneal extravasation on nephrostogram and this was managed with a ureteral stent and a nephrostomy tube for two additional days. One patient had a persistent leak from the nephrostomy site which resolved after stent placement. Stone-free status was achieved in all cases in single or 2 sessions. Matlaga and co-authors reported on 8 patients with congenital pelvic kidneys who underwent PCNL.(45) Six of these patients had laparoscopic assisted procedures for large stone burdens (Figure 16.2). A three port approach was used and overlying bowel loops were mobilized from the kidney. An 18gauge needle was advanced into the targeted calyx under direct and fluoroscopic guidance. The tract was then balloon dilated to 30F and standard PCNL was performed. All patients were stone free in a single procedure. Following PCNL, a Council tip or Cope loop nephrostomy can be left or suture closure of the nephrostomy site on the Gerota's fascia can be performed. In another case, a patient with myelomeningocele had an iliac osteotomy site adjacent to the pelvic kidney and PCNL was performed successfully via this defect.(45) An approach via the greater sciatic foramen has also been described in a patient with a left pelvic kidney and a 12 mm calculus.(64–65) A 5F open ended catheter was first placed for retrograde pyelography followed by trans-sciatic puncture of the calyx with a 21 gauge needle under fluoroscopic guidance. Access is obtained through the greater sciatic foramen, the boundaries of which are the sacrum posteriorly, the ischium anteriorly and the ileum superiorly. Care should be taken to stay close to the sacrum to avoid vascular and neural structures. The transgluteal distance to the pelvic kidney is greater than via the flank approach and this approach may not be feasible in obese patients. In this case, the patient weighed 59kg and required the full length of the 18 cm Amplatz sheath to reach the kidney. The tract was balloon dilated to 30F and the stone was fragmented with lithotripsy and all stone fragments were removed. The nephrostomy tube was kept in place for 2 days and the stent was removed three weeks post-operatively.(65) Suffice it to say, each case must be individualized to determine the optimal approach for the patient with stones in the pelvic kidney.

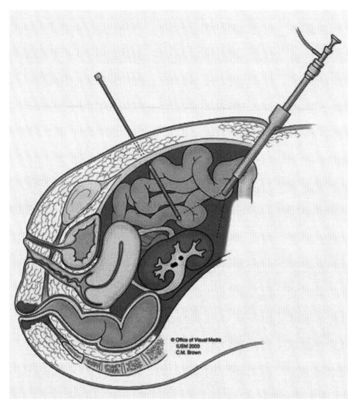

Figure 16.2 Laparoscopic assisted PCNL. Bowel is displaced prior to percutaneous access. **Awaiting permission from IUSM**

Laparoscopy

In the rare patient that open surgery is considered, the advent of laparoscopy has nearly eliminated the need for this approach. In 1985 Eshghi et al. first described a case report of the technique of percutaneous access to a pelvic kidney by retrograde nephrostomy and direct visualization of tract dilation via laparoscopy. Two ports were used and intervening bowel loops were displaced. A 160 cm 20 gauge curved needle (Hunter-Hawkins retrograde percutaneous nephrostomy needle) was placed beside a guidewire through a 5F angiographic catheter within a 9Fr sheath to the desired calyx. Under fluroscopy the calyx was punctured and under direct vision the stylet was grasped through the right lower quadrant trocar exiting the abdominal cavity. The needle was removed and the nephrostomy tract was dilated to 34F under laparoscopic and fluoroscopic vision. Standard PCNL was then performed. Intraperitoneal fluid was suctioned at the case end and a JP drain placed through the umbilical incision. The drain was removed on post-operative day 2 after nephrostogram showed no extravasation or residual stone. The nephrostomy tube was removed 3 days postoperatively.(51) Laparoscopic pyelolithotomy has also been performed as an alternative to PCNL for large stone burdens. Intervening bowel loops can be displaced followed by pyelotomy and stone extraction under direct vision.(66–68) Important in the success of this approach is appropriate imaging to delineate the vascularity relative to calyceal anatomy, use of the Trendelenburg position to assist with bowel displacement, and the ability to suction intraperitoneal fluid at the case end and the ability to perform the procedure in a single stage. The authors have found a tri-pronged stone grasper used for PCNL as a useful tool during laparoscopic pyelolithotomy. Large stones can be entrapped in a laparoscopic specimen bag and intracorporeal lithotripsy within the bag can be performed under laparoscopic vision before extracting the bag with stone fragments through a small skin incision.

Laparoscopic-based approaches have been shown to offer exceptional stone-free rates with minimal morbidity (Table 16.3). Since its introduction, stone-free rates with laparoscopic assisted PCNL of 100% with minimal morbidity have been reported.(54, 56) Holman and Toth reported on their experience with laparoscopic assisted PCNL in 15 patients. All patients were rendered stone-free and there was only one complication of a prolonged urine leak.(54) Maheshwari (6) and Goel et al. (58) have also reported 100% stone-free rates with laparoscopic assisted PCNL in pelvic ectopic kidneys that had previously failed open pyelolithotomy.

Transplant Kidney

Transplanted kidneys deserve special mention as they may be classified as pelvic kidneys. Nephrolithiasis in the transplanted kidney is rare with a reported incidence of 0.4%–1% and can occur after transplantation or be present in the donor kidney. Donor transplant stones can be managed pre-operatively or intra-operatively by bench techniques.(69–72) The composition of most of these stones is calcium oxalate and risk factors specific to renal transplantation include secondary hyperparathyroidism and foreign body such as nonabsorbable sutures or ureteral stents.(73) Other risk factors are similar to those in the general population including obstruction, urinary tract infection and metabolic abnormalities.(74) Patients typically present with fever, elevated creatinine, and hematuria; complete obstruction results in anuria.(75) Patients may report discomfort due to capsule distension and stretching the overlying fascia, but because of denervation during transplantation, most patients do not experience renal colic.(72) These patients require aggressive management to decrease the risk of obstruction and loss of function.(69, 72) Treatment protocols should follow those for a solitary kidney. Expedient recognition and relief of obstruction are required before definitive stone management. Patients with stones less than 4 mm without renal impairment may be observed but require close follow up for renal function as they are frequently asymptomatic. This requires close monitoring of urine output, weekly measurements of serum creatinine and renal ultrasonography, although diagnosis with ultrasound may be unreliable. Excellent patient compliance is mandatory with this approach and the patient must be counseled appropriately.(76)

For stones less than 1.5 cm, ESWL is recommended.(69, 73, 76) As with pelvic kidneys, they can be treated in the prone position to avoid the bony pelvis. Additional procedures may be required such as stent placement, percutaneous nephrostomy tube placement or repeat ESWL sessions. In a series of 19 patients, seven were treated with ESWL, three of them requiring percutaneous nephrostomy tube placement during treatment and all of them were rendered stone free.(76) Challacombe et al. reported on 13 patients treated with ESWL; 8 required multiple sessions, 8 had ureteral stents placed prior to the second procedure, and 4 had nephrostomy tubes placed for obstruction. All were rendered stone free with combined treatment methods.(69) Ureteral stents should be placed if there is potential for obstruction. Likewise, patients should be closely observed for steinstrasse, obstruction, and oliguria.

Ureteroscopy with use of holmium laser and stone extraction is an option for small stones (< 2 cm) refractory to ESWL.(77) Retrograde access may be challenging due to the location and orientation of the transplanted ureter. The use of angled catheters or hydrophilic-coated guidewires has been described to access the transplant ureteral orifice. Del Pizzo et al. reported on seven transplant patients treated ureteroscopically for a ureteral stone in 4 and a stent migration in 3 patients with success in 6 out of seven cases. In these cases access was obtained using a 6.5F curved Cobra open-ended catheter and a 0.035 inch Glidewire. The glidewire was then exchanged for an Amplatz super-stiff guidewire and the ureteral orifice was balloon dilated. An 8F semirigid ureteroscope was used for patients with ureteral calculi and a 7.5F flexible ureteroscope was used for other cases. All of the stones were extracted successfully and one stent had to be retrieved by percutaneous endoscopy.(75) Although transplant ureteroscopy is less well-established than percutaneous and antegrade intervention and may be technically challenging, ureteroscopy can be performed with minimal morbidity and acceptable outcomes. This approach is an advantageous alternative to PCNL in this population of patients who have delayed wound healing and increased susceptibility to infection. However, endoscopic stone extraction is not without its potential complications with possible ureteric damage or impaired healing because of decreased vascularity compared to that of a native ureter.(78)

PCNL should be used for stones larger than 2 cm.(69, 73) It is the most commonly used technique and provides superior access for removing pelvic and calyceal stones.(79, 80) The patient is typically placed supine and the ipsilateral side may be positioned slightly oblique with the use of a bolster under the hip. Ultrasound can be used to guide the puncture to avoid injury to intervening bowel loops. Although the transplant kidney is easier to access than the pelvic kidney due to close proximity to the skin, dilation may be more difficult due to scarring around the kidney and significant bleeding may ensue. Balloon dilation has been used with success to create a nephrostomy tract as well as coaxial metal dilators.(73, 77) The use of rigid nephroscopy may also be limited due to the fibrous sheath surrounding the kidney and a flexible ureteroscope or cystoscope may be required.(71, 72)

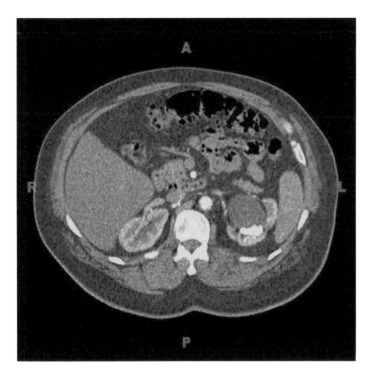

Figure 16.3 UPJ obstruction with renal calculi.

Calyceal Diverticula

Calyceal diverticula are nonsecretory, transitional cell epithelium lined cystic cavities within the renal parenchyma. Invariably they have a narrow neck and are in direct communication with the collecting system, allowing passive influx of urine.(81) The incidence on routine intravenous pyelography ranges from 2 to 4/1,000. True pathogenesis is controversial, but most agree that they are congenital in nature. These diverticula are prone to stone formation due to urinary stasis and incidence has been reported to occur between 10% and 50%.(82) Calculi can cause inflammation and subsequent fibrosis and narrowing of the neck of the diverticulum.(83) Although they may be asymptomatic, flank pain, recurrent infection, and hematuria prompt intervention. Metabolic analysis should be performed as abnormalities may also contribute to stone formation. In a retrospective study of 37 patients, all were found to have metabolic abnormalities similar to random stone-forming patients.(84) These were corrected with medical therapy and the remission rate was 83%. The role of stasis versus metabolic factor towards stone formation is controversial, however metabolic evaluation should be performed to determine risk factors for stone formation.(85) Open surgical procedures such as nephrotomy, marsupiliazation, fulguration of the diverticular cavity and partial nephrectomy is historical. Minimally invasive therapies used for treating calyceal diverticular stones include PNL, ureteroscopy, laparoscopic surgery and ESWL. CT scan and IVU/retrograde urography are useful guides to assess the cortical thickness over the stone, approach to the diverticulum and presence of communication with the main collecting system (Figure 16.3).

ESWL

The use of ESWL to treat these stones is debatable as to prevent recurrence the diverticulum must be obliterated. The stone-free rate with ESWL treatment ranges from 4–58% with a poor average of 21%.(86–90) However, approximately 60% of patients (36% to 86%) were reportedly symptom free. Better success rates may be related to short follow up (3–6months), small stone burden (< 1.5 cm) and patent diverticular neck.(90) While adequate fragmentation may occur, the narrow neck of the diverticulum may prevent passage of stone fragments. However, if stone-free status is necessary because of recurrent infection or when diverticular ablation is required, other treatment options must be considered.(91)

PCNL

The percutaneous approach to diverticular stones allows for stone extraction as well as incision of the diverticular neck and eradication of the diverticulum to prevent recurrence and has been the treatment of choice. Direct puncture can be challenging because of a small diverticular cavity and the frequent presence of diverticulum in the upper pole of the kidney. Following successful puncture, directing the guide wire into the renal pelvis can be difficult either because of a very narrow diverticular neck or stones filling the calyx. Additionally, if the parenchyma overlying the diverticulum is thin, stabilization of the Amplatz sheath can be a problem. In view of the above issues related to the diverticulum, modification of some of the typical access techniques is required. Direct puncture into the diverticulum is preferable as it allows use of rigid instruments for better visualization for identifying the neck of the diverticulum and easy fulguration of the urothelium with a rollerball electrode. If the direct puncture fails, indirect puncture by perforating the wall of the diverticulum or retrograde fashion through the diverticular neck can be achieved. However, the efficacy with the indirect puncture is inferior to the direct puncture. Typically, after percutaneous access is obtained, a guidewire is coiled into the diverticular cavity to assist with stability during tract dilation. This is followed by standard PCNL.(91) If the overlying renal parenchyma is thin, the roof of the diverticulum should be resected and the neck should be fulgurated so that granulation and obliteration of the diverticula can occur. With thicker parenchyma surrounding the diverticulum, the neck should be dilated, the wall fulgurated and nephrostomy tube left in place for 3 to 4 weeks to allow the neck to heal open and prevent new stone formation.(86) Kim and co-workers (2005) reported a single-stage procedure that does not require ureteral catheter placement or entrance into the renal collecting system. Two guide wires are coiled in the diverticular cavity after direct puncture and the track is balloon dilated and once the stone is removed, the cavity is fulgurated.(92)

With percutaneous approach stone-free rates with this approach are reported to be greater than 80%. In addition, symptomatic improvement as well as a decrease in infection rates can be expected.(86, 87, 93, 94) Bellman et al. reported a stone-free rate of 95% in a series of 19 patients treated with percutaneous management.(94) Shalhav et al. reported a 93% stone-free rate with an 85% resolution of symptoms at a mean follow up of 3.5 years.(95) In addition, 76% had no further evidence of a diverticulum. In the single stage procedure described by Kim et al. CT scan obtained on post-operative day one showed a stone-free rate of 85.7%. Intravenous pyelography obtained three months post-operatively showed a decrease in the diverticular size in all cases and complete resolution of the diverticula in 87.5%.(92) Auge et al. in a retrospective review, compared the ureteroscopic approach to PCNL and found a stone-free rate of 19% for ureteroscopy and 78% using PCNL. Although the hospital stay and complication rate was higher with PCNL, the symptom free rate was 86% compared with 35% for those treated endoscopically.(96)

Ureteroscopy

Although percutaneous management yields excellent results and allows treatment of the diverticular neck, stones in small diverticulae, those with a narrow neck, and those that are anteriorly located are problematic for the percutaneous approach. In these cases, a retrograde approach may be employed for smaller (< 1 cm) stone burdens or a combined approach for those with larger stone burden.(97) With flexible uretero-renoscopy, the diverticular neck may be visualized and opened by balloon dilation or laser incision. The calculi may then be extracted or fragmented depending on stone size.(91, 98, 99) Ureteroscopy to identify narrow intrarenal segments followed by dilation and either stone extraction or pretreatment ESWL under the same anesthesia has also been described. In this series, 11 of 15 patients were rendered stone free and two of four with residual stone were asymptomatic. The remaining two reported nonspecific back pain that was nevertheless decreased compared to symptoms at presentation. There were no complications with this method.(93) As with percutaneous management, the retrograde approach allows simultaneous treatment of the diverticulum. After stone retrieval, the neck can be obliterated using laser or electrocautery; in many cases this results in granulation and obliteration of the diverticular cavity.

Laparoscopy

More recently, laparoscopy has been used in the management of calyceal diverticular calculi. Several cases have been reported to date and access can been retroperitoneal or transperitoneal. (100–104) The diverticula were managed with excision and fulguration as well as using perinephric fat or gelatin resorcinol formaldehyde glue to fill the cavity and obliterate the diverticular neck.(102–103) Miller et al. reported on a series of five patients with symptomatic calculi within calyceal diverticulae using a three port retroperitoneal approach. This was preceded by ureteral stent placement into the renal pelvis to aid in identification of the diverticular neck. Indigo carmine was injected through the ureteral catheter in one case and this was visualized laparoscopically through the thinned renal parenchyma. Calculi were identified with the use of fluoroscopy or laparoscopic ultrasound. An incision was made over the thinnest area of parenchyma using electrocautery or scissors and the stones were extracted using laparoscopic or tripronged PCNL grasper. The stones were placed into an endoscopy bag followed by copious irrigation with antibiotic solution to avoid contamination of the retroperitoneal space. Diverticulum with a narrow neck was fulgurated or ablated with argon beam. Larger diverticular necks can be oversewn and the cavity can be fulgurated. A Jackson Pratt drain as well as a double J stent was left in place. In this report, a treatment algorithm was recommended, guided by the amount of overlying renal parenchyma, size of diverticulum and stone, location of the diverticulum and ability to obtain retrograde access. Laparoscopy is recommended for diverticula with thin overlying parenchyma, those that are anteriorly located or those that are inaccessible via endoscopic techniques. Posteriorly located diverticula with adequate renal cortex should be managed via PCNL.(98) Using this algorithm, Wong et al. reported on a case in which an anteriorly located calyceal diverticulum with a narrow neck and complex branched calculi was treated with laparoscopic assisted PCNL. The patient was placed in a modified lithotomy position, the ipsilateral side elevated 30 degrees and three 10 mm trocars were placed and the colon was mobilized medially. A 12 mm trocar was then placed to assist in transperitoneal PCNL. Using laser lithotripsy and graspers, the stones were extracted and the neck of the diverticulum was ablated with the laser.(105) The laparoscopic approach has been shown to be safe and effective for the treatment of calculi within calyceal diverticula in select patients.

Ureteropelvic Junction Obstruction

Ureteropelvic junction obstruction is frequently associated with renal calculi (Figures 16.3 & 16.4). The extent of obstruction, urinary stasis and metabolic abnormalities contributing to the stone formation is not clear. Husmann and colleagues found that 71% of nonstruvite stone formers in patients with UPJ obstruction had metabolic abnormalities.(106) Also, >60% of recurrence stones in the above group of patients were seen in the contralateral kidney, suggesting the importance of evaluating metabolic stone risk factors for stone metaphylaxis. In general, treatment should address both stones and obstruction. Ideally, the treatment should be minimally invasive, have a high success rate and allow concomitant treatment of the UPJ obstruction and stone removal.(107) Patients have traditionally been treated with open pyeloplasty and stone extraction. Advances in laparoscopic and endoscopic technology allow a less invasive approach. PCNL with antegrade endopyelotomy in patients with no crossing vessels addresses both issues and has success rates ranging from 64–85%.(106–113) CT scan with contrast can identify crossing vessels (Figure 16.4). Laparoscopic pyeloplasty with pyelolithotomy offers >90% success rates for UPJ obstruction and stone-free rate of over 90%. Ramakumar et al. reported on a series of 19 (20 renal units) patients with stones and ureteropelvic junction obstruction.(114) A small endopyelotomy was made prior to repair and this was later incorporated into the final incision. Stones within the renal pelvis were extracted with rigid graspers and a flexible cystoscope was used for stones inaccessible by this means. Large stone burdens were treated with laser lithotripsy or placed in a specimen retrieval bag and fragmented within the bag using intracorporeal lithotripsy using ultrasonic device with careful laparoscopic visualization for any disintegration of the bag and removed at the end of the case. It was emphasized that transection of the ureter should not precede complete stone removal as this stabilizes the pyelotomy for retrieval. There were two cases of recurrent stone disease at a mean follow up of 12 months for a long-term stone-free rate of 80%. In a larger series of 147 laparoscopic pyeloplasties performed, 21 patients (22 renal units), underwent lithotomy and had a 98% stone-free rate and successful repair of UPJ obstruction.(115) Whelan and Wiesenthal used a flexible ureteroscope to retrieve stones during laparoscopic pyeloplasty.(116) Ball et al. reported on laparoscopic pyeloplasty and flexible nephroscopy. It was found that this is most effective in patients with a limited stone burden (5–20 mm).(117) Atug and co-workers have reported on the use of robotic-assisted laparoscopic pyeloplasty (RALP) along with stone extraction in 8 patients.(118) All patients were stone free with no intra or post-operative complications related to the procedure. The stones were extracted with robotic pyelolithotomy or by flexible

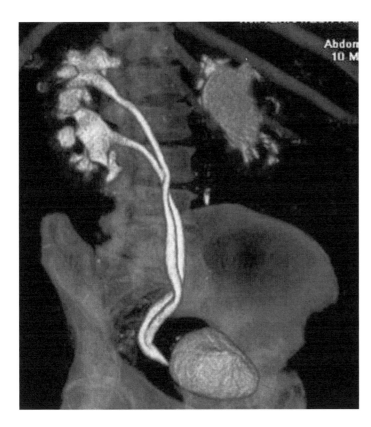

Figure 16.4 3D Reconstruction of UPJO of above patient.

nephroscope after undocking one of the robotic arms to introduce a flexible scope. Suction through the assistant port was used to aspirate irrigant fluid during nephroscopy. Basket or a stone grasper was used to extract stones from the calyces. If there is a large stone or multiple stones, then they can be placed within a specimen bag before retrieval.. The present study showed no significant impact of concomitant stone removal on the duration of stay, estimated blood loss, anastomosis times, complications, or success rates when RALP was used. Moon et al. reported on 11 patients who underwent successful extraction of coexisting renal calculi along with pyeloplasty.(115) Overall, success rates for the treatment of concomitant renal calculi and UPJO with laparoscopic techniques is promising and can be used to treat complex stone disease as well as provide optimal treatment of the patient with UPJO.

SUMMARY

The management of calculous disease in anomalous kidneys must be individualized to achieve a stone-free status using minimally invasive treatment strategies. Abnormal renal position, calyceal anatomy, ureteral insertion, and aberrant vascularity make imaging of paramount importance to plan surgical intervention. Stone-free status should be the most important goal along with the correction of associated abnormalities that might predispose to stone formation or compromise clearance of stone fragments. The treatment principles used for the stones in normal renal units can be applied to anomalous kidneys with the currently available tools and techniques including PCNL, flexible ureterorenoscopy, laparoscopy or a combination to achieve the above goals. Lastly, metabolic stone risk evaluation should be performed in all patients to guide preventative management in this challenging group of patients.

REFERENCES

1. Gleason PE, Kelalis PP, Husmann DA et al. Hydronephrosis in renal ectopia: incidence, etiology and significance. J Urol 1994; 151: 1660–1.

2. Drach GW, Dretler S, Fair W et al. Report of the United States cooperative study of extracorporeal shock wave lithotripsy. J Urol 1986; 135(6):1127–33.

3. Winfield HN, Clayman RV, Chaussy CG et al. Monotherapy of staghorn renal calculi: a comparative study between percutaneous nephrolithotomy and extracorporeal shock wave lithotripsy. J Urol 1988; 139(5): 895–9.

4. Bauer SB. Anomalies of the upper urinary tract. In: Wein, Kavoussi, Novick, Partin, Peters, editors. Campbell-Walsh urology, 9th edition. Philadelphia: W.B. Saunders Co; 2007: 3287–9.

5. Lampel A, Hohenfellner M, Schultz-Lampel D et al. Urolithiasis in horseshoe kidneys: therapeutic management. Urology 1996; 47: 182–6.

6. Raj GV, Auge BK, Assimos D, Preminger GM. Metabolic abnormalities associated with renal calculi in patients with horseshoe kidneys. J Endourol 2004; 18(2): 157–61.

7. Jenkins AD, Gillenwater JY. Extracorporeal shock wave lithotripsy in the prone position: treatment of stones in the distal ureter or anomalous kidney. J Urol 1988; 139: 911–5.

8. Gupta M, Lee MW. Treatment of stones associated with complex or anomalous renal anatomy. Urol Clin N Am 2007; 34: 431–41.

9. Madorsky M, Finlayson B. Geometrical considerations to optimize use of Dornier blast path. J Urol 1986; Part 2, 135: 160A, abstract 227.

10. Smith JE, Van Arsdalen KN, Hanno PM, Pollack HM. Extracorporeal shock wave lithotripsy treatment of calculi in horseshoe kidneys. J Urol 1989; 142: 683–6.

11. Locke DR, Newman RC, Steinbock, GS, Finlayson B. Extracorporeal shock wave lithotripsy in horseshoe kidneys. Urology 1990; 35: 407–11.

12. Serrate R, Regue R, Prats J, Rius G. ESWL as the treatment for lithiasis in horseshoe kidney. Eur Urol 1991; 20: 122–5.

13. Vandeursen H, Baert L. Electromagnetic extracorporeal shock wave lithotripsy for calculi in horseshoe kidneys. J Urol 1992; 148: 1120–2.

14. Bhatia V, Biyani CS. Urolithiasis with congenital upper tract anomalies: a 4-year experience with extracorporeal shock wave lithotripsy. J Endourol 1994; 8: 5–8.

15. Kirkali Z, Esen AA, Mungan MU. Effectiveness of extracorporeal shock wave lithotripsy in the management of stone-bearing horseshoe kidneys. J Endourol 1996; 10: 13–5.

16. Lampel A, Hohenfellner M, Schultz-Lampel D et al. Urolithiasis in horseshoe kidneys: therapeutic management. Urology 1996; 47: 182–6.

17. Sheir KZ, Madbouly K, Elsobky E, Abdelkhalek M. Extracoporeal shock wave lithotripsy in anomalous kidneys: 11-year experience with two second-generation lithotripters. Urology 2003; 62: 10–6.

18. Tunc L, Tokgoz H, Tan MO et al. Stones in anomalous kidneys: results of treatment by shock wave lithotripsy in 150 patients. Int J Urol 2004; 11: 831–6.

19. Jenkins AD, Gillenwater JY. Extracorporeal shock wave lithotripsy in the prone position: treatment of stones in the distal ureter or anomalous kidney. J Urol 1988; 139: 911–5.

20. Theiss M, Wirth MP, Frohmuller HG. Extracorporeal shock wave lithotripsy in patients with renal malformations. BJU Int 1993; 72: 534–8.

21. Semerci B, Verit A, Nazli O et al. The role of ESWL in the treatment of calculi with anomalous kidneys. Eur Urol 1997; 31: 302–4.

22. Al-Tawheed AR, Al-Awadi KA, Kehinde EO et al. Treatment of calculi in kidneys with congenital anomalies: an assessment of the efficacy of lithotripsy. Urol Res 2006; 34(5): 291–8.

23. Chaussy C, Schmiedt E. Extracorporeal shock wave lithotripsy (ESWL) for kidney stones. An alternative to surgery? Urol Radiol 1984; 6(2): 80–7.

24. Taherimahmoudi M, Purmand G, Mehrsai A. Extracorporeal shock wave lithotripsy in horseshoe kidneys [abstract]. J Endourol 2006; 20(Suppl 1): A255.

25. Singal RK, Denstedt JD. Contemporary management of ureteral stones. Urol Clin North Am 1997; 24: 59–70.

26. Abdel-Razzak OM, Bagley DH. The 6.9F semirigid ureteroscope in clinical use. Urology 1993; 41: 45–8.

27. Grasso M, Bagley DH. A 7.25/8.2 French actively deflectable, flexible ureteroscope: a new device for both diagnostic and therapeutic upper urinary tract endoscopy. Urology 1994; 43: 435–41.

28. Stein RJ, Desai MM. Management of urolithiasis in the congenitally abnormal kidney (horseshoe and ectopic). Curr Opin Urol 2007; 17: 125–31.

29. Andreoni C, Portis AJ, Clayman RV. Retrograde renal pelvic access sheath to facilitate flexible ureteroscopic lithotripsy for the treatment of urolithiasis in a horseshoe kidney. J Urol 2000; 164: 1290–1.

30. Tawfiek ER, Bagley DH. Management of upper urinary tract calculi with ureteroscopic techniques. Urology 1999; 53: 25–31.

31. Weizer AZ, Springhart WP, Ekeruo WO et al. Ureteroscopic management of renal calculi in anomalous kidneys. Urology 2005; 65(2): 265–9.

32. Lakmichi MA, Labou I, Niang L et al. Ureteroscopic management of renal calculi in kidneys with abnormality of fusion [abstract]. J Endourol 2006; 20(Suppl 1): A117.

33. Lingeman JE, Matlaga BR, Evan AP. Surgical management of upper urinary tract calculi. In: Wein, Kavoussi, Novick, Partin, Peters, editors. Campbell-Walsh urology, 9th edition. Philadelphia: W.B. Saunders Co; 2007: 1443.

34. Al-Otaibi K, Hosking DH. Percutaneous stone removal in horseshoe kidneys. J Urol 1999; 162: 674–7.

35. Shokeir AA, El-Nahas AR, Shoma AM et al. Percutaneous nephrolithotomy in treatment of large stones within horseshoe kidneys. Urology 2004; 64(3): 426–9.

36. Goswami AK, Shrivastava P, Mukherjee A, Sharma SK. Management of colonic perforation during percutaneous nephrostomy in horseshoe kidney. J Endourol 2001; 15: 989–91.

37. Janetschek G, Kunzel KH. Percutaneous nephrolithotomy in horseshoe kidneys. Applied anatomy and clinical experience. Br J Urol 1988; 62: 177–22.

38. Raj GV, Auge BK, Weizer AZ et al. Percutaneous management of calculi within horseshoe kidneys. J Urol 2003; 170(1): 48–51.

39. Matlaga BR, Shah OD, Zagoria RJ et al. Computerized tomography guided access for percutaneous nephrostolithotomy. J Urol 2003; 170(1): 45–7.

40. Al-Kohlany KM, Shokeir AA, Mosbah A et al. Treatment of complete staghorn stones: a prospective randomized comparison of open surgery compared with percutaneous nephrolithotomy. J Urol 2005; 173(2): 469–73.

41. Janetschek G, Kunzel KH. Percutaneous nephrolithotomy in horseshoe kidneys. Applied anatomy and clinical experience. Br J Urol 1988; 62: 177–22.

42. Jones DJ, Wickham JE, Kellet MJ. Percutaneous nephrolithotomy for calculi in horseshoe kidneys. J Urol 1991; 145: 481–3.

43. Salas M, Gelet A, Martin X et al. Horseshoe kidney: the impact of percutaneous surgery. Eur Urol 1992; 21: 134–7.

44. Desai MR, Jasani A. Percutaneous nephrolithotomy in ectopic kidneys. J Endourol 2000; 14: 289–92.

45. Matlaga BR, Kim SC, Watkins SL e t al. Percutaneous nephrolithotomy for ectopic kidneys: over around or through. Urology 2006; 67: 513–7.

46. Gupta RC, Desai MR, Anil R et al. Role of percutaneous nephrolithotomy in pelvic ectopic kidneys – 17 years experience [abstract]. J Endourol 2006; 20(Suppl 1): A22.

47. Saagar VR, Singh K, Sarangi R. Retroperitoneoscopic heminephrectomy of a horseshoe kidney for calculus disease. Surg Laparosc Endosc Percutan Tech 2004; 14: 172–4.

48. Obek K, Porter J. Laparoscopic pyelolithotomy in a horseshoe kidney. J Endourol 2004; S18: MP27.

49. Ghevariya JD, Wani K, Shrivastav P et al. Laparoscopic pyelolithotomy in horseshoe kidney-a case report. J Endourol 2004; S18: V23, p. A229.

50. Chammas M Jr, Feuillu B, Coissard A et al. Laparoscopic robotic-assisted management of pelviureteric junction obstruction in patients with horseshoe kidneys: technique and 1-year follow up. BJU Int 2006; 97: 579–83.

51. Eshghi AM, Roth JS, Smith AD. Percutaneous transperitoneal approach to a pelvic kidney for endourological removal of staghorn calculus. J Urol 1985; 134: 525–7.

52. Valdivia-Uria JG, Abril Baquero G, Monzon Alebesque F et al. Laparoscopic management of complex lithiasis in horseshoe kidneys. Actas Urol Esp 1994; 18(Suppl): 346–50.

53. Hoenig DM, Shalhav AL, Elbahnasy AM et al. Laparoscopic pyelolithotomy in a pelvic kidney a case report and review of the literature. JSLS 1997; 1: 163–5.

54. Holman E, Toth C. Laparoscopically assisted percutaneous transperitoneal nephrolithotomy in pelvic dystopic kidneys: experience of 15 successful cases. J Laproendosc Adv Surg Tech 1998; 8: 431–5.

55. Ramakumar S, Lancini V, Chan DY et al. Laparoscopic pyeloplasty with concomitant pyelolithotomy. J Urol 2002; 167(3): 1378–80.

56. Maheshwari PN, Bhandarkar DS, Andankar MG et al. Laparoscopically guided transperitoneal percutaneous nephrolithotomy for calculi in pelvic ectopic kidneys. Surg Endosc 2004; 18: 1151.

57. Maheshwari PN, Bhandarkar DS, Shah RS et al. Laparoscopy-assisted transperitoneal percutaneous nephrolithotomy for recurrent calculus in ishthmic calix of horseshoe kidney. J Endourol 2004; 18: 858–61.

58. Goel R, Yadav R, Gupta NP, Aron M. Laparoscopic assisted percutaneous nephrolithotomy (PCNL) in ectopic kidneys: two different techniques. Int Urol Nephrol 2006; 38: 75–8.

59. Talic RF. Extracorporeal shock-wave lithotripsy monotherapy in renal pelvic ectopia. Urology 1996; 48: 857–61.

60. Kupeli B, Isen K, Biri H et al. Extracorporeal shock-wave lithotripsy in anomalous kidneys. J Endourol 1999; 13: 349–52.

61. Jenkins AD, Gillenwater JY. Extracorporeal shock wave lithotripsy in the prone position: treatment of stones in the distal ureter or anomalous kidney. J Urol 1988; 139: 911–5.

62. Theiss M, Wirth MP, Frohmuller HG. Extracorporeal shock wave lithotripsy in patients with renal malformations. BJU Int 1993; 72: 534–8.

63. Semerci B, Verit A, Nazli O et al. The role of ESWL in the treatment of calculi with anomalous kidneys. Eur Urol 1997; 31: 302–4.

64. Watterson JD, Cook A, Sahajpal R et al. Percutaneous nephrolithotomy of a pelvic kidney: a posterior approach through the greater sciatic foramen. J Urol 2001; 166: 209–10.

65. Butch RJ, Mueller PR, Ferrucci JT Jr et al. Drainage of pelvic abscesses through the greater sciatic foramen. Radiology 1986; 158: 487–91.

66. Zafar FS, Lingeman JE. Value of laparoscopy in the management of calculi complicating renal malformations. J Endourol 1996; 10: 379–83.

67. Kamat N, Khandelwal P. Laparoscopic pyelolithotomy- a technique for the management of stones in the ectopic pelvic kidney. Int J Urol 2004; 11: 581–4.

68. Chang TD, Dretler SP. Laparoscopic pyelolithotomy in an ectopic kidney. J Urol 1996; 156: 1753.

69. Challacombe B, Dasgupta P, Tiptaft R et al. Multimodal management of urolithiasis in renal transplantation. BJU Int 2005; 96: 385–9.

70. Mundy AR, Podesta ML, Bweick M et al. The urological complications of 1000 renal transplants. Br J Urol 1981; 53: 397–402.

71. Rhee BK, Bretan PN Jr, Stoller ML. Urolithiasis in renal and combined pancreas/renal transplant recipients. J Urol 1999; 161: 1458–62.

72. Crook TJ, Keoghane SR. Renal transplant lithiasis: rare but time-consuming. BJU Int 2005; 95: 931–3.

73. Benoit G, Blanchet P, Eschwege P et al. Occurrence and treatment of kidney graft lithiasis in a series of 1500 patients. Clin Transplant 1996; 10: 176–80.

74. Lancina Martin JA, Garcia Buitron JM, Diaz Bermudez JA et al. Urinary lithiasis in transplanted kidney. Arch Esp Urol 1997; 50: 141–50.

75. Del Pizzo JJ, Jacobs SC, Sklar GN. Ureteroscopic evaluation in renal transplant patients. J Endourol 1998; 12: 125–38.

76. Klinger HC, Kramer G, Lodde M et al. Urolithiasis in allograft kidneys. Urology 2002; 59: 344–8.

77. Francesca F, Felipetto R, Mosca F et al. Percutaneous nephrolithotomy of transplanted kidney. J Endourol 1999; 16: 225–7.

78. Caldwell TC, Burns JH. Current operative management of urinary calculi after renal transplantation. J Urol 1988; 140: 1360–3.

79. Abott KC, Schenkman N, Swanson SJ, Agodoa LY. Hospitalized nephrolithiasis after renal transplantation in the United States. Am J Transplantation 2003; 3: 465–70.

80. Bailey IS, Griffin P, Evans C, Matthews PN. Percutaneous surgery of the transplanted kidney. Br J Urol 1989; 63: 327–3

81. Lingeman JE, Matlaga BR, Evan AP. Surgical management of upper urinary tract calculi. In: Wein, Kavoussi, Novick, Partin, Peters, editors. Campbell-Walsh urology, 9th edition. Philadelphia: W.B. Saunders Co; 2007: 1442.

82. Middleton AW Jr, Pfister RC. Stone-containing pyelocaliceal diverticulum: Embryogenic, anatomic, radiologic and clinical characteristics. J Urol 1974; 111: 2–6.

83. Burns JR. Calyceal diverticulum. AUA Updates Series XL, 1992: 421.

84. Auge, BK, Maloney ME, Mathias BJ, Pietrow PK, Preminger GM. Metabolic abnormalities associated with calyceal diverticular stones. BJU Int 2006; 97(5): 1053–6.

85. Matlaga BR, Miller NL, Terry C et al. The pathogenesis of calyceal diverticular calculi. Urol Res 2007; 35(1): 35–40.

86. Hendrikx AF, Bierkens AF, Bos R, Oosterhof GO, Debruyne FM. Treatment of stones in caliceal diverticula: Extracorporeal shock wave lithotripsy versus percutaneous nephrolitholapaxy. Br J Urol 1992; 70: 478–82.

87. Jones JA, Lingeman JE, Steidle CP. The roles of extracorporeal shock wave lithotripsy and percutaneous nephrostolithotomy in the management of pyelocaliceal diverticula. J Urol 1991; 146: 724–7.

88. Pshramis KE, Dretler SP. Extracorporeal shock wave lithotripsy of caliceal diverticula calculi. J Urol 1987; 138: 707–11.

89. Ritchie AW, Parr NJ, Moussa SA, Tolley DA. Lithotripsy for calculi in caliceal diverticula? Br J Urol 1990; 66: 6–8.

90. Streem SB, Yost A. Treatment of caliceal diverticular calculi with extracorporeal shock wave lithotripsy: Patient selection and extended followup. J Urol 1992; 148: 1043–6.

91. Cohen TD, Preminger GM. Management of calyceal calculi. Urol Clin North Am 1997; 24(1): 81–96.

92. Kim SC, Kuo RL, Tinmouth WW, Watkins S, Lingeman JE. Percutaneous nephrolithotomy for caliceal diverticular calculi: a novel single stage approach. J Urol 2005; 173(4): 1194–8.

93. Hulbert JC, Reddy PK, Hunter DW et al. Percutaneous techniques for the management of caliceal diverticula containing calculi. J Urol 196; 135: 225–7.

94. Bellman GC, Silverstein JI, Blickensderfer S, Smith AD. Technique and follow-up of percutaneous management of caliceal diverticula. Urology 1993; 42: 21–5.

95. Shalhav AL, Sble JJ, Nakada SY et al. Long-term outcome of caliceal diverticula following percutaneous endosurgical management. J Urol 1998; 160: 1635.

96. Auge BK, Munver R, Kourambas J, Newman GE, Preminger GM. Endoscopic management of symptomatic caliceal diverticula: a retrospective comparison of percutaneous nephrolithotripsy and ureteroscopy. J Endourol 2002; 16(8): 557–63.
97. Grasso M, Lang G Loisedes P et al. Endoscopic management of the symptomatic caliceal diverticular calculus. J Urol 1995; 153: 1878–81.
98. Miller SD, NG CS, Streem SB, Gill IS. Laparoscopic management of caliceal diverticular calculi. J Urol 2002; 167: 1248–52.
99. Fuchs GL, David RD. Flexible ureterorenoscopy, dilation of narrow caliceal neck and ESWL: a new, minimally invasive approach to stones in caliceal diverticula. J Endourol 1989; 3: 255–63.
100. Ruckle HC, Segura JW. Laparoscopic treatment of a stone-filled, caliceal diverticulum: a definitive, minimally invasive therapeutic option. J Urol 1994; 151: 122–4.
101. Gluckman GR, Stoller M, Irby P. Laparosopic pyelocaliceal diverticula ablation. J Endourol 1993; 7: 315–17.
102. Harewood LM, Agarwal D, Lindsay S et al. Extraperitoneal laparoscopic caliceal diverticulectomy. J Endourol 1996; 10: 425–30.
103. Hoznek A, Herrard A, Ogiez N et al. Symptomatic caliceal diverticula treated with extraperitoneal laparoscopic marsupialization fulguration and gelatin resorcinol formaldehyde glue obliteration. J Urol 1998; 160: 352–5.
104. Curran MJ, Little AF, Bouyounes B et al. Retroperitoneoscopic technique for treating symptomatic caliceal diverticula. J Endourol 1999; 13: 723–5.
105. Wong C, Zimmerman RA. Laparoscopy-assisted transperitoneal percutaneous nephrolithotomy for renal caliceal diverticular calculi. J Endourol 2005; 19(6): 608–13.
106. Husmann DA, Milliner DS, Segura JW. Ureteropelvic junction obstruction with a simultaneous renal calculus: Long term follow up. J Urol 1995; 153: 1399–402.
107. El-Shazly MA, Moon DA, Eden CG. Laparoscopic pyeloplasty: status and review of literature. J Endourol 2007; 21: 673–8.
108. Arun N, Kekre NS, Nath V, Gopalakrishan G. Is open pyeloplasty still justified? Br J Urol 1997; 80: 379–81.
109. O'Reilly PH, Brooman PJ, Mak S et al. The long-term results of Anderson-Hynes pyeloplasty. BJU Int 2001; 8: 287–9.
110. Brooks JD, Kavoussi LR, Preminger GM, Schuessler WW, Moore RG. Comparison of open and endourologic approaches to the obstructed ureteropelvic junction. Urology 1995; 46: 791–5.
111. Cassis AN, Brannen GE, Bush WH, Correa RJ, Chambers M. Endopyelotomy: review of results and complications. J Urol 1991; 146(6): 1492–5.
112. Meretyk I, Meretyk S, Clayman RV. Endopyelotomy: comparison of ureteroscopic retrograde and antegrade percutaneous techniques. J Urol 1992; 148(3): 775–82.
113. Motola JA, Badlani GH, Smith AD. Results of 212 consecutive endopyelotomies: an 8-year followup. J Urol 1993; 149(3): 453–6.
114. Ramakumar S, Segura JW. Laparoscopic surgery for renal urolithiasis: pyelolithotomy, caliceal diverticulectomy, and treatment of stones in a pelvic kidney. J Endourol 2000; 14(10): 829–32.
115. Moon DA, El-Shazly MA, Chang CM, Gianduzzo TR, Eden CG. Laparoscopic pyeloplasty: evolution of a new gold standard. Urology 2006; 67: 932–6.
116. Whelan, JP, Wiesenthal JD. Laparoscopic pyeloplasty with simultaneous pyelolithotomy using a flexible ureteroscope. Can J Urol 2004; 11: 2207–9.
117. Ball AJ, Leveillee RJ, Patel VR, Wong C. Laparoscopic pyeloplasty and flexible nephroscopy: simultaneous treatment of ureteropelvic junction obstruction and nephrolithiasis. JSLS 2004; 8(3): 223–8.
118. Atug F, Castle EP, Burgess SV, Thomas R. Concomitant management of renal calculi and pelvi-ureteric junction obstruction with robotic laparoscopic surgery. BJU Int 2005; 96: 1365–68.

17 | Pediatric urolithiasis

Bruce Slaughenhoupt

INCIDENCE OF PEDIATRIC UROLITHIASIS

Although urolithiasis is still not as prevalent among children as it is among adults, over the past several years we have seen an increasing incidence of children with stones.(1, 2, 3, 4) Although not yet conclusive, epidemiological studies are suggesting this is due to a change in social conditions and eating habits.(5)

In 1951, Lattimer reported no cases of urolithiasis in 21,835 children at the Babies Hospital in New York.(6) More recently, the literature has become populated with many series of children who have urolithiasis. The actual incidence of pediatric urolithiasis and the predominant types of stones produced in children varies throughout the world. In the United States, the reported incidence of children admitted to the hospital for management of a stone has ranged from 1 per 1,000 to 1 per 7,6000 pediatric hospital admissions in 1989.(7, 8) However, since many children with stones are not admitted for their treatment, this is a poor estimation of the actual incidence of stones in this country. A 1973 study from the United Kingdom cited an annual incidence of pediatric urolithiasis of two per one million children.(9) A very inclusive 2005 Icelandic study reported a much higher incidence of heritable genetic mutations which contribute to stones in their children at a higher rate of 6 per 100,000. These children accounted for approximately 1 per 1,000 pediatric hospital admissions.(10) In most parts of the developed world, children are still believed to represent only 2% to 3% of the overall population of stone formers.(11, 12) In parts of the Middle East and Southeast Asia, pediatric urolithiasis is endemic.(13) These stones, however, are much more likely to develop in the bladder, as opposed to the upper urinary tract, and are believed to be due to malnutrition and a low-protein, high-starch diet.(7, 13, 14, 15)

Historically, adult males develop significantly more stones than females. However in children, the ratios of boys to girls with urolithiasis appear to be more equal at 1–1.5 boys to 1 girl. A 2005 review of urolithiasis in India demonstrated a male to female ratio of 1.5: 1.(16) A 2002 report from the Vanderbilt group identified a 1: 1 ratio. And a multi-institutional study from Michigan and Virginia cited a 1.1:1 male to female ratio.(17, 18) In 2007, the Pittsburgh group reported a female preponderance of 1.4 girls to each boy.(3) In Iceland, the incidence in girls is also higher than in boys at 1.4 girls to 1 boy.(10)

Familial Inheritance

Although most children with stones do not have a family history of urolithiasis, many studies report at least a 20 to 40% incidence of a first- or second-degree relative with a history of stones.(19, 20, 21) In Iceland, where there is a higher than normal incidence of Adenine Phosphoribosyltransferase deficiency (APRT), 33% of the children had a first- or second-degree relative with a past history of stones.(10) In a 2002 report, 34% of children in Brazil had a first-degree family member with a history of stones.(20)

The genetic causes of urolithiasis have been well studied but are still inconclusive. The only conclusive findings are that the etiology is usually polygenic and partially penetrative.(22, 23) Fewer than 2% of children who form stones can be identified with a monogenic abnormality.(24)

Just as there are various kinds of kidney stones, there are also various genetic causes for stone formation. Various chromosomal loci have been recognized as playing a part in the development of stones.(17, 25) For example, more frequent polymorphisms in the vitamin D-receptor (VDR) gene have been identified in children with a history of stones when compared to normal control children without stones.(26) Dent's disease is an X-linked spectrum of entities comprised of hypercalciuria, urolithiasis, nephrocalcinosis, proteinuria, and in some patients, renal failure. A mutation of the renal-specific chloride channel gene *CLCN-5* on chromosome Xp11.22 has been identified as a contributor to this disease spectrum.(27) This mutation impairs expression of the chloride transport channel in the proximal tubule, thick ascending limb of Henle, and proximal collecting ducts.(28)

Cystinuria is a recessively inherited aminoaciduria caused by a defect in the transport of cystine, arginine, lysine, and ornithine in the renal tubular and intestinal epithelium. At least two genes, *SLC3A1* and *SLC7A9*, are known to be responsible for this defect. A Chinese study from 2006 identified heterogeneous mutations in these genes that lead to different cystine concentrations in the urine of patients.(29) Cystinuria's prevalence varies throughout the world. Newborn screening programs have estimated it to be 1:15,000 in the United States, 1:2,000 in the United Kingdom, 1:4,000 in Australia, and 1:2,500 in Libyan Jews.(30)

Another genetically linked illness that often leads to the development of stones during childhood is the autosomal recessively inherited primary hyperoxaluria (PH). Type 1 PH is caused by a mutational error on chromosome 2, which leads to a deficiency of hepatic alanine-glyoxalate aminotransferase. Type 2 PH involves a deficiency of glyoxalate reductase/hydroxypyruvate reductase. Through a series of hepatic enzymatic deficiencies, this leads to an overproduction of oxalate. Hyperoxaluria then can lead to renal failure, which in turn leads to increased serum oxalate levels and deposition of calcium oxalate throughout solid organs and bone. Although most affected individuals develop renal failure during adolescence, some do so during infancy.(31)

A 2006 study of the genetic inheritability of urinary stone risk in identical twins revealed interesting findings. The authors found a high heritability coefficient (H^2 of 90% or greater) indicating a significant genetic component for urinary levels of calcium (94%), oxalate (94%), citrate (95%), and uric acid (96%). In contrast urinary pH and sodium levels had low degrees of heritability. The authors concluded that since urinary calcium, oxalate, and citrate had a high heritability coefficient, they might be associated with specific genes that impact stone risk. They also felt that since urinary pH and sodium may be weakly linked genetically, improvement in these lithogenic risk factors might be more amenable to dietary or pharmacologic intervention.(19)

Stone Recurrence Rates

Stone recurrence rates in the pediatric literature have covered quite a range (16%–48%).(21, 32, 33) Some reports also show a close association between recurrence rates and metabolic abnormalities or recurrent urinary tract infections (UTIs).(33) In 1989, Diamond published a 27-year review of 270 children with stones from Massachusetts and Liverpool with an overall recurrence rate of 16%. He found the children with a lithogenic metabolic abnormality had a higher 30% chance of recurrence, while the children with an anatomic abnormality had a 27% chance. The children with infection as well as the idiopathic stone formers each had only a 14% recurrence rate.(32) Since some of their patients did not develop their recurrent stones for 7–13 years, they recommended prolonged follow up for children with stones.(32) The Vanderbilt group reported a recurrence rate of 19% for all children evaluated. This rate approached 50% when reviewing only those children younger than 10 years of age with an identifiable metabolic abnormality. The recurrence rate was less than 10% if no metabolic abnormality was identified.(18)

Presenting Symptoms

While typically the adult with urolithiasis presents with unilateral colicky flank pain, the signs and symptoms of urolithiasis in children are more varied and likely to be different for different age groups.(4) Most of the literature concerning pediatric urolithiasis suggests that the clinical presentation is often more subtle and not as likely to be pain-related when compared to their adult counterparts. Younger children are more likely to have their calculi diagnosed after undergoing an evaluation for hematuria, urinary tract infections, or vague abdominal pain, whereas it is the older children who are more likely to present with classic renal colic.(4, 34, 35) However, in Milliner's 1993 landmark study the chief presenting complaint was most often pain in 47%, gross or microscopic hematuria in 33%, UTI in 15%. Asymptomatic stones were found incidentally 15% of the time.(21) Similarly in a 2002 report, 92% of the children presented with flank pain, 40% had hematuria, 20% had UTI, 44% had nausea and/or vomiting, and 12% were azotemic.(17) Even in the retrospective review of Icelandic children, 80% presented with abdominal pain and /or irritability. Thirty one percent each had gross hematuria and/or dysuria.(10)

Imaging Techniques

Because of a low clinical suspicion for urolithiasis in the younger child with vague abdominal pain, primary care physicians are more likely to initially diagnose the presence of a renal stone by ultrasonographic imaging (US). Stones seen by US are usually hyperechoic and may have a shadowing effect. Newer ultrasound technology may cause the stone to produce more of a twinkling effect. Ureteral stones may not be seen by US, but if hydronephrosis is present, it should be visible. Palmer found that US failed to detect a stone in 41% of patients that presented with colicky pain. US's ability to detect a stone was dependent on the stone's location (kidney 90%, kidney and ureter 75%, and ureter alone 37%). Noncontrast computerized tomography (CT) was much more sensitive in detecting a stone in children with colicky pain regardless of the stone's location (96–100%). He therefore concluded that although US was a reasonable screening tool, it should be followed by a noncontrast CT if the child's symptoms persist.(36) Further, now that more community emergency departments have CT scanners available for the evaluation of abdominal pain, more children may have their initial stone diagnosed by CT. CT can identify renal and ureteral stones in children as well as in adults. However, most are hesitant to obtain many scans due to possible harmful long-term effects from exposing children to the ionizing radiation.

Plain abdominal radiographs of the kidneys, ureter, and bladder (KUB) are often used to monitor the size and location of a stone. However in some pediatric studies, only 64% of the stones were radiopaque.(10) Therefore this is not always a useful tool. In Pietrow's 2002 Vanderbilt report of 129 children with stones, the vast majority were seen on US or CT. Intravenous pyelography (IVP) was rarely performed, although plain radiography (KUB) was used to monitor stones that were radiopaque for size and location.(18)

Stone Location

In children, the location of stones found within the urinary tract differs significantly in different parts of the world. In North American and most European countries with high protein diets, the predominance of stones in children are seen in the upper urinary tract.(14) But, in certain parts of the Mid-East and Southeast Asia, bladder stones are much more common.(7, 13, 15)

In Milliner's report of 221 children with urolithiasis, 78% of the stones were present in one or both kidneys. Only 5% were ureteral, and 4% of the children had both renal and ureteral stones. A total of 9% had bladder stones, and of these children, the vast majority had undergone prior bladder augmentation and had prior urinary tract infections. Four of the 221 patients had urethral stones, and of these, 2 were found in urethral diverticula.(21) In a more contemporary series, stones were almost equally distributed between kidneys 54%, and ureters 46%.(3)

There was also an increase in the number of ureteral stones diagnosed in a 2002 report. Only 41% of the stones were renal while 59% were ureteral.(18) Of note, the younger children, aged 0–5 years, were much more likely to present with renal stones during an evaluation for hematuria. The older children aged 11–18 years, more often presented in the emergency department. with abdominal pain and were then found to have ureteral stones.(18) The increased incidence of ureteral stones being diagnosed is most likely due to the increased availability of CT scanning in community emergency departments.

Bladder calculi are endemic in the pediatric population in some developing countries. In the U.S., most bladder calculi are seen in association with prior bladder augmentation and continent urinary diversion. In this group of children, the incidence of bladder calculi may reach as high as 50%.(16) Depending on the child's prior operative history, these can usually be managed with a transurethral approach, or a percutaneous suprapubic approach. Cain extracted bladder stones successfully from 92% of the children in his series with a percutaneous approach.(37)

Common Stone Types

Stone compositions in pediatric series are very similar to those in the adult literature. A large review by Stapleton in 2002 found that the majority of stones in children are comprised of calcium oxalate (45–65%), or calcium phosphate (14–30%), whereas uric acid, struvite, and cystine stones usually comprise only 5 to 10%.(38) A total of 45% of the Mayo's patients' stones were calcium oxalate; 24%were calcium phosphate; 17% were struvite; 8% were cystine; 2% were uric acid, while the remaining 4% were described as mixed.(21) In 2002, a U.S. study reported 71% of stones contained calcium oxalate. 14% contained cystine, while 10% were struvite, and 5% contained uric acid.(17) Similarly in 2005, Tan published that 52% of his patients' stones were calcium oxalate, 17% cystine, and 4% each of uric acid and calcium carbonate, while 20% could not be assessed.(39) In 2007, the Pittsburgh group published their series with similar results. There data showed: calcium oxalate monohydrate (30%), calcium oxalate dihydrate (16%), calcium carbonate (7%), cystine (6%), struvite (5%), and uric acid (4%).(3) Even in a report from the United Arab Emirates, 60% of renal calculi were calcium oxalate and 40% were struvite.(7)

The bladder stones endemic to parts of the Mid-East and Southeast Asia are usually comprised of ammonium acid urate and uric acid.(13) These are attributed to malnutrition and a diet low in protein and refined carbohydrates.(7, 13, 14, 15)

MEDICAL ABNORMALITIES MOST OFTEN CONTRIBUTING TO STONE FORMATION

Hypercalciuria is the most common metabolic abnormality detected in children with stones.(18, 20, 21, 40) Milliner found 52% of the children in her study had an identifiable metabolic predisposition to urolithiasis. The most common of these was hypercalciuria (34%) hyperoxaluria (20%), hypocitraturia (9%), and hyperuricosuria (8%). 19% had infection-related stones, and of these children, 36% also had metabolic abnormalities.(21) In a more recent study, a very similar 50% of the children were found to have a metabolic abnormality. The most common of these was again hypercalciuria (26%), followed by hypocitraturia (5.4%), a history of furosemide use in the newborn unit (4%), hyperuricosuria (2.3%), renal tubular acidosis (2.3%), cystinuria (1%), and enteric hyperoxaluria (1%).(18) In a Brazilian study, 66% of the children were found to have hypercalciuria.(20)

A very high 96% of the children who formed stones in Iceland had a metabolic abnormality. Hypercalciuria was the most common (78%), hyperoxaluria and hypocitraturia were also present (13% each). That study also had two patients with Adenine Phosphoribosyltransferase deficiency (APRT) deficiency that has a relatively high prevalence in Iceland.(10)

Unfortunately, the literature concerning stone development in children lags significantly behind that for adults. Recent articles mention that we are handicapped in our management of children with stones by not having well-established normal values for urinary metabolite concentrations or supersaturation indices in children.(21, 41–44) There is not yet universal agreement on what constitutes a normal value for many of the concentrations and supersaturation indices. Recent articles in the pediatric literature have begun to address this void by calling for contemporary studies which assess true urinary metabolite concentrations and supersaturation indices in healthy children of various ages.(41, 42, 45) In our preliminary studies, we have found that the urinary concentrations of many metabolites vary with age and sex. (Slaughenhoupt BS, unpublished work) Further work needs to be done to establish age- and sex-specific reference ranges for metabolite concentrations and urinary supersaturation indices.

Since children seem to only comprise 2–3% of all patients that form stones, most agree that they are unique and should undergo a full metabolic evaluation. Others perform a metabolic evaluation only after a child has formed his or her second stone, or for those with a family history of urolithiasis. The American Urologic Association Ureteral Calculi guidelines do not comment specifically whether or not all children with stones should undergo a metabolic evaluation.(46) The European Association of Urology (EAU) Guidelines on Pediatric Urology state that all children that present with urolithiasis should undergo a full metabolic evaluation.(47)

Anatomic Abnormalities Associated With Stones

Urologic structural abnormalities have been reported in association with pediatric stone formers 19 to 30% of the time.(10, 21) Anatomic abnormalities are more commonly found in the younger children.(4) In one study, obstruction and hydronephrosis was present 26% of the time: vesicoureteral reflux (VUR) 25%, and bladder exstrophy or neurogenic bladder 25%. The remaining 24%included patients who had undergone urinary diversion, or had ureteral anomalies such as a ureterocele, megaureter, ureteral duplication, horseshoe kidney, caliceal or bladder diverticula, or urethral stricture.(21) In a 2006 report from Canada, 17% of the children had an anatomic abnormality contributing their stone formation. These included myelomenigocoele, developmental delay with immobilization, exstrophy, and VUR.(48) In the Icelandic study with the high incidence of genetic inborn errors of metabolism, only 19% of the children also had a structural urologic anomaly. These included UPJ (11%), VUR in one child, and history of augmentation cystoplasty for bladder exstrophy in one child.(10)

Spontaneous Passage

Van Savage was one of the first to report on the similar spontaneous passage rates for distal ureteral stones in children as in adults. No stones greater than 4 mm passed, whereas 55% of smaller stones passed. He suggested distal ureteral stone intervention guidelines for children similar to the AUA guidelines for adults.(49) The Vanderbilt group reported a poor spontaneous passage rate of only 27% for all renal stones. They generally allowed at least two weeks for passage as long as there was no evidence of infection, severe pain, or a solitary kidney. Their older children between 11 and 18 years of age had a higher passage rate of 50%. Roughly two-thirds of all ureteral stones passed without intervention.(18) If the stone reached a size of 4 mm, the spontaneous passage rate dropped significantly. Only 1 of the 129 children evaluated passed a stone larger than 5 mm. This three-year old boy's 7 mm stone then became lodged in his urethra and required endoscopic extraction.(18) In another report, 35% of the children aged 5 to 15 years passed their stones with the largest being 5 mm in diameter.(10) The Pittsburgh group reported that they allowed their children a 3–4 week period of observation for possible spontaneous passage, as long as they were not in debilitating discomfort or had a UTI.(3)

In the adult literature, medical expulsive therapy (MET) is being strongly advocated as it has led to a higher spontaneous passage rate than hydration alone. To date, this has not yet received wide publication in the pediatric literature. However, just as pediatric urologists have been quick to adopt the surgical practices used in adult stone management, I have no doubt, that the literature will soon start to report on the safety and efficacy of MET in children.

SURGICAL PROCEDURES

SWL

Due to a lack of lithotriptors and appropriately sized endoscopic equipment, early reports of pediatric stone surgery advocated open surgical management.(50, 51) However, in the mid-1980s, extracorporeal shock wave lithotripsy (SWL) replaced open surgery as the predominate form of surgical management used for treating children with stones smaller than 2 cm.(3, 52, 53)

Contemporary stone-free rates for children after SWL for renal stones range from 50% for stones larger than 2 cm to 92% for smaller ones.(52, 54, 55) Some of the higher rates required more than one treatment.(55) DeFoor reported stone-free rates of only 68% after one treatment and 74% after two treatments for stones of a mean size of 6.1mm. Their success rates were greater for stones smaller than 6mm. They noted no change in success whether or not a stent had been placed at the time of the procedure.(56) Although no patients were said to have a complication, two (2.3%) required ureteroscopy and stenting for obstructing fragments.(56) These and other reports also commonly cite the need for further ancillary procedures such as stent placement or high re-treatment rates Table 17.1.(52)

Table 17.1 Results of SWL.

Author	Number of Patients	Lithotriptor Used	Stone Free	Mean Stone Size
(52) Raza	85	Piezolith 2300	53%	2.6 cm
			76%	1.3 cm
			84%	0.7 cm
	35	Dornier Compact Delta	50%	2.9 cm
			82%	1.3 cm
			92%	0.6 cm
(53) Braun	46	Lithostar Plus Modulith SL20/SLX SLK	81%	staghorn 20% renal > 1.5 cm 34% calyceal 0.3 - 2 cm 29%
(56) DeFoor	88	Dornier Compact Delta	68% after 1 treatment	
			74% after 1 treatment	0.61 cm

Gofrit compared renal SWL fragment clearance rate in children to that of adults for stones 1cm or smaller. He found a 95% stone-free rate in children compared to a 79% rate for adults. (54) Others have also found a higher passage rate of fragments in children than in adults.(53) In 2001, the EAU recommended SWL as the first-line treatment for pediatric nephrolithiasis.(47)

Although there were initial concerns about the safety of SWL use in the pediatric population, it soon gained widespread acceptance due to its minimally invasive nature. Recommended precautions for children include the use of extra foam cushioning to protect their lungs from pulmonary contusion as well as lower power settings during treatment.(4) Although many adults tolerate this modality well with sedation or only local anesthesia, the vast majority of children undergoing SWL require general anesthesia. Petechial bruising of the skin and tenderness over the site of treatment are commonly the result of SWL in children. With proper precautions, more severe complications such as pulmonary contusion, hemoptysis, or perirenal hematoma are exceedingly rare.

In a report of 40 consecutive children that underwent SWL, US performed immediately after treatment revealed six small hematomas (15%). These all resolved on follow up. Further, no change in glomerular filtration rate was detected on post-procedure nuclear imaging.(57) One series reported an 8% rate of fever associated with recurrent UTI's in their patients treated with SWL. Some of them needed to undergo post-SWL stenting or a percutaneous procedure. (53) Other short-term studies also showed it to be an effective and safe mode of treatment of stones in children without any apparent deleterious effect on renal function, renal growth, or blood pressure.(58, 59, 60)

It was not until 2006 that a long-term follow up study raised the possibility of an increased incidence in diabetes and hypertension in children who had previously undergone SWL. Krambeck reported an association between prior SWL treatment and the development of diabetes mellitus and hypertension.(61) The group from Mayo Clinic retrospectively questioned 578 patients who underwent SWL in 1985. They found that diabetes mellitus and hypertension were more commonly identified in those patients who underwent SWL when compared to controls who had not. They also found that bilateral SWL treatment was more likely to be associated with hypertension than was unilateral treatment.(61)

PCNL

While SWL was playing an ever-increasing role in the management of smaller stones, percutaneous nephrolithotomy (PCNL) became the procedure of choice for larger stones. In 1985, Woodside reported the first series of PCNL in children.(62) Although it was initially reserved for children older than 8 years of age, in 1987, Boddy, and later in1993 Callaway demonstrated that it was also safe for younger children.(63, 64) In 1999, Desai showed that intraoperative hemorrhage during PCNL was related to the size of the endoscopic equipment and could be reduced with smaller instruments.(65) Smaller pediatric percutaneous access sheaths and working instruments have been developed. Jackman reported successful use of an 11Fr sheath for pediatric PCNL.(66)

Various success rates have been reported including 68–90% stone-free rates. Ancillary procedures are required from 37 to 45% of the time.(16, 52, 67) Re-treatment rates of 7% and complications including infection, hemorrhage, and pneumothorax have been reported 6% of the time.(16, 52) One report cites a 68% stone free rate after a single procedure. And a 92% free rate after either repeat PCNL or SWL. No late complications were noted.(67) Today, PCNL is usually reserved for larger stones, or stones associated with anatomic variations such as ureteropelvic junction (UPJ) obstruction.

Ureteroscopy

Although the first report of ureteroscopy in a child was in 1929 when a 2-week old boy with posterior urethral valves underwent ureteroscopy of his dilated ureters with the pediatric cystoscope (68), it was not until 1988 when Ritchey and Shepard first described ureteroscopy for distal ureteral stones in children.(69, 70) Segura and others then reported their successful use of rigid ureteroscopy in the pediatric population.(71, 72) Larger series reported stone-free rates of 86% to 100% in select patients with rigid and semi-rigid scopes.(73, 74) With the advent of smaller, flexible scopes, pediatric ureteroscopy became more popular. Since report of the successful ureteroscopic use of the Holmium:YAG laser (HO:YAG) in children, basket extraction with or without laser lithotripsy has become the first line of treatment for many pediatric ure-teral and renal stones.(3, 75, 76) The holmium laser has been described as the most effective and safest method of stone fragmentation for children.(77)

Success rates for ureteroscopy in children closely match those reached in adults. However, working with children offers some unique obstacles that must be overcome. The infant urethra may not be large enough to accommodate the pediatric endoscopic equipment. This is true espe-cially in males. Similarly, the child's ureteral orifice may not be large enough to allow passage of the ureteroscope. Rapid dilation of the ureteral orifice with either a balloon or serial dilator could be performed, or a JJ stent could be passed for gradual dilation. Concerns have been raised about ureteroscopy and rapid dilation of the ureteral orifice and its possible contribution to ureteral trauma, ureteral perforation with urinary extravasation, vesicoureteral reflux (VUR), stricture formation and ureteral avulsion. A 2005 meta-analysis of 185 ureteroscopic cases revealed a 1.6% incidence of ureteral perforation.(16) Most ureteral injuries are associated with the use of either an electrohydraulic or ultrasonic lithotriptor, although there are also rare reports of small ureteral perforations associated with the use of a laser. It is reports such as these as well as the develop-ment of improved, flexible ureteroscopes that have caused electrohydraulic lithotriptors to no longer be as commonly used for pediatric ureteroscopy in the U.S.(17, 49, 77, 78)

The published incidence of the more serious ureteral stricture post-ureteroscopy is also exceedingly rare at 0.0% to 1.7 %.(1, 3, 17, 77) Some feel serial dilators may cause an even lower complication rate than balloons due to the tactile feedback they give the operator.(3) The Cincinnati group recommends serial dilators over balloon dilators as they refer to their one-of-three patients who underwent balloon dilation and subsequently developed the only stricture in their series.(1)

Despite these very low complication rates associated with active ureteral orifice dilation, some still advocate for a more passive dilation obtained by placing a JJ ureteral stent for a week or two. Hubert first described this practice in children in 2005.(79) All children for whom ure-teroscopy could not initially be performed had stents placed for 2 to 8 weeks (median 3). All subsequently underwent successful ureteroscopy without post-procedure hydronephrosis.(79) Some have reported stricture formation even after passive dilation.(3)

More recently, ureteral access sheaths are being used for pediatric ureteroscopy. They have been shown to decrease operative time, improve stone-free rates, and reduce intrarenal pressures in the adult population.(80) Singh reported a 100% stone-free rate and no postopera-tive ureteral strictures in a pediatric population followed for 10 months after a ureteral access sheath was used.(81) Smaldone, Thomas, and others reported similar successes, and recom-mend using a 12Fr or 14 Fr sheath when doing prolonged flexible ureteroscopic cases.(3, 82) The Cincinnati group recommends a 9.5 Fr sheath.(1)

Another concern raised historically as pediatric ureteroscopy became more popular was its possible contribution to the development of vesicoureteral reflux (VUR). Many were par-ticularly concerned about this in the face of active ureteral dilation. Some initially advocated that voiding cysto-urethrograms (VCUG's) routinely be performed after ureteroscopy.(71) This fell out of favor after it was demonstrated that if reflux was present, it was most often transient and asymptomatic.(83) Minevich recommended post-ureteroscopy renal ultrasound to insure hydroureteronephrosis has not occurred after instrumentation.(84) He does not advocate rou-tine VCUG to rule out reflux.

Stenting after ureteroscopy in the pediatric population remains controversial. The rela-tive indications for placement of a ureteral stent after a ureteroscopic procedure are edema of the ureteral orifice or extensive ureteral manipulation. Most pediatric urologists prefer to stent after ureteral manipulation.(2)

In 2002, ureteroscopy was described as safe and effective for treatment of stones in pre-pubertal children.(17) A review of 25 children from Michigan and Virginia with a mean age of 9.2 years were treated. 6.9 and 8 Fr flexible or rigid ureteroscopes were used. Some ureters were dilated passively with a stent while others were dilated with a balloon. They had a 92% stone-free rate after the first procedure, and a 100% stone-free rate after two procedures. One case was complicated by post-operative pyelonephritis while another stent migrated proximally and required ureteroscopic extraction.(17)

In 2005, the Cincinnati group reported their series of ureteroscopic stone management. (1) The mean patient age was 7.5 years and the mean follow up was 2.8 years. They used a holmium:YAG (HO:YAG) laser in 72%, and extracted or basketed the stone in 38%. Their stone-free rate, based on post-operative ultrasound at 4–6 weeks was 98%. One patient who underwent balloon dilation of her ureteral orifice developed a distal ureteral stricture that was treated successfully with ureteroscopic laser incision.(1)

In 2006, Lesani reported that proximal rigid ureteroscopy and limited pyeloscopy could be performed safely in prepubertal children.(73) Tortuosity of the ureter required conversion to a flexible ureteroscope in 17%. All were stone free based on direct endoscopic conclusions. None developed hydronephrosis with a mean of 1.9-year follow up. The authors hypothesized that the pre-adolescent ureter may be better able to accept the ureteroscope than in the adult, but they offered no explanation for this.(73)

In 2007, the Pittsburgh group reported their series of 100 children with a mean age of 13.2 years and a mean stone size was 8.3mm. Half of the children had stents placed preoperatively. 8Fr and 10Fr ureteral coaxial dilators were used to dilate the orifice in 70% of the children while 9.5Fr and 12 Fr ureteral access sheaths were used to dilate the orifice in 24% of the children. They had an overall stone-free rate of 91% based on follow-up US, KUB or CT. Patients younger than 13 were stone free 96% of the time while the children older than 13 had an 86% stone-free rate. 7 % required staged ureteroscopic procedures in order to be stone free. They had no major intraoperative complications, but 5 children had a ureteral perforation or extravasation that required a stent for healing. Only one patient, 1%, required a ureteral reimplant for a distal ureteral stricture. That child's ureteral orifice had been dilated passively with a JJ ureteral stent prior to undergoing ureteroscopy.(3)

In summary, ureteroscopy is felt by all trained in the technique to be the first line of treatment for children with symptomatic ureteral stones.(2, 3, 39, 82) With its very high stone-free rates, it has already replaced SWL as first line treatment for stones in some communities. (3, 39, 82) Complications from ureteroscopy in the pediatric population are very rare, and usually quite manageable.

Laparoscopic Surgery

It is still unclear what role the ever-expanding uses of laparoscopic surgery may play in the treatment of urolithiasis in children. In 2004, Casale successfully performed laparoscopic pyelolithotomy in eight children after failed percutaneous access.(85) In 2007, Lee reported on five children who underwent robot assisted laparoscopic lithotomy. Four patients had staghorn cystine stones who had already undergone either SWL or PCNL, and one had an associated UPJ obstruction and also underwent pyeloplasty at the same time. One patient required conversion to an open procedure and also subsequently required three more procedures to be stone free.(86) The role of laparoscopic surgery in the management of pediatric urolithiasis remains unclear.

What I Do

When an asymptomatic renal stone is discovered during an evaluation for a completely unrelated issue, I make an initial assessment with ultrasound to ensure there is no hydronephrosis present. The child is seen in our interdisciplinary Pediatric Kidney Stone Clinic. There, I along with a nephrologist and a dietician evaluate the child. In addition to obtaining a complete medical and family history and performing a thorough physical exam, the metabolic evaluation also includes assessment of their serum electrolytes and metabolites including sodium, potassium, bicarbonate, blood urea nitrogen (BUN), creatinine, calcium, phosphorous, magnesium, alkaline phosphatase, uric acid, and intact parathyroid hormone (PTH) levels. They will also contribute a 24-hour urine collection including a measurement of cystine concentration. The frequency of repeat testing depends upon how actively the child is forming stones. Changes in dosages of medications or the addition or deletion of a medication would prompt more frequent testing as well.

If the child is asymptomatic and has two functioning kidneys, I will often recommend expectant management for children with stones 3mm or smaller. Families are also counseled on surgical options including SWL, ureteroscopy or PCNL, depending on the stone burden. Annual US is obtained to ensure that there is no hydronephrosis. KUB is also obtained if the stone is radiopaque.

If the stone is between 4 mm and 2cm, I encourage surgical intervention with ureteroscopy. For some radiopaque stones, I also discuss SWL as an alternative treatment option. All children have been scheduled for general anesthesia for their treatment.

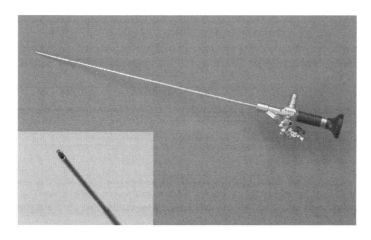

Figure 17.1 Wolf semi-rigid 4.5 Fr Pediatric Ureteroscope with working channel seen in inset.

I obtain a retrograde ureteropyelogram before proceeding with ureteroscopy. For distal ureteroscopy, I begin with a semi-rigid 4.5Fr ureteroscope that graduates to an 8.5 Fr diameter. (Richard Wolf Medical Instruments, Vernon Hills IL) Although the optics are not quite as clear as with the larger scopes, the smaller tip can oftentimes pass through a ureteral orifice that a larger flexible scope could not and therefore makes this a very good scope to start with Figure 17.1.

For mid- and proximal-ureteral stones as well as renal stones, I use a flexible 6.5 Fr scope as my instrument of choice. If the scope will not pass through the ureteral orifice, I usually dilate it with an 8 Fr – 10 Fr semi-rigid ureteral dilator. I usually leave a JJ ureteral stent for a few days after active dilation and ureteroscopy. If the child's entire ureter appears to be narrow, I am more likely to simply pass a stent, and then re-attempt ureteroscopy or nephroscopy with laser lithotripsy and/or extraction in two weeks. We maintain a wide supply of ureteral stents from 3 to 6 Fr wide and from 4 to 26 cm long to accommodate the many different sizes of children we treat. (Cook Medical Inc, Bloomington IN) Often, even if the ureteral orifice can be dilated to accept the ureteroscope, the ureter itself is too narrow to allow passage of the scope more proximally. Although stents have generally been well tolerated in my patients, they have occasionally been associated with urinary tract infections and some of the children have required anti-cholinergic medication for management of bladder spasms. Their subsequent ureteroscopic procedure is usually uneventful and successful. I will usually leave a ureteral stent after passive dilation, only if the stone burden has been large and the procedure has required extensive ureteral manipulation.

I reserve PCNL for larger renal stones, or those associated with inaccessible ureteral anatomy. After consultation, our interventional radiologists help me gain access to the collecting system. We usually use an 11 or 14 Fr access sheath to minimize renal trauma. A small nephrostomy tube is left in place for a few days. A nephrostogram is obtained and either the tube removed, or a second-look procedure is scheduled.

I perform an imaging study within one month after any stone procedure. I usually obtain an US to assess for residual stone fragments as well as to check for the development of new hydronephrosis.

REFERENCES

1. Minevich E, DeFoor W, Reddy P et al. Ureteroscopy is safe and effective in prepubertal children. J Urol 2005; 174: 276–9.
2. Minevich E, Sheldon CA. The role of ureteroscopy in pediatric urology, Curr Opin Urol 2006; 16: 295–8.
3. Smaldone MC, Cannon GM Jr, Wu H-Y et al. Is ureteroscopy first line treatment for pediatric stone disease?. J Urol 2007; 178: 2128–31.
4. Durkee CT, Balcom A. Surgical management of urolithiasis. Pediatr Clin North Am 2006; 53: 465–77.
5. Srivastava T, Alon US. Urolithiasis in adolescent children, Adolesc Med 2005; 16: 87–109.
6. Lattimer JK, Hubbard M. Pediatric urologic admissions. J Urol 1951; 66: 289–93.
7. Ghafoor M, Majeed I, Nawaz A, Al-Salem A, Halim A. Urolithiasis in the pediatric age group. Ann Saudi Med 2003; 23: 201–4.

8. Pearle MS, Calhoun EA, Curhan GC. Urologic Diseases in America, US Government Publishing Office, Washington DC; 2004.

9. Ghazali S, Barratt TM, Williams DI. Childhood urolithiasis in Britain, Arch Dis Child 1973; 48: 291–5.

10. Edvardsson V, Elidottir H, Indridason OS, Runolfur P. High incidence of kidney stones in Icelandic children. Pediatr Nephrol 2005; 20: 940–4.

11. Malek RS, Kelalis PP. Pediatric nephrolithiasis. J Urol 1975; 113: 451–4.

12. Polinsky MS, Kaiser BA, Baluarte HJ. Urolithiasis in childhood. Pediatr Clin North Am 1987; 34: 683–710.

13. Sarica K. Pediatric urolithiasis: etiology, specific pathogenesis and medical treatment. Urol Res 2006; 34: 96–101.

14. Stapleton FB. Nephrolithiasis in children. Pediatr Rev 1989; 11: 21–30.

15. Ali SH, Rifat UN. Etiological and clinical patterns of childhood urolithiasis in Iraq. Pediatr Nephrol 2005; 20: 1453–7.

16. Desai M. Endoscopic management of stones in children. Curr Opin Urol 2005; 15: 107–12.

17. Schuster TG, Russell KY, Bloom DA, Koo HP, Faerber GJ. Ureteroscopy for the treatment of urolithiasis in children. J Urol 2002; 167: 1813–6.

18. Pietrow PK, Pope JC IV, Adams MC, Shyr Y, Brock JW III. Clinical outcome of pediatric stone disease. J Urol 2002; 167: 670–3.

19. Monga M, Macias B, Groppo E, Hargens A. Genetic heritability of urinary stone risk in identical twins. J Urol 2006; 175: 2125–8.

20. Perrone HC, dos Santos DR, Santos MV. et al. Urolithiasis in childhood: metabolic evaluation. Pediatr Nephrol 1992; 6: 54–6.

21. Milliner DS, Murphy ME. Urolithiasis in pediatric patients. Mayo Clin Proc 1993; 68: 241–8.

22. Hemant KB, Himanshu C, Rama DM. Association of vitamin-D and calcitonin receptor gene polymorphism in pediatric nephrolithiasis. Pediatr Nephrol 2005; 20: 773–6.

23. Reed BY, Gitomer WL, Heller HJ et al. Identification and characterization of a gene with base substitutions associated with the absorptive hypercalciuria phenotype and low spinal bone density. J Clin Endocrinol Metab 2002; 87: 1476–85.

24. Goldfarb DS, Fischer ME, Keich Y, Goldberg J. A twin study of genetic and dietary influences on nephrolithiasis: a report from the Vietnam Era Twin (VET) Registry. Kidney Int 2005; 67: 1053.

25. Goodman HO, Holmes RP, Assimos DG. Genetic factors in calcium oxalate stone disease. J Urol 1995; 153: 301–7.

26. Seyhan S, Yavascaoglu I, Kilicarslan H, Dogan HS, Kordan Y. Association of vitamin D receptor gene Taq I polymorphism with recurrent urolithiasis in children. Int J Urol 2007; 14: 1060–2.

27. Lloyd SE, Pearce SHS, Fisher SE et al. A common molecular basis for three inherited kidney stone diseases. Nature 1996; 379: 445–9.

28. Thakker RV. Pathogenesis of Dent's disease and related syndromes of X-linked nephrolithiasis. Kidney Int 2000; 57: 787–93.

29. Yuen YP, Lam CW, Lai CK et al. Heterogeneous mutations in the SLC3A1 and SLC7A98 genes in Chinese patients with cystinuria. Kidney Int 2006; 69: 123–8.

30. Shekarriz B, Stoller ML. Cystinuria and other noncalcareous calculi. Endocrinol Metab Clin North Am 2002; 31: 951–77.

31. Milliner DS. Stones, bones, and heredity. Acta Paediatr Suppl 2006; 452: 27–30.

32. Diamond DA, Menon M, Lee PH et al Etiological factors in pediatric stone recurrence. J Urol 1989; 142: 606.

33. Marquardt H, Nagel R. Urolithiasis in childhood. Urology 1977; 9: 627.

34. Stapleton FB. Childhood stones. Endocrinol Metab Clin North Am 2002; 31: 1001–15.

35. Hulton SA. Evaluation of urinary tract calculi in children. Arch Dis Child 2001; 84: 320–3.

36. Palmer JS, Donaher ER, O'Riordan MA, Dell KM. Diagnosis of pediatric urolithiasis: role of ultrasound and computerized tomography. J Urol 2005; 174: 1413–6.

37. Cain MP, Casale AJ, Kaefer M. et al. Percutaneous cystolithotomy in the pediatric augmented bladder. J Urol 2002; 168: 1881.

38. Stapleton FB, Childhood stones. Endocrinol Metab Clin North Am 2002; 31: 1001–15.

39. Tan AHH, Al-Omar M, Denstedt JD, Razvi H. Ureteroscopy for pediatric urolithiasis: an evolving first-line therapy. Urology 2005; 65: 153–6.

40. Alon US, Zimmerman H, Alon M. Evaluation and treatment of pediatric idiopathic urolithiasis—revisited. Pediatr Nephrol 2004; 19: 516–20.

41. Battino BS, DeFoor W, Coe F et al. Metabolic evaluation of children with urolithiasis: are adult references for supersaturation appropriate?. J Urol 2002; 168: 2568–71.

42. Pietrow PK, Pope JC IV, Adams MC, Shyr Y, Brock JW III. Clinical outcome of pediatric stone disease. J Urol 2002; 167: 670.

43. Tekin A, Tekgul S, Necmettin A et al. A study of the etiology of idiopathic calcium urolithiasis in children: hypocitruria is the most important risk factor. J Urol 2000; 164: 162–5.

44. Hoppe B, Langman CB, Akcay T. Hypocitraturia in patients with urolithiasis/reply, Arch Dis Child 1997; 76: 174–5.

45. DeFoor W, Asplin J, Jackson E et al. Urinary metabolic evaluations in normal and stone-forming children. J Urol 2006; 176: 1793–6.

46. Preminger GM, Tiselius H-G, Assimos DG et al. 2007 Guideline for the management of ureteral calculi. J Urol 2007; 178(6): 2418–34.

47. Riedmiller H, Androulakakis P, Beurton D, Kocvara R, Gerharz E. EAU guideline on paediatric urology. Eur Urol 2001; 40: 589–99.

48. Schwarz R. Pediatric kidney stones. Urology 2006; 67: 812–6.

49. Van Savage JG, Palanca LG, Andersen RD, Rao GS, Slaughenhoupt BL. Treatment of distal ureteral stones in children: similarities to the American Urological Association guidelines in adults. J Urol 2000; 164: 1089.

50. Paulson DF, Glenn JF, Hughes J, Roberts LC, Coppridge AJ. Pediatric urolithiasis. J Urol 1972; 108: 811.

51. Bennett AH, Colodny AH. Urinary tract calculi in children. J Urol 1973; 109: 318.

52. Raza A, Turna B, Smith G, Moussa S, Tolley D. Pediatric Urolithiasis: 15 years of local experience with minimally invasive endourological management of pediatric calculi. J Urol 2005; 174: 682–5.

53. Braun PM, Seif C, Jünemann KP, Alken P. Urolithiasis in children. Int Braz J Urol 2002; 28: 539–44.

54. Gofrit ON, Pode D, Meretyk S et al. Is the pediatric ureter as efficient as the adult ureter in transporting fragments following extracorporeal shock wave lithotripsy for renal calculi larger than 10 mm?. J Urol 2001; 166: 1862–4.

55. Muslumanoglu AY, Tefekli A, Sarilar O et al. Extracorporeal shock wave lithotripsy as first line treatment alternative for urinary tract stones in children: a large scale retrospective analysis. J Urol 2003; 170: 2405–8.

56. DeFoor W, Dharamsi N, Smith P et al. Use of mobile extracorporeal shock wave lithotripter: experience in a pediatric institution. Urology 2005; 65: 778–81.

57. Goel MC, Baserge NS, Babu RV et al. Pediatric kidney: functional outcome after extracorporeal shock wave lithotripsy. J Urol 1996; 155: 2044–6.

58. Lottmann H, Archambaud F, Traxer O, Mercier-Pageyrai B, Helal B. The efficacy and parenchymal consequences of extracorporeal shock wave lithotripsy in infant. Br J Urol 2000; 85: 311–5.

59. Lottmann H, Archambaud F, Helal B, Mercier Pageyrai B. 99mTechnetium-dimercapto-succinic acid renal scan in the evaluation of potential long term renal parenchymal damage associated with extracorporeal shock wave lithotripsy in children. J Urol 1998; 169: 521–4.

60. Vlajković M, Slavković A, Radovanović M et al. Long-term functional outcome of kidneys in children with urolithiasis after SWL treatment. Eur J Pediatr Surg 2002; 12: 118–23.

61. Krambeck AE, Gettman MT, Rohlinger AL et al. Diabetes Mellitus and Hypertension associated with shock wave lithotripsy of renal and proximal ureteral stones at 19 years of followup. J Urol 2006; 175: 1742–7.

62. Woodside JR, Stevens GF, Stork GF et al. Percutaneous stone removal in children. J Urol 1985; 134: 1166–67.

63. Boddy SM, Kellett MJ, Fletcher MS et al. Extracorporeal shock wave lithotripsy and percutaneous nephrolithotomy in children. J Ped Surg 1987; 22: 223.

64. Callaway TW, Lingardh G, Basata S, Sylven M. Percutaneous nephrolithotomy in children. J Urol 1992; 148: 1067–8.

65. Desai M, Ridhorkar V, Patel S et al. Pediatric percutaneous nephrolithotomy: assessing impact of technical innovations on safety and efficacy. J Endourol 1999; 13: 359–64.

66. Jackman SV, Hedican SP, Peters CA et al. Percutaneous nephrolithotomy in infants and preschool age children: experience with a new technique. Urology 1998; 52: 697.

67. Mor Y, Elmasry YET, Kellett MJ, Duffy PG. The role of percutaneous nephrolithotomy in the management of pediatric renal calculi. J Urol 1997; 158: 1319–21.

68. Young HH, McKay RW. Congenital valvular obstruction of the prostatic urethra. Surg Gynecol Obstet 1929; 48: 509.

69. Ritchey M, Patterson DE, Kelalis PP, Segura JW. A case of pediatric ureteroscopic lasertripsy. J Urol 1988; 139: 1272.

70. Shepard P, Thomas R, Harmon EP. Urolithiasis in children: innovations in management. J Urol 1988; 140: 790.

71. Hill DE, Segura JW, Patterson DE, et al. Ureteroscopy in children. J Urol 1990; 144: 481–3.

72. Cajone P, De Gennaro M, Capozza N et al, Endoscopic manipulation of ureteral calculi in children by rigid operative ureterorenoscopy. J Urol 1990; 144: 484.

73. Lesani OA, Palmer JS. Retrograde proximal rigid ureteroscopy and pyeloscopy in prepubertal children: safe and effective. J Urol 2006; 176: 1570–3.

74. Dogan HS, Tekgul S, Akdogan B, Keskin MS, Sahin A. Use of the holmium: YAG laser for ureterolithotripsy in children. BJU Int 2004; 94: 131.

75. Wollin TA, Teichman JMH, Rogenes VJ et al. Holmium: YAG lithotripsy in children. J Urol 1999; 162: 1717.

76. Reddy PP, Barrieras DJ, Bägli DJ et al. Initial experience with endoscopic holmium laser lithotripsy for pediatric urolithiasis. J Urol 1999; 162: 1714.

77. Raza A, Smith G, Moussa S, Tolley D. Ureteroscopy in the management of pediatric urinary tract calculi. J Endourol 2005; 19: 151–8.

78. al Busaidy SS, Prem AR, Medhat M. Paediatric ureteroscopy for ureteric calculi: a 4-year experience. Br J Urol 1997; 80: 797.

79. Hubert KC, Palmer JS. Passive dilation by ureteral stenting before ureteroscopy: eliminating the need for active dilation. J Urol 2005; 174: 1079–80.

80. L'Esperance JO, Ekeruo WO, Scales CD Jr et al. Effect of ureteral access sheath on stone-free rates in patients undergoing Ureteroscopic management of renal calculi. Urology 2005; 66: 252.

81. Singh A, Shah G, Young J et al. Ureteral access sheath for the management of pediatric renal and ureteral stones: a single center experience. J Urol 2006; 175: 1080–2.

82. Thomas JC, DeMarco RT, Donohoe JM et al. Pediatric Ureteroscopic stone management. J Urol 2005; 174: 1072–4.

83. Thomas R, Ortenberg J, Lee BR et al Safety and efficacy of pediatric ureteroscopy for management of calculous disease. J Urol 1993; 149: 1082.

84. Minevich E, Rousseau MB, Wacksman J et al. Pediatric ureteroscopy: technique and preliminary results. J Pediatr Surg 1997; 32: 571.

85. Casale P, Grady RW, Joyner BD et al. Transperitoneal laparoscopic pyelolithotomy after failed percutaneous access in the pediatric patient. J Urol 2004; 172: 680–3.

86. Lee RS, Passerotti CC, Cendron M, Estrada CR, Borer JG. Early results of robot assisted laparoscopic lithotomy in adolescents. J Urol 2007; 177: 2306–10.

Index

Page numbers in *italics* refer to tables; those in **bold** to figures.

Printed and bound by CPI Group (UK) Ltd, Croydon, CR0 4YY

29/10/2024

01780630-0001